Josl[illegible]
O'Connor

joconnor@csulb.edu

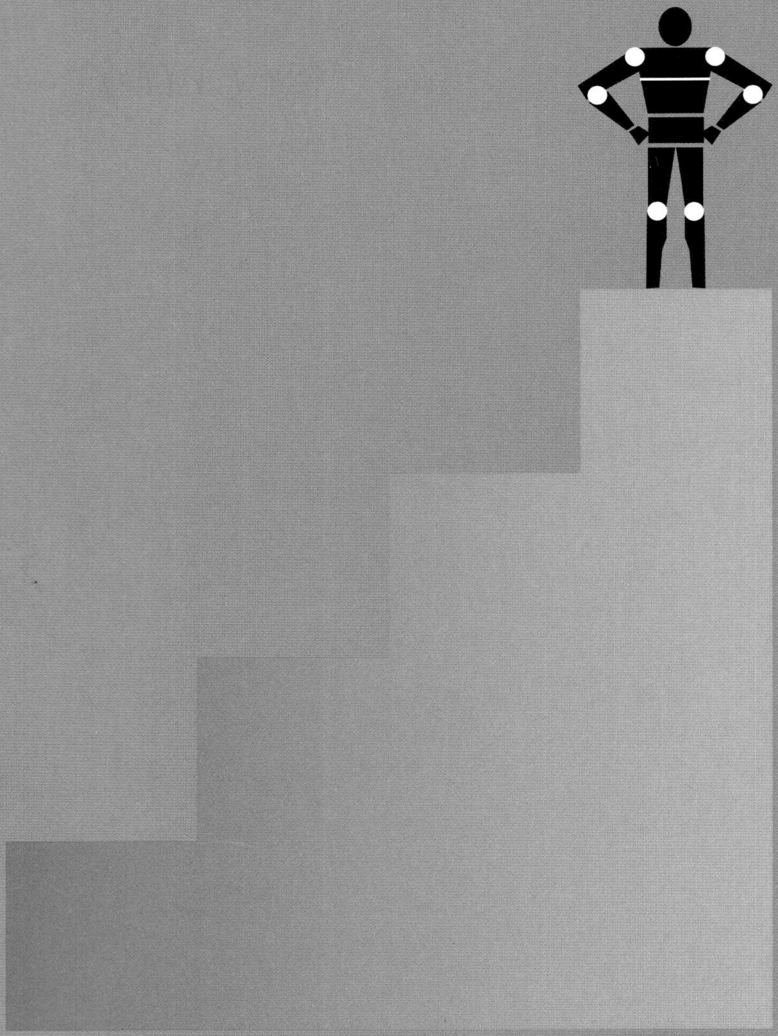

Weight Training for Life

Sixth Edition

James L. Hesson
Black Hills State University

THOMSON
WADSWORTH

Australia • Canada • Mexico • Singapore • Spain • United Kingdom • United States

THOMSON
WADSWORTH

Publisher: Peter Marshall
Associate Editor: April Lemons
Assistant Editor: John Boyd
Editorial Assistant: Andrea Kesterke
Marketing Manager: Jennifer Somerville
Marketing Assistant: Mona Weltmer
Advertising Project Manager: Shemika Britt
Project Manager, Editorial Production: Sandra Craig
Print/Media Buyer: Tandra Jorgensen
Permissions Editor: Joohee Lee
Production and Composition: Ash Street Typecrafters, Inc.
Text and Cover Design: Harry Voigt
Copy Editor: Carolyn Acheson
Cover Images: Large Photo: ©2002 David Madison/Getty Images/Stone; inset: ©2002 Stephen Simpson/Getty Images/FPG
Printer: Transcontinental Printing

Printed in Canada
1 2 3 4 5 6 7 06 05 04 03 02

For more information about our products, contact us at:
Thomson Learning Academic Resource Center
1-800-423-0563
For permission to use material from this text, contact us by:
Phone: 1-800-730-2214
Fax: 1-800-730-2215
Web: http://www.thomsonrights.com

Library of Congress Cataloging-in-Publication Data

Hesson, James L.
Weight training for life / James L. Hesson.—6th ed.
p. cm.
Includes index.
ISBN 0-534-57854-3
1. Weight training. I. Title

GV546 .H48 2003
613.7'13—dc21

2001057458

Wadsworth/Thomson Learning
10 Davis Drive
Belmont, CA 94002-3098
USA

Asia
Thomson Learning
60 Albert Street, #15-01
Albert Complex
Singapore 189969

Australia
Nelson Thomson Learning
102 Dodds Street
South Melbourne, Victoria 3205
Australia

Canada
Nelson Thomson Learning
1120 Birchmount Road
Toronto, Ontario M1K 5G4
Canada

Europe/Middle East/Africa
Thomson Learning
Berkshire House
168-173 High Holborn
London WC1 V7AA
United Kingdom

Latin America
Thomson Learning
Seneca, 53
Colonia Polanco
11560 Mexico D.F.
Mexico

Spain
Parafino Thomson Learning
Calle/Magallenes, 25
28015 Madrid, Spain

Contents

Preface ix

Part I Getting Started 1

1 ***What, Who, and Why*** 1
What is Weight Training? 1
Who Trains with Weights? 1
Who Should Participate in Weight Training? 2
Why Weight Training? 4

2 ***Questions, Concerns, and Answers*** 7

3 ***Muscle Structure and Function*** 11
Characteristics of Muscle Tissue 11
Types of Muscle Tissue 12
The Musculoskeletal System as a Lever System 12
The Structure of Skeletal Muscle 12
Muscle Contraction and Exercise Movements 13
Motor Unit 14
Muscle Atrophy and Hypertrophy 15
Basic Principles of Muscle Development 16

4 ***Warm-Up, Flexibility, and Stretching*** 17
Warm-Up 17
Flexibility 18
Stretching 18
Weight Room Stretching Routine 20

5 ***Safe and Effective Weight Training*** 21
Medical Clearance 21
Clothing 21
Performing a Weight Training Exercise 22
Additional Considerations for Machine Exercises 24
Training Partner 26
Spotting 26
Safety 27

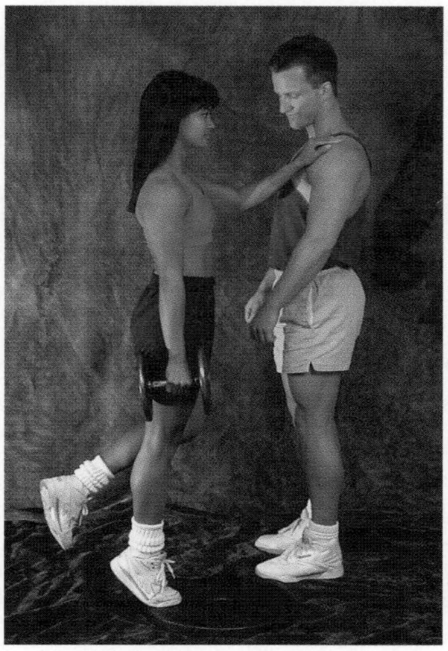
Eric Risberg

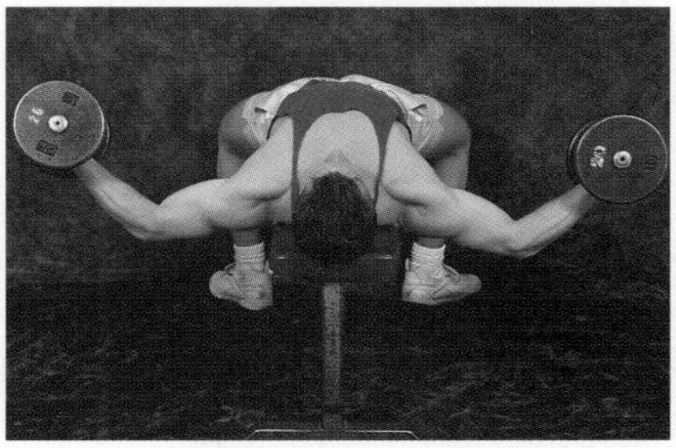
Eric Risberg

6 ***A Beginning Weight Training Program*** 29
Free Weights or Machines? 29
Grips 30
Getting in Position 31
Basic Exercises 32
Frequency and Resistance 32
The First Six Weeks 33
Guidelines for Productive Training 34

7 ***Nutrition, Rest, and Drugs*** 39
Nutrition 39
The "Secret" Weight Training Diet 43
Nutrient Supplementation 45
Weight Gain 47
Weight Loss 47
Rest 48
Drugs 49

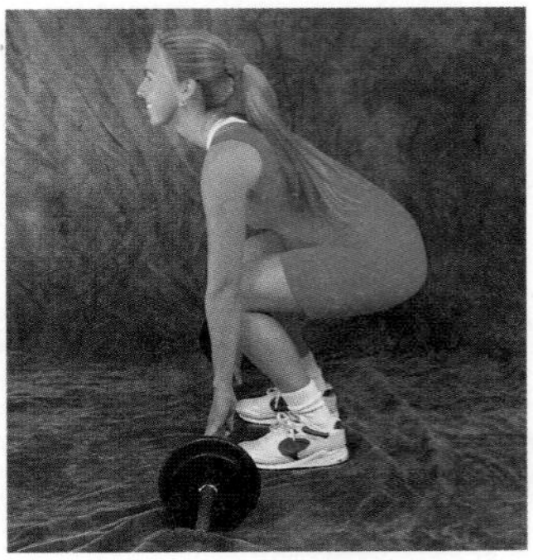

Eric Risberg

Part II
Learning More Weight Training Exercises 57

Major Muscles of the Human Body 58

8 ***Chest Exercises*** 59
Chest (Pectoralis major) 60
Chest/Back 66

9 ***Back Exercises*** 69
Back (Latissimus dorsi) 70
Upper Back (Trapezius) 74

10 ***Shoulder Exercises*** 77
Shoulder (Deltoid) 78

11 ***Arm Exercises*** 87
Upper Arm (Elbow Flexion, Biceps) 88
Upper Arm (Elbow Extension, Triceps) 92
Forearm (Wrist flexors and Wrist extensors) 98

12 ***Leg Exercises*** 101
Hip and Knee Extension 102
Hip Extension 108
Hip Flexion (Iliopsoas) 109
Knee Extension (Quadriceps) 110
Knee Flexion (Hamstrings) 111
Ankle Plantar Flexion 112

13 ***Trunk Flexion and Extension Exercises*** 117
Trunk Flexion (Abdominals) 118
Trunk and Hip Flexion (Abdominals and Hip Flexors) 120
Trunk Extension (Erector Spinae) 124
The Ab Solution 126

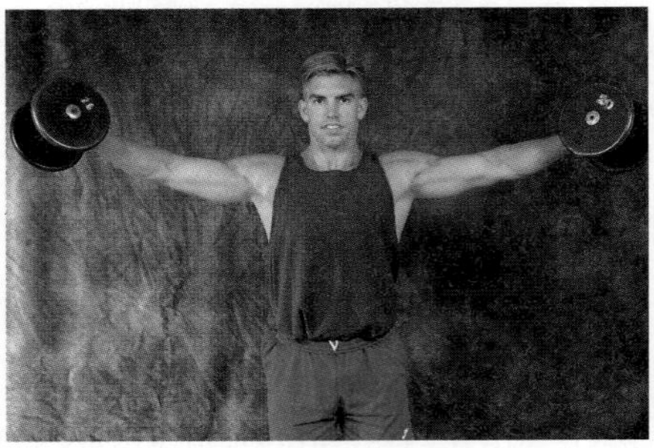

Eric Risberg

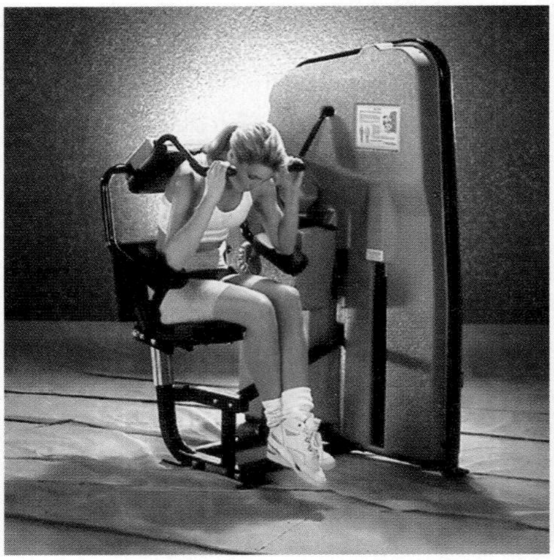

© Nautilus Sports/Medical Industries, Inc.

Part III
Getting the Most Out of Weight Training 127

14 ***Record Keeping and Measuring Progress*** 127
Record Keeping 127
Measuring Progress 128
Evaluating Progress 131

15 ***Success*** 139
A Formula for Success 139
Writing Weight Training Goals 141

16 ***Planning Your Personal Weight Training Program*** 145
Basic Weight Training Principles 145
Considerations in Planning Your Weight Training Program 145
Suggested Lifetime Fitness Weight Training Programs 147
A Simple Home Training Program for Busy People 148

17 ***Advanced Weight Training*** 153
Progressive Overload 153
Increasing Exercise Intensity 154
Total Body and Split Routines 154
Fixed Systems 155
Variable Systems 155
Training Equipment 156

18 ***Weight Training for Life*** 157
Transtheoretical Model of Behavior Change 157
Tips for Sticking With It 158

Internet Sites 161
References and Suggested Readings 163
Index 165

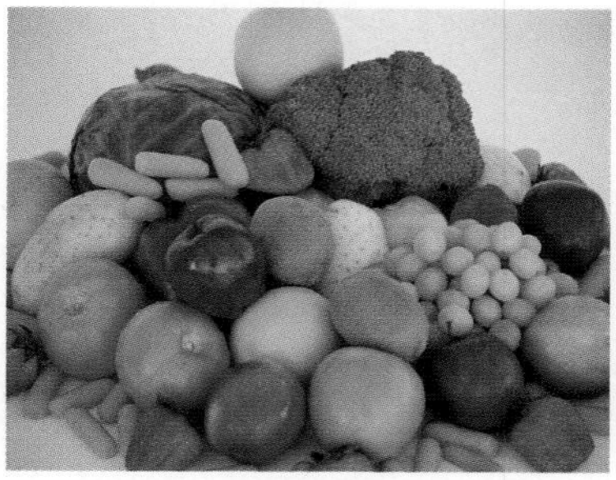
© Fitness & Wellness, Inc.

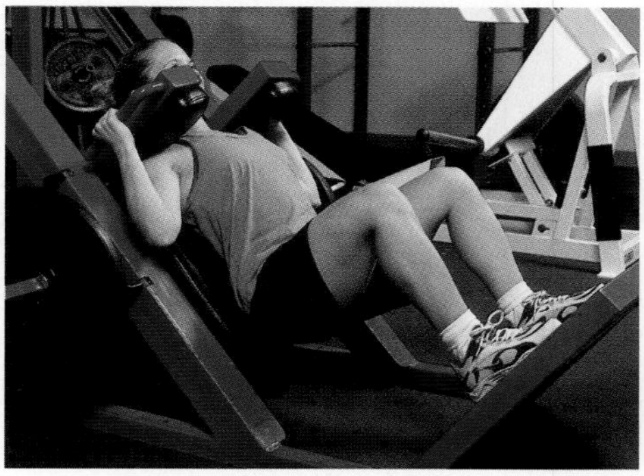
Jon Kelley

Dedication

To the wind beneath my wings, the creator of all that is, the source of my inspiration and strength, the source of my knowledge and wisdom, the great spirit that lives within all of us, and the great spirit through which we are all joined as one in the endless cycle of life.

To Margie, Jennifer, and David, with love.

To all of the teachers, coaches, friends, and colleagues who have shared their time, energy, and knowledge with me.

To all of my students who have taught me, and who continue to teach me, how to help them learn.

To my parents, Jack and Gladys Hesson, who taught me the basic values and attitudes that have made all other learning and accomplishment possible.

Preface

To the Student

Weight Training for Life has been written to you and for you. Learning about weight training by the trial-and-error method can be difficult, embarrassing, and confusing. We hope this book will make learning simple, easy, and fun. The purpose of this book is to help you build a solid foundation of current knowledge and practice in beginning weight training. All of the exercise information in this book is consistent with the recommendations of the National Strength and Conditioning Association (NSCA) and the American College of Sports Medicine (ACSM).

This book does not attempt to include everything there is to know about weight training. It is a book for beginners, not for exercise physiologists or strength coaches or advanced-strength athletes although one chapter is devoted to advanced weight training. This is a book to help you get started *weight training for life*.

To the Teacher

Weight Training for Life has been written to help you and to help your students. It does not attempt to cover everything you know about weight training, but it does attempt to organize some basic information for you and your students.

One common challenge for most weight training teachers is time. Answer the following questions quickly.

- Do you have enough class time to tell your students all that you wish you could about weight training?
- Are your students always present, on time, and alert for your weight training lectures?
- Do you have other classes to prepare for?
- Are you paid for talking or for helping students learn?
- Do you ever get bored presenting the same beginning weight training information year after year and class after class?
- Have you ever forgotten to mention some basic information you wanted your students to know?
- Could you be more productive if you didn't have to repeat the same basic information again and again?
- Would your students learn more effectively if they were required to actively seek information?
- Do you have enough class time to lecture and lift?
- Do you teach more than one weight training class?
- Have you ever noticed how the right tool can help you complete a task easier, faster, and better?

This book is a tool that can help you perform your task of teaching weight training. It can make your performance of this task better and, at the same time, easier. A book will never replace you as a teacher because your role is much more important, dynamic, and complex. Your responsibility is to create a stimulating learning environment, to motivate, to provide direction, and to give feedback.

The material in this book can be covered in any order you choose. You also are encouraged to add or delete any material you wish. Based on the feedback I have received, there seems to be an infinite variety of ways to help beginners learn about weight training.

This tool can be more effective if we work together. As you use the book, let me know how we can improve it to help you and your students. To those of you who used the first five editions and sent your suggestions for improvements, you will find most of these in this sixth edition. Thank you for making this revision possible and for making it better.

Acknowledgments

I would like to thank everyone who helped make this sixth edition possible. Special appreciation is given to the following individuals.

Margie Hesson for serving as a contributing author of this book. Her professional and personal knowledge of exercise and healthy lifestyles brought valuable changes to this new edition. Margie's careful proofreading of the manuscript, in addition to her writing contributions, brought the female perspective to the presentation of the material making this a more balanced text for men and women.

Dr. Larry Tentinger for serving as a contributing author.

To all of the **Weight Training Teachers** who answered our questions and helped to shape this new edition.

- **James Gustafson**, Messiah College
- **David W. Hunter**, Hampton University
- **Joe Peoples**, Coastal Georgia Community College
- **L. Kristi Sayers**, University of Montevallo
- **William C. Whiting**, California State University-Northridge

Kristin Dilworth, Jon Kelley, and **Eric Risberg** for their excellent photography.

Josh Cooper, Doug Duran, and **Erik Berger** for their expert advice and help during photo sessions.

Andre Morrow for all he did to make this book possible. Andre, you are the greatest.

Leslie Araya, Courtney Bennigson, Erik Berger, Sara Brinkley, Grant Conklin, Josh Cooper, Therese Crawford, T.C. Dantzler, Samantha Dompier, Jason Gatson, Sanjuan Jones, Brett McClure, Anna Lissa I. Nool, Chris Parker, and Jason Yeske for their time, energy, ideas, encouragement, and patience as models.

Jeff Boyle for allowing us to take photographs in Gold's Gym of Colorado Springs.

Werner and **Sharon Hoeger** for being generous and caring to share their knowledge and material with us so we can share it with you.

Nautilus and **Universal Gym Equipment, Inc**. for the excellent photographs.

David Hesson for his help in selecting photographs.

Kristi Willenberg for her help with internet sites and proofreading.

Jim Bryant for his friendship and helpful attitude as well as everything he did for me to make the earlier editions of this book possible.

Milton Wilder for his support, encouragement, and friendship. As you know Milton, this book never would have happened without you. Thank you.

Tom Kidd for his early encouragement and support of an extremely thin and weak young boy. He supported my early weight training at a time when weight training was not popular and was not recommended by most coaches. It took a lot of courage to stand up for what you believed to be right, when all of the other coaches thought you were wrong. Scientific research has since proven that you were right and they were wrong.

Jake Geier for teaching me the difference between "producers" and "excusers."

Phil Allsen for his friendship as well as his continuing faith in me and support of my professional and personal development.

Joanne Saliger for making this such an attractive and functional book.

JLH

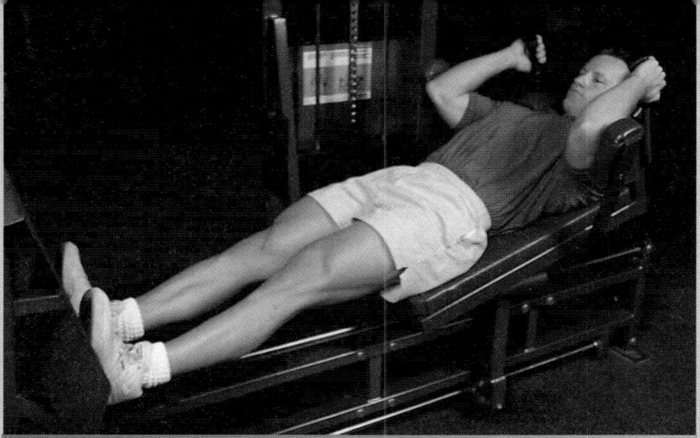
Eric Risberg

1

What, Who, and Why

You have an opportunity to participate in your own creation. The process of your creation did not end with your birth; it continues throughout your life. All of the living cells in your body have a time limit. Millions of your cells die and are replaced every day. In terms of living cells, you are not the same person you were last year, yesterday, an hour ago, or even 5 minutes ago. You are in a continual process of changing, and being re-created. What will you be like tomorrow, next week, or next year?

Your attitude, behavior, and lifestyle choices have a significant impact on who you are and who you will become. Through weight training and healthy eating you start to change your body. You will find, however, that as your body changes, your life begins to change. I challenge you to follow a well-planned weight training program, along with a healthy eating program, for one year and see for yourself. After a year of disciplined weight training and healthy eating, you will see such a dramatic difference, I believe, that you also will believe in *weight training for life*.

What Is Weight Training?

Weight training is a form of progressive resistance exercise. Weight can be added to, or taken from, the total load to arrive at the correct resistance for you for each exercise and each muscle group. Weight training exercises are done for different reasons. The categories of weight trainers discussed next will help you understand why there are so many different kinds of weight training programs.

Who Trains with Weights?

Those who train with weights include Olympic lifters, power lifters, body builders, athletes, medical patients, physical fitness enthusiasts, and weight trainers.

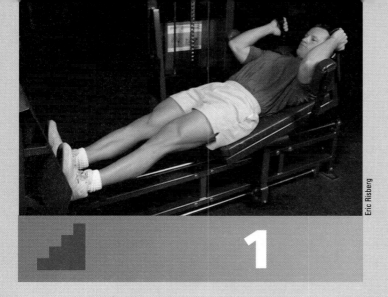

Olympic Lifters

Olympic-style weight lifting is a competitive sport. The objective in Olympic-style lifting is to see who can lift the most total weight overhead using two different lifts: the snatch and the clean-and-jerk.

1. The *snatch lift* requires lifting the weight in one continuous movement from the floor to a position in which the weight is overhead and both arms are straight. The lifter may drop below the weight to catch it overhead but must rise to a stationary standing position to complete the lift.

2. In the *clean-and-jerk lift* the weight must first be brought from the floor to a position on the upper chest and shoulders. Then, from a standing position the weight is thrust overhead to a straight-arm finish.

The winner is the individual with the highest total when the snatch and the clean-and-jerk lifts are added together. The competitors are grouped into different body weight classifications so they are competing against others who are approximately the same size.

Power Lifters

Power lifters compete in three lifts: the *bench press*, the *squat*, and the *dead lift*. The winner is the lifter with the highest total for the three lifts. The competitors are grouped by body weight so they are competing against other lifters who are approximately the same size.

Body Builders

Body builders participate in competition that is more art than sport. Through weight training they create a living sculpture using the human body as the clay. Body builders attempt to develop maximum muscular size while maintaining a balanced appearance (symmetry) and a high degree of muscular visibility (definition). In this competition the appearance of the body is most important.

Athletes

Ever since the rehabilitation work of Dr. Thomas DeLorme following World War II, progressive resistance exercise has gradually gained acceptance by the medical profession and the coaching profession. This form of exercise has changed dramatically during the last 50 years. In the 1950s and early 1960s most coaches told their athletes that they should not lift weights. During the 1970s lifting became more acceptable for athletes. In the 1980s and 1990s most coaches required their athletes to lift weights.

Most top-level athletes now use some form of weight training to improve their sports performance and to recover from sports injuries. Because skeletal muscles are responsible for voluntary human movement, athletes who increase the functional ability of their muscular system almost always improve their sports performance.

Recently there has been increased focus on opposing muscle groups. In the early years of weight training to improve athletic performance, much of the emphasis was placed on the muscles that produce the successful sports movements. Although the training did strengthen the desired muscles and improve performance, this type of training often created an imbalance of strength surrounding a joint. Occasionally the more strongly developed muscles on one side of the joint overpowered and injured the weaker, undeveloped muscles on the other side of the joint. Good weight training programs for athletes now include exercises for balanced development to improve performance and reduce the risk of injury.

Patients

Physicians and physical therapists frequently prescribe progressive resistance exercise as a part of the rehabilitation program for people who have been injured. By training with weights, these patients regain strength, muscle size, and functional ability after an injury.

Physical Fitness Enthusiasts

Many people who exercise for health and physical fitness have discovered the benefits of weight training. The people in this category want to look better, feel better, and be healthier.

Weight training to increase muscle tissue should be an important part of any fat-loss program. Many people have overlooked the benefits of weight training for fat loss because of the attention to calories spent during an exercise session. Although you might spend more calories during an aerobic training session than a weight training session, the increased muscle mass from weight training increases your metabolic rate.

You might use as many as 75 calories per day to support the energy needs of 1 pound of muscle tissue. You might use as few as 3 calories per day to support the energy needs of 1 pound of fat tissue. Because muscle is active tissue that burns calories and fat is inactive tissue that stores calories, those who are trying to lose body fat should increase their muscle mass.

Weight Trainers

Anyone who trains with weights could be considered a weight trainer. This book has been written primarily for those who are just beginning to lift weights and for the physical fitness enthusiast, with the hope that if they get off to a good start, they will participate in *weight training for life*.

Who Should Participate in Weight Training?

Everyone who has a muscular system can benefit from a regular program of progressive resistance exercise. Therefore, almost everyone should participate in *weight training for life*—men, women, and children of all ages, including people with disabilities.

Men and Women

The benefits of weight training for men and women include greater strength, increased muscle size, greater muscle endurance, improved appearance, higher self-esteem, and better sports performance. The location and function of the skeletal muscles is the same in men and women. Research during the last three decades has indicated that the weight training principles, methods, programs, and exercises that have worked well for men work equally well for women.

Weight training exercises are the same for men and women. There are no "men's exercises" or "women's exercises." Men and women, however, may choose to develop different muscle groups in different ways, which may affect their selection of exercises. As a result of a well-planned weight training program, men and women alike develop a strong, firm, healthy, attractive appearance.

Is weight training an appropriate activity for girls and women? Absolutely! All women achieve increases in muscular strength when they participate in properly planned weight training programs. Most women, however, do not experience as much of an increase in muscle size as most men on the same training program. This seems to be related to lower levels of the hormone testosterone and a lower number of muscle fibers in women.

Weight training will not make a woman appear masculine or cause a woman to develop any secondary male characteristics such as a deeper voice, facial hair, or thicker body hair. Secondary gender characteristics are caused by hormones. During puberty boys begin producing higher levels of male hormones, which produce the secondary gender characteristics we associate with males. At puberty girls begin producing higher levels of female hormones, which produce the secondary gender characteristics we associate with females. This hormone production varies from one person to another.

Although weight training can be beneficial during pregnancy for both mother and baby, there are some cautions. Any kind of exercise during pregnancy should be discussed with your doctor. When weight training is done during pregnancy, you should avoid

- holding your breath and straining to lift a heavy weight
- exercises that include excessive compression of the abdomen
- exercises that cause an increase in core body temperature
- high-intensity exercise
- long-duration exercise
- high-impact exercise

In other words, exercise during pregnancy should be light to moderate in intensity and duration, and regular in frequency.

Children

Children can gain important benefits through a carefully planned and closely supervised weight training program. Those who participate in weight training can gain strength, improve their self-image, increase their level of physical fitness, improve their sports performance, and possibly reduce their risk of youth sport injury.

The risk of injury from weight training during participation in a carefully planned and closely supervised weight training program for children is low. The few injuries that have been reported usually have occurred during improperly performed overhead lifts. Contributing factors include too much weight, improper technique, poorly planned programs, and a lack of supervision.

Those responsible for planning and supervising weight training programs for children must be trained and qualified in this area. Each exercise, along with the spotting techniques for that exercise, must be taught and demonstrated correctly. Young weight trainers should not be allowed to train alone without proper adult supervision and a trained spotter. The training area should be clean, bright, attractive, and large enough for the child to perform each lift safely. Training programs for children should focus on all-around physical development, not just strength training. Strength is only one aspect of physical development.

Children should train with moderate to light weights with which they can handle a fairly high number of repetitions. The National Strength and Conditioning Association recommends 6 to 15 repetitions in each set. This means that a child should not be allowed to lift a weight unless he or she can complete at least 6 correct repetitions using that weight. One-repetition maximum lifts are not recommended for children.

Weight training for children should be on a voluntary basis. If young children are forced to participate in weight training, they are more likely to develop a negative attitude toward this beneficial activity. If they develop a negative attitude, they probably will not participate in *weight training for life.*

After puberty and during adolescence, with the accompanying hormonal changes, children begin to undergo greater physical changes as a result of a weight training program. During this time they should maintain strict exercise form, and close qualified adult supervision is critical. Boys at this age seem to have an overwhelming urge to find out who can lift the most weight one time. Of course, what they often find out is how much they cannot lift one time. The risk of injury is too high.

As young people approach full growth and full physical maturity, weight training can have its most dramatic positive effects on physical performance, appearance, and self-confidence. This is a time when they can handle heavier exercise loads and more intense exercise programs. To maximize safety and progress, however, the emphasis must remain on correct exercise technique. Many young men resort to poor exercise technique to move a heavier weight. This can result in injury. Weight training exercises performed correctly rarely result in injury.

Adults

During the aging process, strength and muscle mass decline. How much of this decrease is a result of aging and how much is a result of a sedentary lifestyle? Very little of the decline in strength during the adult years is a result of aging. Individuals living in societies that are advanced in technology and automation reveal a much greater loss of strength and mobility as they get older. This is usually the result of inactivity and failure to maintain the muscular system.

Many individuals in the wage-earning adult years think they don't have time for weight training. Weight training actually is an efficient form of exercise. With weight training, a muscle group can be isolated and worked very hard in an extremely short time. A stimulus strong enough to maintain strength, or to cause a gain in the strength of a muscle group, may be achieved in about a minute with some weight training programs. This can be a greater strength gain stimulus than the same muscle group would achieve in hours of participating in some adult recreational activities.

All of the major muscles in the body can be exercised in 15 to 20 minutes. If a person adheres to this weight training program two or three times each week, it is an investment of 30 to 60 minutes a week. Each week has 168 hours, and you could maintain your strength during your adult years by investing approximately 1 hour per week in weight training. If you have limited time for exercise, weight training is one of the fastest ways to maintain or increase the functioning of your muscular system. It is important for adults to continue *weight training for life*.

Older Adults

At what age should adults stop weight training? Never! Humans should not use age as an excuse to stop weight training. Some physicians advise older adults to stop weight training because of medical problems, but as long as a person has no medical reason to quit, there is no reason to stop weight training at any certain age. Weight training programs, however, do have to be modified with age.

Sometime in their 60s, 70s, 80s, or 90s, most older adults undergo a more rapid decline in physical performance. How much of this decline is a result of the decrease in physical activity that often accompanies retirement and how much relates to a person's deciding that it is time to get old and to act old is difficult to determine. In either case, older adults must maintain their muscular system if they wish to retain their freedom and mobility. Therefore, older adults should participate in *weight training for life*.

People with Disabilities

Many people with disabilities are able to participate in weight training if they focus on their abilities. There certainly are exercises they cannot do; however, there are often exercises they can do. Each person with a disability needs to find out what he or she can do.

Everyone

Weight training is an efficient form of exercise to develop and maintain your muscular system. Though your goals and training programs will change as you progress through life, weight training is a valuable lifetime activity that you should continue. Everyone should participate in some form of *weight training for life*.

Why Weight Training?

The need for exercise has been underscored by the Office of the Surgeon General. The benefits are many and affect all areas of human development—physical, mental, social, emotional, and spiritual.

Surgeon General's Report

The Centers for Disease Control and Prevention (CDC) released *Physical Activity and Health: A Report of the Surgeon General* in 1996. One of the findings reported was that "Approximately 15 percent of U.S. adults engage regularly (3 times a week for at least 20 minutes) in vigorous physical activity during leisure time." This means, of course, that 85% do not. One of the major conclusions in the report was that "people of all ages, both male and female, benefit from regular physical activity." Also, "significant health benefits can be obtained by including a moderate amount of physical activity on most, if not all, days of the week."

According to the Surgeon General's report, regular physical activity that is performed on most days of the week reduces the risk of developing or dying from some of the leading causes of illness and death in the United States. Regular physical activity improves health by

- reducing the risk of dying prematurely
- reducing the risk of dying prematurely from heart disease
- reducing the risk of developing diabetes
- reducing the risk of developing high blood pressure
- helping to reduce blood pressure in people who have high blood pressure already
- reducing the risk of developing colon cancer
- reducing feelings of depression and anxiety
- helping to control weight
- helping to build and maintain healthy bones, muscles, and joints
- helping older adults become stronger and better able to move about without falling
- promoting psychological well-being

Regular physical activity should include cardiovascular exercise, resistance exercise (weight training), and flexibility exercise.

Personal Development

Personal development encompasses physical, mental, social, emotional, and spiritual development. Weight training can contribute to all of these areas of personal development.

Physical Development

Weight training makes its most obvious contributions in the area of physical development. All of the following can be improved with a well-planned weight training program:

muscle strength
tendon strength
ligament strength
bone strength
muscle size
muscle tone
appearance
posture
flexibility
metabolism
joint stability
muscle endurance
power
sports performance
lean body mass
physical fitness
health

Weight training is a lifetime activity that can help you to maintain fitness, reduce body fat, and reduce the risk and rate of injury.

Mental Development

A successful weight training program requires:

- knowledge about how your body functions
- knowledge about how your body responds to exercise
- knowledge about correct exercise technique
- knowledge about which exercises develop which muscles
- intelligent exercise program planning
- consistent self-discipline to follow your plan
- continual analysis of your progress and your plan
- insightful, intelligent problem solving

Social Development

Weight training is an activity that can be done alone, with one training partner, or with a group. Positive social qualities can be developed through weight training with others—among them, sharing, caring, encouraging, and helping. The workouts provide a time to participate with others in an activity that produces positive results for all participants. In contrast to many recreational games, which must result in a winner and a loser, everyone is a winner in weight training.

Weight training provides a common activity in which to participate and a common topic to discuss, as well as a time to be together. It can be an excellent activity for family members or friends because everyone can be together while performing their own individual training program at their own level without interfering with anyone else's progress.

A good weight training program includes the achievement of goals. Sharing your goals with others and helping others achieve their goals is rewarding. A bond often develops among those who do difficult activities together.

Emotional Development

Weight training can help a person release emotional stress and tension. A measurable decrease in neuromuscular tension occurs following a weight training session. It also provides an opportunity to release anger and frustration in a socially acceptable and healthy manner—intense physical activity that is not directed at another person.

Because weight training involves overcoming physical challenges during each training session, some regular participants seem to adopt a more objective and positive approach to other challenges in their lives. This produces greater emotional stability.

Measurable and noticeable changes in physical appearance result from a well planned weight training program. Increased muscle size or muscle tone, or both, create a firm, shapely appearance for men and women alike. That firm, trim, athletic look can never be achieved by diet alone. Also, posture improves. These physical improvements tend to be accompanied by an enhanced self-image and greater self-esteem. Those who lift weights often look better and feel better about themselves.

Spiritual Development

The spirit refers to the soul or the life force within each living human. It is one of the intangible and invisible things in life that cannot be accurately measured or adequately described. Yet, somehow you know the life force is there. Those who increase the strength of their body and their mind also seem to become stronger in spirit. Stronger people have greater resiliency, a greater life force, a stronger spirit. Many can "talk the talk" but few can "walk the walk." *Weight training for life* can help you become a "can do" person with a strong spirit.

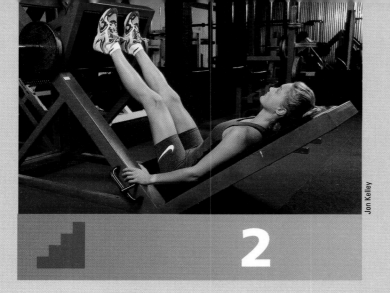

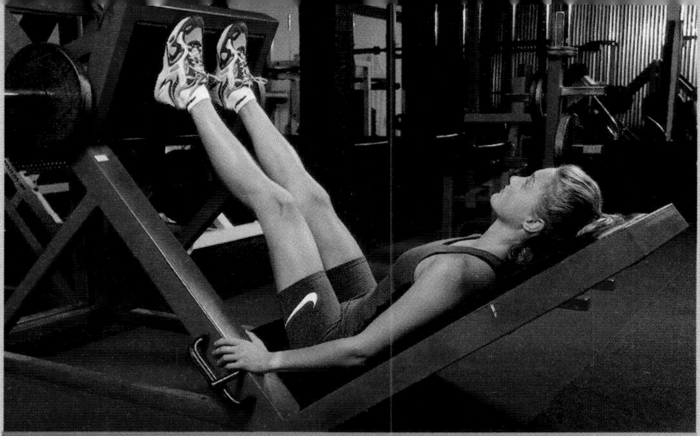

Jon Kelley

2

Questions, Concerns, and Answers

I don't want to get too big, so can I just tone my muscles?

Yes. You can design your training program so you don't get too big. If you use moderate to light resistance (60% to 80% of your 1 repetition maximum) for relatively high repetitions (12 to 15 repetitions) and relatively few sets (1 or 2 sets) of relatively few exercises (1 exercise per muscle group) performed relatively few days per week (2 or 3 days per week), your strength and muscle tone will improve and your muscles will not increase much in size. Actually, a lot of hard work is necessary for most men and women to increase the size of their muscles.

If I build muscle, will it turn to fat when I stop weight training?

No. Muscle tissue and fat tissue are two distinctly different kinds of tissue in the human body, and muscle tissue cannot become fat tissue. If you stop training, however, you could accumulate more body fat.

Muscle tissue adapts to the demands placed upon it. When you stop training, your muscles will adapt to the new demand. If the new demand is much less than it was before, the muscles will respond by getting smaller and weaker (*atrophy*). If you continue eating the same as you did when you were training hard every day, the extra calories will now be stored as body fat. Even if you manage to stay at the same body weight, you will have less muscle and more fat, leaving you with the outward appearance that your muscles have turned to fat. Because fat tissue is not as dense as muscle tissue, you can expect to gain inches in your body circumference measurements.

To make matters worse, as you lose metabolically active muscle tissue, your ability to use calories is reduced. Muscle cells are active calorie-burning cells. As these calorie-burning cells atrophy, your metabolic rate slows down and you need even fewer calories than before. To think you can maintain a trim, muscular, shapely appearance by diet alone is foolish. Are you beginning to realize the importance of *weight training for life*?

Are nutrition and rest important for weight training progress?

Yes. Weight training workouts provide a stimulus for positive changes to occur in your body, but without adequate nutrition and rest the changes may be slow or may not occur at all. Your weight training workouts could be a waste of time if you do not eat and sleep properly. For more details, read the Chapter 7 discussion on nutrition and rest.

Will weight training make a woman look masculine?

No. Hormones, not weight training, determine if a person appears more masculine or more feminine. Men usually produce much more testosterone than women. The higher levels of testosterone contribute to the secondary characteristics we generally consider as masculine. Women who participate in weight training develop healthy, shapely, trim female figures.

Will weight training make me muscle-bound?

No. If you follow correct weight training principles, weight training will not make you muscle-bound. "Muscle-bound" people have a limited range of joint motion. One weight training principle is to train each muscle through a full range of motion. Each muscle should be exercised from full extension to full contraction. Another principle is that opposing muscles should receive an equal amount of exercise so the muscles on one side of a joint do not develop more than muscles on the other side. When these principles are followed, flexibility and joint mobility will tend to increase rather than decrease. The United States has many more "fat-bound" people than "muscle-bound" people. Their range of motion is limited by an excessive accumulation of stored body fat.

Athletes can become muscle-bound as a result of the unbalanced muscular development resulting from their participation in sports training. When some athletes train with weights to improve their sports performance, they train only those muscles that already are overdeveloped and ignore balanced development. As a consequence, athletes sometimes see weight training as the reason for their muscle-bound condition when their condition actually is the result of a poorly planned weight training program.

Weight trainers can develop a high level of strength and a high level of flexibility, but they have to work on both. A good example of a high level of strength development accompanied by a high level of flexibility is the gymnast.

Will weight training "shape up" a specific part of my body?

Yes and no. Exercises for a specific body part will firm up weak, sagging muscles and may result in a trimmer appearance but will not effectively reduce excess body fat stored in that area. The idea of losing body fat from a specific body part is known as *spot reducing*. Examples of spot reduction are sit-ups to lose fat from the abdomen and hip extensions to lose fat from the hips. The research in this area indicates that spot reduction does not work. To lose fat from a specific area requires a reduction in total body fat. This is best accomplished by reducing caloric intake while increasing caloric expenditure.

Is aerobic exercise the best way to lose excess body fat?

No. The best way to lose body fat is a combination of aerobic exercise, weight training, and healthy eating. Aerobic exercise is a good way to burn calories and develop your cardiovascular system. Weight training is a good way to build muscle tissue, which increases your ability to burn calories and reshape your body. Healthy eating is necessary to avoid excess caloric intake and ensure an adequate supply of the nutrients you need to rebuild your body. The combination of these three is the best way to lose body fat.

Weight training is an important component of the fat-loss process. The increase in muscle tissue will help with fat loss by building more active muscle tissue that is capable of using calories and by increasing your resting metabolic rate so you will use more calories even when you are resting. If you want to improve the shape of your body, you need to include *weight training for life*.

Will weight training make me slower?

No. I hope this myth is no longer around. Coaches used to tell their athletes not to lift weights because it would make them slower. The research in this area indicates that the opposite is true. Weight training can increase your speed. Muscle contraction is responsible for human movement. If your strength increases more than your body weight, you should be able to move faster. Muscular weakness and excess body fat will make you slower.

Will weight training damage my joints?

No. If done correctly, weight training exercises will increase joint strength. Exercises should be performed in a smooth, continuous manner. Weight training exercises done improperly could damage your joints.

What if I don't have time for weight training?

Everyone has 168 hours a week; nobody gets more or less. "Having time" is really about prioritizing. What is most important to you? If you don't have time for weight training, you either have set your weight training goals too high (requiring too much time) or too many things in your life are more important to you. Keep a time log for a week and see where you are spending time, investing time, and wasting time. Many

Americans watch television 3 to 4 hours a day but don't have time to exercise.

Does weight training require hours of training each week?

No. Weight training is an efficient form of exercise. All of the major muscle groups in your body can be trained in 15 to 20 minutes two or three times each week. This is a minimal program, but it may be more than you are doing now and it is certainly better than doing nothing. The amount of time you need to spend training with weights is related to the goals you set for yourself. Body builders, Olympic lifters, and power lifters do spend many hours each week training with weights; however, that is what they enjoy doing and they have set some very high goals.

Will weight training ruin my coordination?

No. This is another myth that I hope has disappeared. Although some neuromuscular adjustment accompanies an increase in strength, most people make this minor adjustment with no problem. Athletes in a sport in which "touch," or fine motor coordination, is critical might be advised to increase their strength during the off-season and maintain a constant strength level through the competitive season. For weak and untrained individuals, weight training will often improve coordination.

Can I just play sports instead of weight training to gain strength?

No. Most sports do not provide the proper type, intensity, duration, or frequency of exercise to increase strength effectively. Weight training can produce in a short time a strength-gain stimulus that is greater than a muscle would receive from hours of participation in most sports. Many recreational sports injuries are the result of placing an unfit body in a competitive situation. You should gain strength to participate in sports, not participate in sports to gain strength.

Could heavy lifting cause a hernia?

Yes. A hernia, or a rupture in the abdominopelvic cavity, occurs when any of the internal organs is pushed through the wall that surrounds it. If you hold your breath and strain to lift an object that is too heavy, the pressure in the abdominal cavity increases to a high level and could cause a hernia. This happens more often to individuals who do not train on a regular basis. They do not know correct lifting technique or how much they can lift safely. The unfit person moving furniture is a classic example.

It is possible, but highly unlikely, that a person would incur a hernia during a well-planned weight training program using correct lifting techniques. Correct weight training procedures require that you not hold your breath and strain to lift a weight. Exhaling as you exert force is generally best. In weight training you should learn about, and practice, correct lifting mechanics and breathing. These two factors, along with knowing how much weight you can lift safely, should reduce your risk of getting a hernia while you are weight training. Start light and progress slowly. This is a lifetime fitness activity. Hernias occur approximately 20 times less often among weight trainers than among non-weight trainers!

Is weight training for only the young and athletic?

No. Weight training is a healthy lifetime fitness activity for males and females of all ages. Young athletes do use weight training to improve athletic performance, but that is certainly not the only use.

When is a person too old to start weight training?

Never. A person is never too old to start a sensible weight training program. Some people may be too unhealthy, but never too old. *Weight training for life* can be beneficial for anyone who has a muscular system to maintain. Each person should have an individualized training program. Your individual goals, training programs, and results will be different, but weight training can be beneficial at any age. Research has shown that individuals who are more than 90 years old gain strength and muscle mass after they begin weight training.

What if I miss a workout?

You will miss a workout—everyone does. Just get back on your training schedule as soon as possible, and keep going. A lifetime of exercise is a lifetime of starting over again and again and again. Keep interruptions to a minimum, and get back on schedule as soon as possible. Over many years a few missed workouts will not make much difference. Weight training is a lifetime fitness activity, and the benefits come from years of regular training.

Why should I spend my time and energy lifting weights?

Most people lift weights to improve their appearance, health, and movement. *Weight training for life* can add more life to your years and maybe more years to your life.

Can weight training develop total health-related physical fitness?

Yes. A well-planned circuit weight training program can develop all aspects of health-related physical fitness. Total health-related physical fitness involves the development of cardiovascular endurance, healthy body composition, muscular strength, muscular endurance, and flexibility (Table 2.1). Most weight training programs are designed to develop strength or muscular endurance, but they can be designed to develop all aspects of health-related physical fitness.

	Type of Exercise (What Kind of Exercise?)	Intensity (How Hard?)	Duration (How Long?)	Frequency (How Often?)
Cardiovascular	Large muscle groups Rhythmic Continuous	Exercise at 60 to 90% of Maximum Heart Rate	20 to 60 Minutes	3 to 5 Days Per Week
Body Composition (For Loss of Excess Body Fat)	Large muscle groups Low Impact Rhythmic Continuous	Exercise at 60 to 80% of Maximum Heart Rate*	30 to 60 Minutes	5 to 7 Days Per Week
Strength	Isotonic Exercise Full Range of Movement Against Resistance	85% to 100% of Maximum Voluntary Contraction** 1 to 6 RM***	1 to 6 Repetitions 1 to 3 Sets	2 to 3 Days Per Week
Muscular Endurance	Isotonic Exercise Full Range of Movement Against Resistance	Low to Moderate Resistance 50% to 70% of Maximum Voluntary Contraction** 12 to 20+ RM	12 to 20+ Repetitions 1 to 3 Sets	2 to 3 Days Per Week
Flexibility	Static Stretch	Moderate Discomfort	Hold for 10 to 30 Seconds 1 to 3 Times	3 to 7 Days Per Week

* Estimated Maximum Heart Rate = 220 minus age
** Maximum Voluntary Contraction = One Repetition Maximum
*** Repetition Maximum (RM) = The heaviest weight you can lift for a specific number of repetitions
Developed by: Dr. James Hesson, Professor of Biology and Biokinetics, Black Hills State University

Table 2.1 Exercise Guidelines for Health-Related Physical Fitness

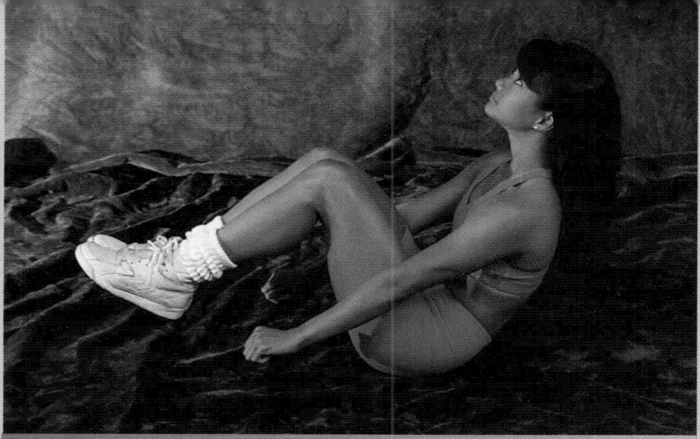

Eric Risberg

3

Muscle Structure and Function

Your body has approximately 600 muscles, making up about 50% of your total body weight. Skeletal muscles account for about 40% of your total body weight, and the other 10% is primarily involuntary muscle of the circulatory and digestive systems. Although muscles vary a great deal in size, shape, arrangement of fibers, and internal characteristics, they all perform the same general function—to provide movement. The importance of muscle tissue cannot be overemphasized. Human movement is made possible by muscle contraction.

Characteristics of Muscle Tissue

Characteristics of muscle tissue include extensibility, elasticity, excitability, and contractility. These four characteristics combine to make muscle tissue a very special kind of tissue. Muscle tissue is responsible for body movement.

Extensibility

Extensibility is the ability of muscle tissue to be stretched. If muscle tissue could not stretch, you would not have the mobility or range of motion you have.

Elasticity

Elasticity is the ability of muscle tissue to return to its normal resting length and shape after being stretched. If muscle tissue did not have elasticity, it would remain at its stretched length.

Excitability

Excitability refers to the ability of muscle tissue to receive a stimulus from the nervous system.

Contractility

Contractility is the quality that really sets muscle tissue apart. When a stimulus is received, muscle tissue can contract.

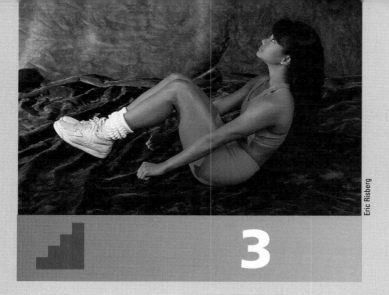

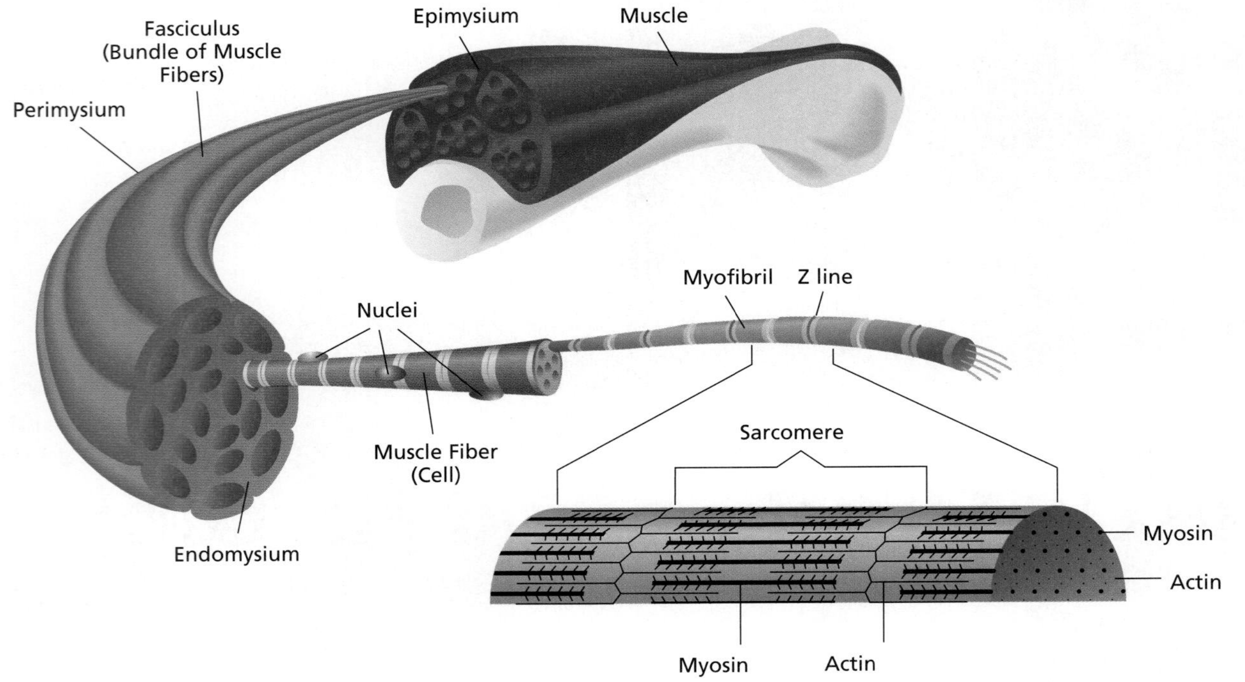

Figure 3.1 Components of skeletal muscle tissue.

Types of Muscle Tissue

The types of muscle tissue are skeletal, smooth, and cardiac. Each of these has specific functions.

Skeletal Muscle

The primary focus of this book is the development of *skeletal muscle*, which is attached to the bones of the skeletal system. Skeletal muscle is voluntary muscle—the contraction of skeletal muscle is a result of conscious voluntary control.

Smooth Muscle

Smooth muscle primarily lines hollow internal structures such as blood vessels and the digestive tract. Smooth muscle is involuntary because its contraction and relaxation phases are automatic and not the result of conscious, voluntary control.

Cardiac Muscle

Cardiac muscle is found only in the heart. This type is classified as involuntary because a person cannot consciously contract the muscle tissue of the heart.

The Musculoskeletal System As A Lever System

The human body has three types of levers and six different classifications of freely movable joints. This combination enables a wide variety of human movements, made possible by skeletal muscle tissue pulling on different bones across joints. Some joints, such as the ball-and-socket joint of your shoulder, offer a wide range of movement possibilities. Others, such as the hinge joint of your elbow, are limited to two movements—flexion and extension.

The Structure of Skeletal Muscle

Each of the skeletal muscles has connective tissue running through it and around it. Where this connective tissue attaches a muscle to a bone, it is called a *tendon*. The tendon is continuous with the connective tissue that encloses the muscle tissue.

The connective tissue that encloses skeletal muscle tissue is divided into three categories:

1. *Epimysium*: connective tissue that surrounds the entire muscle.

2. *Perimysium*: connective tissue that surrounds a bundle of muscle fibers (fasciculus).

3. *Endomysium*: connective tissue that surrounds a muscle fiber. This is the type of tissue you are stretching primarily when you stretch a muscle. The intensity of the stretch has to be sufficient to increase the length of the connective tissue without tearing it.

Inside the muscle are bundles of *muscle fibers* (muscle cells). Skeletal muscle fibers (cells) are generally long and relatively small in diameter. (See Figure 3.1.)

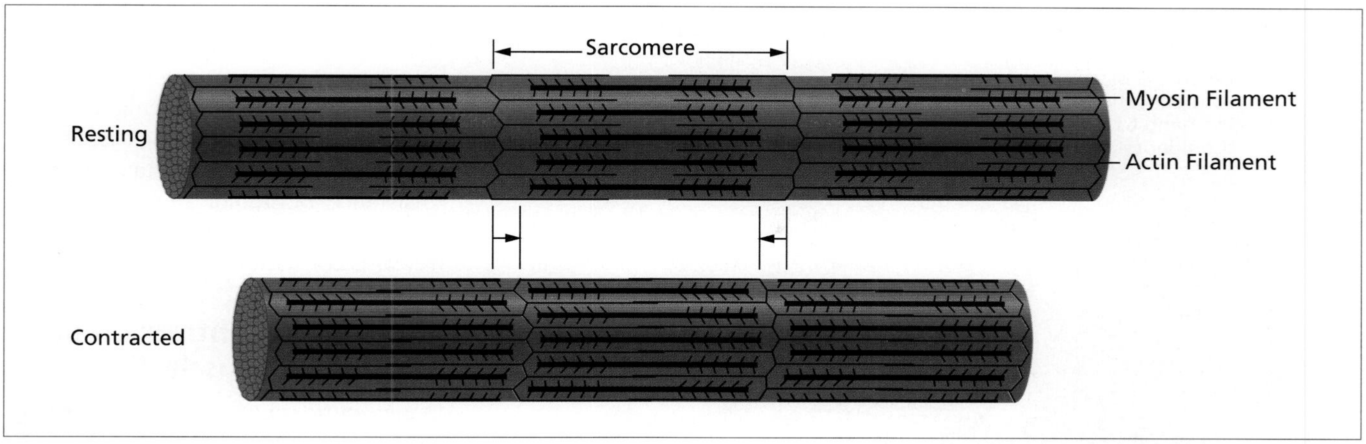

Figure 3.2 During muscle contraction, cross-bridges from the myosin attach to actin filaments and pull the actin filaments toward the center of the sarcomere.

Within each muscle fiber are long, threadlike structures called *myofibrils*, which run lengthwise through the muscle fiber. Each myofibril consists of many *sarcomeres* attached end to end (see Figure 3.1). The sarcomere is the basic contractile unit of skeletal muscle tissue (see Figures 3.1 and 3.2.) Within the sarcomere are *myofilaments*. The thinner myofilaments are called *actin*, and the thicker myofilaments are called *myosin*.

According to the sliding filament theory of muscle contraction, the myosin filaments have cross-bridges that contact the actin filaments. The actin and myosin filaments do not change in length, but the myosin cross-bridges pull the actin filaments toward the center of the sarcomere. Because the actin filaments are attached to the ends of the sarcomere, the sarcomere becomes shorter in length as the actin filaments are pulled toward the center. (See Figures 3.2 and 3.3.)

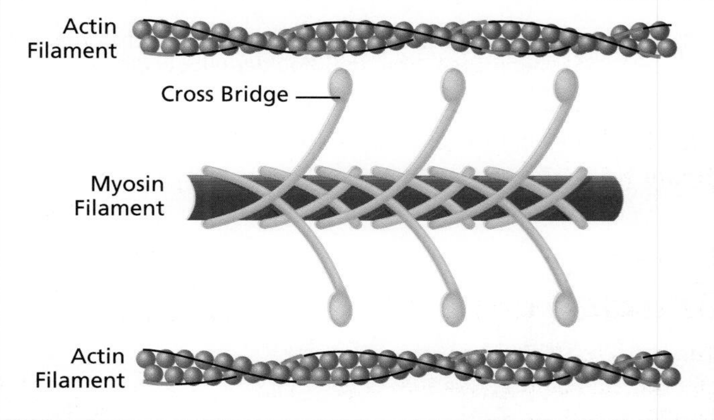

Figure 3.3 At higher magnification, during muscle contraction, cross-bridges from the myosin attach to actin filaments and pull the actin filaments toward the center of the sarcomere.

Muscle Contraction And Exercise Movements

Muscle tissue can contract or relax. Therefore, muscle can pull on bones or stop pulling on bones. Muscle tissue can only pull. It cannot push. In some exercises an object, such as a barbell, is pushed away from the body. A pushing movement during an exercise is accomplished by muscles pulling on bones and causing joints to extend. All exercises involve muscles pulling on bones across a joint. The movement that takes place depends upon the structure of the joint and the position of the muscle attachments involved. (See Figure 3.4.) The types of contraction are isometric, isotonic, concentric, eccentric, and isokinetic.

Isometric Contraction

Iso means equal, and *metric* refers to length or measure. Therefore, an *isometric contraction* is one in which the muscle maintains an equal length. This occurs when contracting a muscle and creating a force against an immovable object. The muscle contracts and tries to shorten but cannot overcome the resistance. An example of an isometric contraction is trying to lift a truck.

Isotonic Contraction

Tonic means tone or tension. Therefore, an *isotonic contraction* is one in which movement occurs but muscle tension remains about the same. An example is a complete barbell curl. Actually, during barbell and dumbbell exercises, while the external resistance remains constant, the muscle does not maintain constant tone throughout the exercise movement because of the continuous change in its angle of pull on the bone.

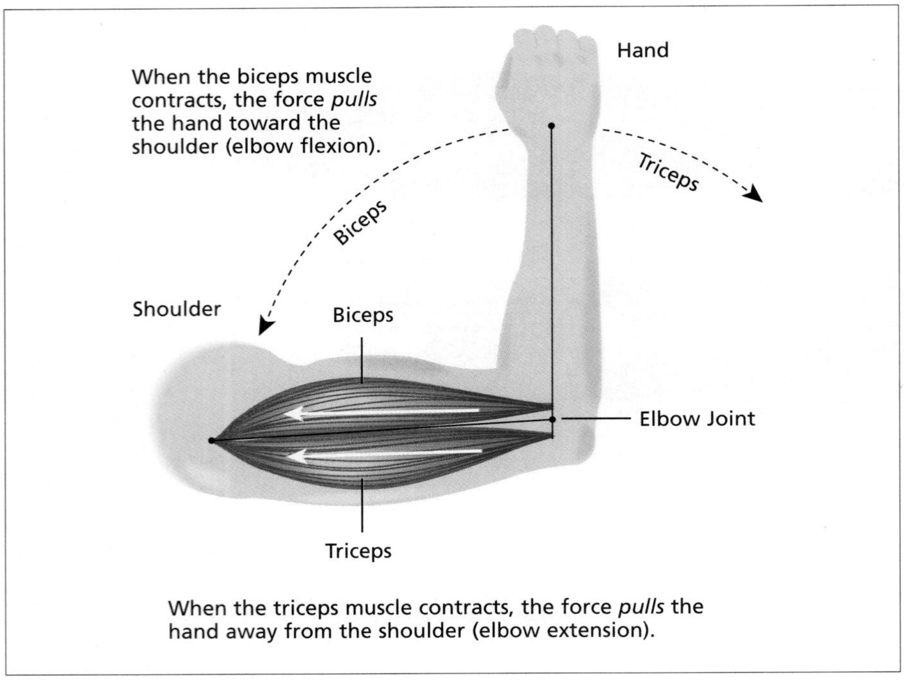
When the biceps muscle contracts, the force *pulls* the hand toward the shoulder (elbow flexion).
Hand
Triceps
Biceps
Shoulder
Biceps
Elbow Joint
Triceps
When the triceps muscle contracts, the force *pulls* the hand away from the shoulder (elbow extension).

Figure 3.4 Two muscles showing pulling characteristics.

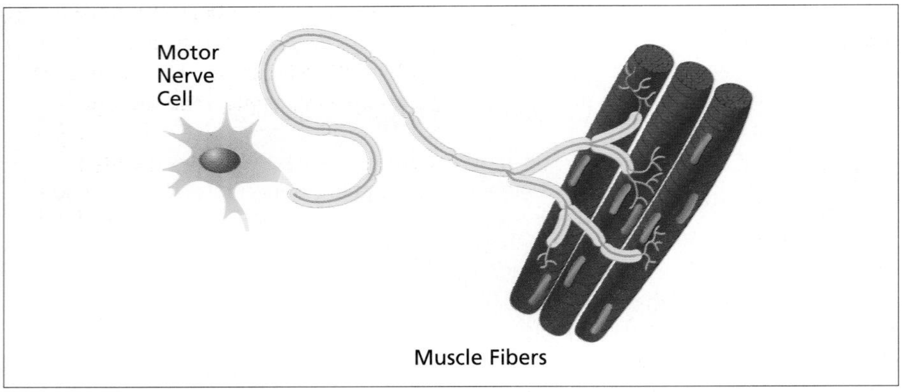
Motor Nerve Cell
Muscle Fibers

Figure 3.5 Motor unit, composed of a motor nerve and muscle fibers.

Consequently, another term is *DCER, dynamic constant external resistance*. This is not a new type of training but, rather, an attempt to be more accurate in describing exercise movements against a constant external resistance. *DCER* indicates that the resistance, not the muscle tone, is what remains constant.

Concentric Contraction or Concentric Muscle Action

A *concentric contraction* is a shortening contraction. The muscle becomes shorter and overcomes the resistance. An example is lifting the weight upward during the barbell curl.

Eccentric Contraction or Eccentric Muscle Action

An *eccentric contraction* is a lengthening contraction. The muscle contracts and tries to shorten but is overcome by the resistance. Eccentric contractions allow you to lower things smoothly and slowly. An example is lowering the weight in a smooth, controlled manner during the barbell curl.

Isokinetic Contraction

Kinetic signifies motion. Therefore, a true *isokinetic contraction* is a constant-speed contraction. The speed is set on the exercise device so the muscle can contract at 100% throughout the full range of motion without causing any acceleration. An example is the leg extension on a Cybex 350 Extremity Testing and Rehabilitation System.

Motor Unit

A *motor nerve* coming from the brain or spinal cord causes a muscle to contract or a gland to secrete. A *sensory nerve* carries information to the spinal cord and brain. A *motor unit* consists of a single motor nerve and all the muscle fibers to which it sends impulses. Although a motor nerve is connected to many muscle fibers, each muscle fiber is controlled by only one motor nerve. (See Figure 3.5.)

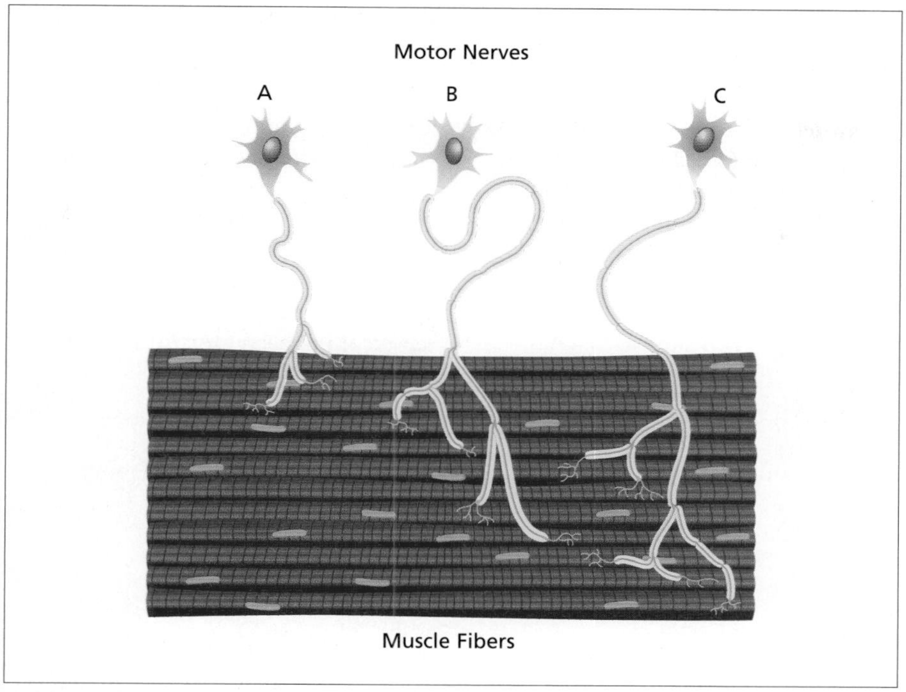

Figure 3.6 Muscle fiber and motor unit recruitment.

A motor nerve that is responsible for very fine movement may be connected to very few muscle fibers, such as those responsible for eye movements. A motor nerve responsible for large or heavy human movements may be connected to many muscle fibers, such as those responsible for hip extension.

All-or-None Principle

A muscle fiber contracts completely or not at all. If a stimulus for contraction is below the threshold value, the muscle does not contract. If the stimulus is above the threshold value, the muscle contracts completely. All of the muscle fibers in a motor unit contract completely or not at all. (See Figure 3.5.)

Recruitment

Each muscle contains hundreds of motor units. The force a muscle exerts is determined primarily by the size and number of motor units recruited for the task. As an example, refer to Figure 3.6. If a small amount of force is necessary, motor unit A may be used. In this case, three muscle fibers contract completely. If a moderate amount of force is required, motor units A and B might both be used. In this case, seven muscle fibers contract completely. If a maximum force is necessary, all three motor nerves may be activated, and they would stimulate 12 muscle fibers to contract completely, thereby producing more force.

Muscle Atrophy and Hypertrophy

Muscles that are not used will shrink—called *atrophy*—to a size that is adequate for the demands placed upon them. A good example of muscle atrophy occurs with a broken leg or arm that is immobilized in a cast during the bone-healing process. When the cast is removed, that arm or leg is much smaller than the active arm or leg. The same thing happens to people who do not train their muscular system, but both limbs are reduced in size and the process is so gradual that it often goes unnoticed.

The opposite is also generally true: Muscles that are forced to work harder than normal generally increase in size—called *hypertrophy*. This muscle growth is much more visible and more pronounced in men than it is in women. The reason for the greater increase in muscle size in men is related to the hormone testosterone, and to a larger number of muscle fibers in a muscle. As your curiosity about muscle structure and function increases, you may want to refer to current human anatomy, human physiology, and exercise physiology textbooks for more detailed information.

Basic Principles of Muscle Development

Three basic principles underlying all weight training progress are specificity, overload, and progression.

Specificity

The principle of *specificity* states that:

1. You must exercise the specific muscles you want to develop.

2. You must follow specific exercise guidelines to produce the specific type of change you desire: muscle strength, muscle size, or muscle endurance.

Overload

The *overload* principle is the basis of all training programs. In weight training the muscle to be developed must be overloaded, or forced to work harder than normal. The overload must be enough to stimulate improvement but not enough to cause injury.

Progression

Once the muscles adapt to a given workload, they no longer are overloaded. The workload must be increased progressively as the muscle adapts to each new demand. The *progression* in workload has to be enough to continue to stimulate improvement but not so much that it causes injury. This is one reason that keeping a written record of each exercise session is important.

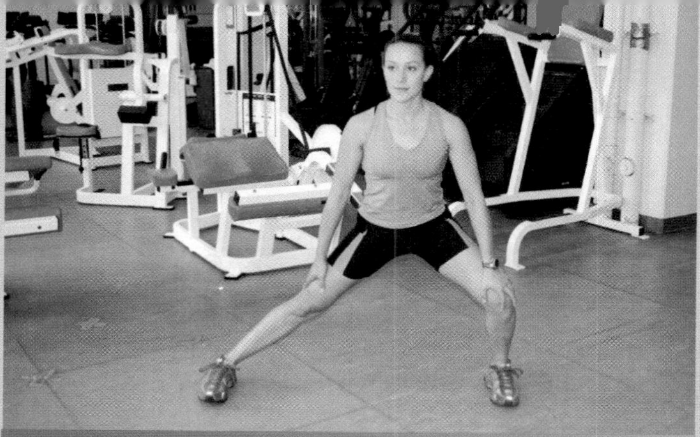

Kristin Dilworth

4

Warm-Up, Flexibility, and Stretching

The concepts of warm-up, flexibility, and stretching are often intermingled and confused in a person's mind. Each, however, has a separate purpose.

Warm-Up

Before participating in vigorous physical activity, many adults prefer to warm up. Warm-up activities usually consist of light muscular activity and some light stretching movements. A good warm-up should improve performance and reduce the risk of injury.

One common and effective way to warm up for weight training is to perform light to moderate warm-up sets for each exercise before progressing to heavier sets. (See Figure 4.1.) Almost all Olympic lifters, power lifters, body builders, and athletes warm up for heavy exercise in this manner. This form of warm-up seems to be beneficial for mental preparation as well as physical preparation to exert greater effort in heavier sets.

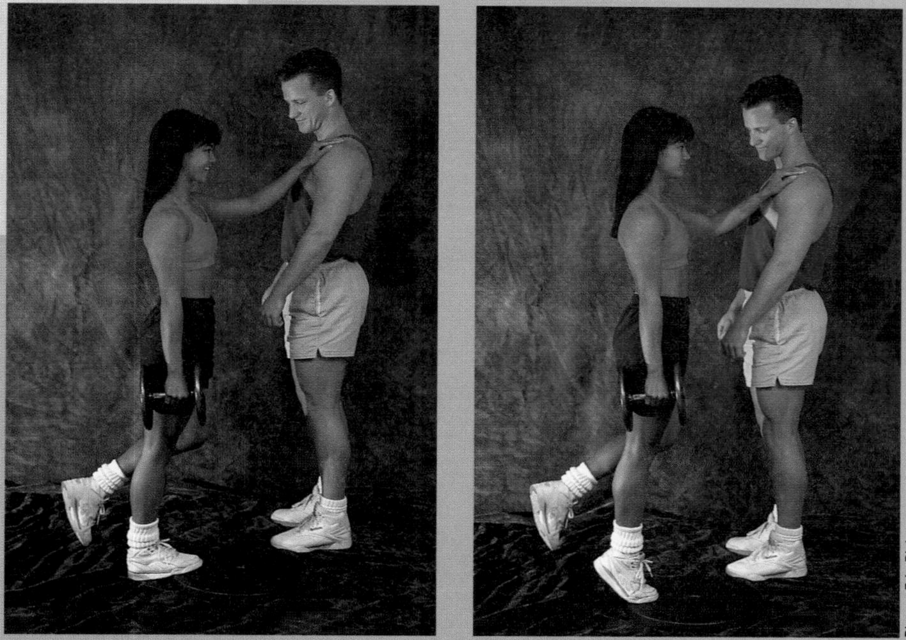

Photos Eric Risberg

Figure 4.1 Light weight warm-up sets.

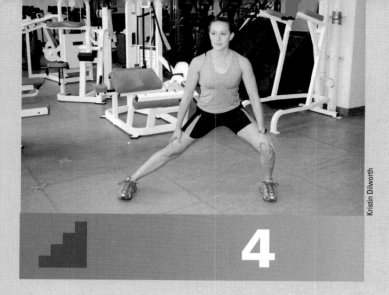

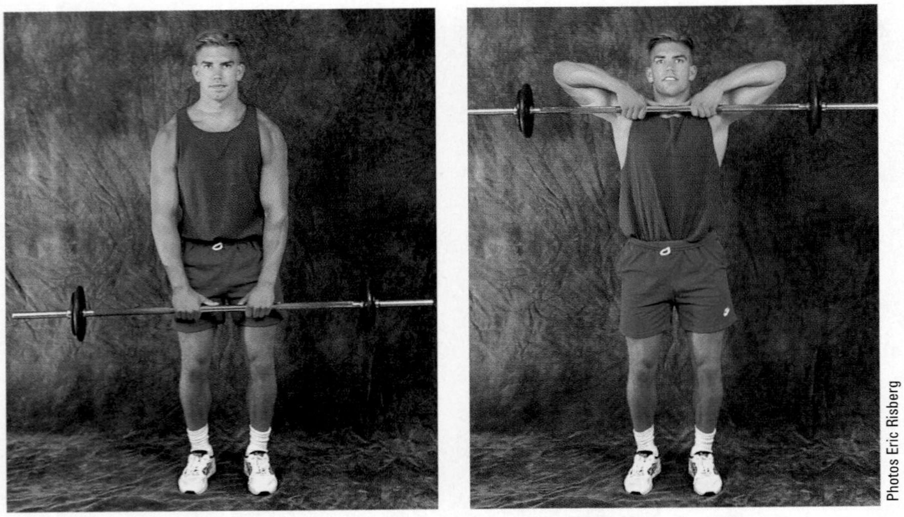

Figure 4.2 Exercising through full range of motion.

Another way to warm up is to perform some type of aerobic activity such as walking, jogging, or cycling, followed by some light stretching exercises to gently increase the range of motion before proceeding to more vigorous exercise.

Flexibility

Flexibility refers to the range of motion available in a joint. It is specific to each joint and each joint movement. Therefore, a person might be flexible in shoulder joint movements and tight in hip joint movements. An individual also could be flexible in hip joint flexion but tight in hip joint extension.

Correct weight training should increase or maintain flexibility. Proper weight training consists of:

1. Exercise through a full range of joint motion in a smooth and continuous manner, and
2. A balanced program of exercises for all opposing muscle groups that surround a joint.

Individuals who do not perform any exercise, those who participate in only one sport, and athletes who have trained with weights but have used partial movements or have neglected to develop opposing muscle groups are frequently less flexible than those who train correctly with weights.

How much flexibility is enough? There are no absolute measurable standards for healthy flexibility. Some charts report population averages, but in an unfit population how useful is that? In general, a joint should move freely in all of the directions appropriate for that joint.

Is more flexibility better? Not always. There is a trade-off between flexibility and joint stability. If a joint has too much flexibility, it is less stable and the individual is more prone to dislocation-type injuries. But if a joint has too little flexibility, it is highly stable but the individual is more likely to incur soft-tissue injuries to the muscles, tendons, and ligaments surrounding the joint.

Weight training can be an ideal exercise to arrive at a healthy amount of flexibility because each joint is moved through a full range of motion and all of the muscles, tendons, and ligaments that surround and support a joint are strengthened. (See Figure 4.2.) One result of correct weight training should be strong, flexible joints.

Equipment can make a difference. Dumbbells generally allow the greatest range of motion and therefore may contribute more to flexibility. (See Figure 4.3.) The range of motion of some exercise machines is not as great as that of the individual using the machine. If this is the case, the individual will not increase flexibility when exercising on that machine.

Stretching

Stretching is a type of exercise used to increase flexibility. The range of motion of a joint is usually restricted by the soft tissue surrounding it—muscles, tendons, and ligaments. Therefore, stretching exercises should gently stretch these soft tissues without damaging them or the joint.

Factors Involved in Stretching

The variables involved in stretching include type, intensity, duration, and frequency.

Type

Stretching exercises can be performed in different ways. *Static stretch* is a method of stretching in which the bones of a joint are moved to the point where the soft tissues surrounding the joint restrict further movement. These soft tissues (muscle, tendon, ligament, and joint capsule) are gently stretched and held in this stretched position for a period of time. Six reasons for recommending static stretch are:

1. It is an effective way to increase flexibility.
2. The risk of injury is low.
3. It is easy to learn.
4. You can stretch alone.
5. Static stretch relieves some types of muscle soreness.
6. If done correctly, static stretch does not cause muscle soreness.

Intensity

To be effective in increasing flexibility, the soft connective tissue surrounding a joint should be stretched to about 10% beyond its normal length. Although this is difficult to measure, we have built-in sensors for judging the intensity of a static stretch exercise. When you are stretching at the correct intensity, you will experience moderate discomfort or moderate tension in the tissues being

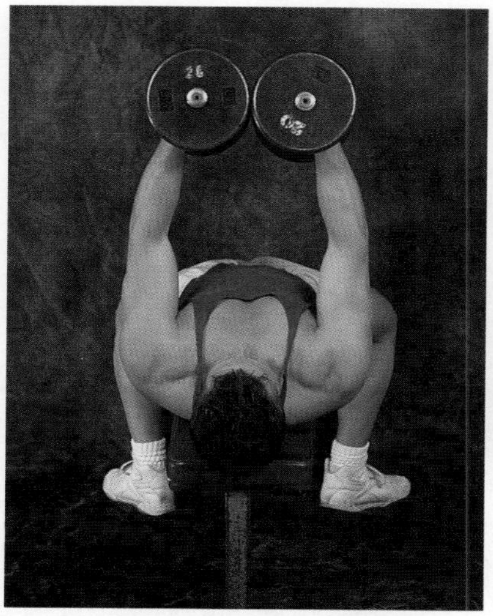

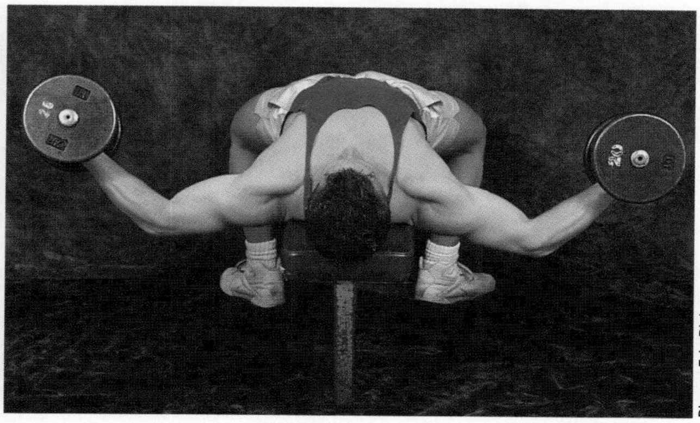

Photos Eric Risberg

Figure 4.3 Using dumbbells to promote range of motion.

Stretching Guidelines

Type	Static Stretch
Intensity	Moderate Discomfort
Duration	10- to 30-second hold 1 to 3 repetitions
Frequency	3 to 7 days per week

stretched. If you can't feel any stretch, you probably have not gone far enough. If you feel pain, you have gone too far. You should ease into each stretch gradually so you don't get to the pain level.

Duration

When you are performing static stretching exercises, you should hold a static stretch position at an intensity level of moderate tension for 10 to 30 seconds. You should perform each stretching exercise one, two, or three times.

Frequency

To be most effective in increasing flexibility, you should repeat static stretching exercises at least 3 days per week. Static stretching exercises can be performed up to 7 days per week.

Joints to Stretch

A stretching exercise can be designed for every muscle and every joint in your body, but stretching the major areas—neck, trunk, shoulders, wrists, hips, knees, and ankles—is more practical. Each of these joints is stretched in each major direction that it can move and is held in that position for 10 to 30 seconds. Your weight training instructor can give you additional advice on safe stretching exercises.

Many good stretching exercises have been said to be potentially harmful. Usually, however, it is not the exercise but, instead, the way it is performed that makes it harmful. You always should be careful when stretching so the exercises produce flexibility and not injury.

When to Stretch

Many people feel better if they stretch their muscles and joints prior to more vigorous exercise such as weight training. This stretching helps to prevent exercise injuries and may improve performance.

Some research has indicated that vigorous stretching of cold muscles may be harmful. Therefore, any stretching before warming the muscles should be done carefully. Stretching cold muscles should consist of light, gentle stretching exercises designed to loosen the movements of those joints.

Vigorous stretching to increase flexibility should be done only after the muscles and joints have been thoroughly warmed up. One good time to do this type of stretching is immediately after your weight training workout. Another good time to stretch is during the rest between sets.

An Example of a Safe Weight Room Stretching Routine

The usual reasons people give for not stretching are that "it takes too long" and "I don't have a good place to stretch." This gentle and safe stretch routine has been developed to counter those reasons. Although the illustrations show only one side, you should stretch both sides of your body.

If you hold each of these 21 stretch positions for 10 seconds, you can complete this stretch routine in 3½ minutes for a quick, light, easy, warm-up stretch.

Weight Room Stretching Routine

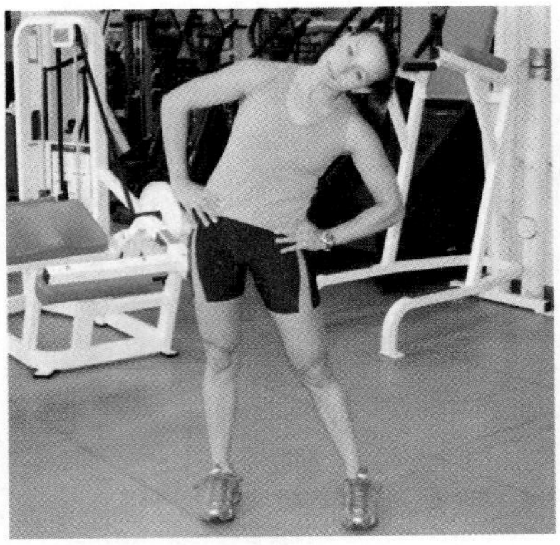

Neck, Trunk, and Hip

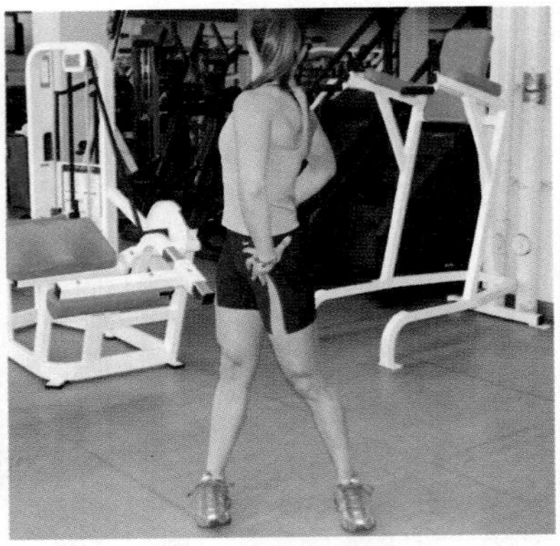

Neck, Trunk, and Hip

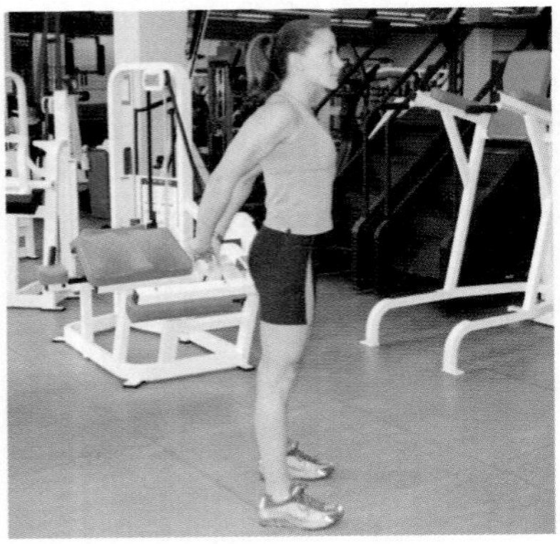

Chest, Shoulders, and Elbows

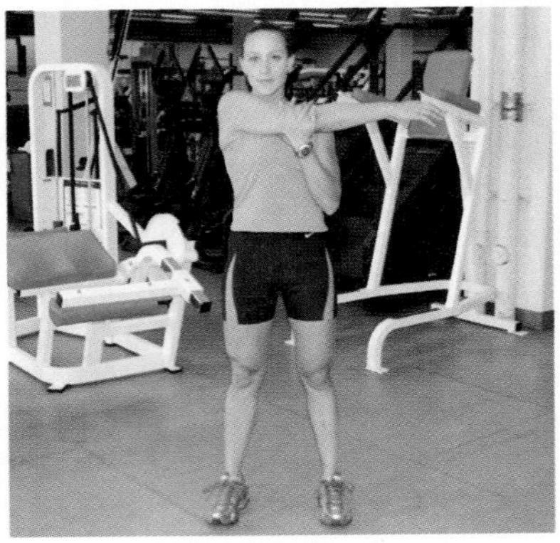

Upper Back and Shoulder

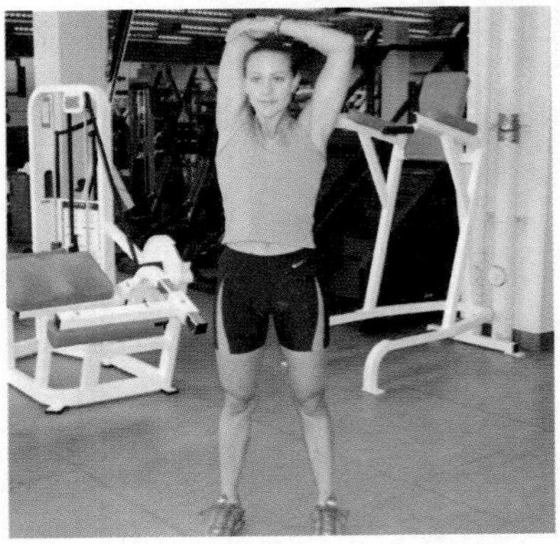

Upper Back and Shoulder

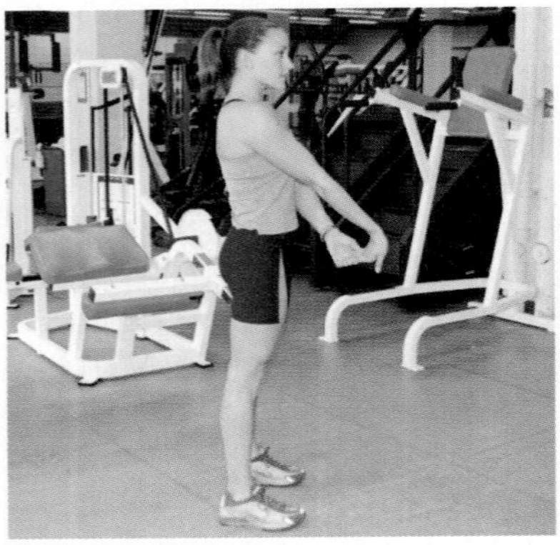

Wrists and Elbows

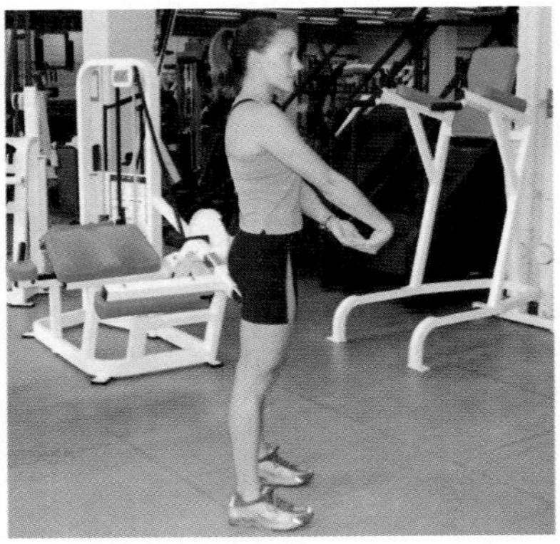

Wrists and Elbows

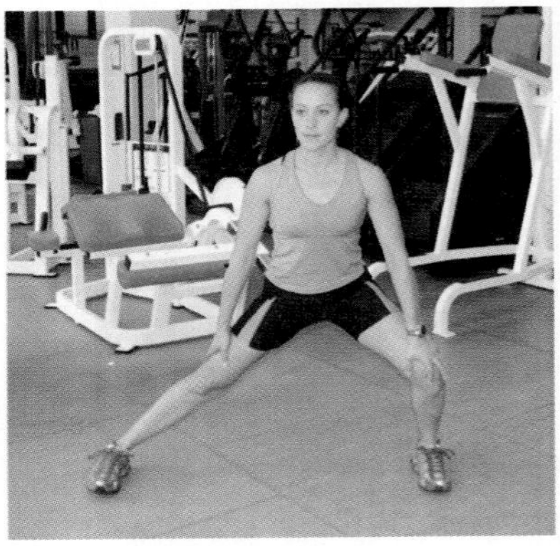

Inside of Thigh

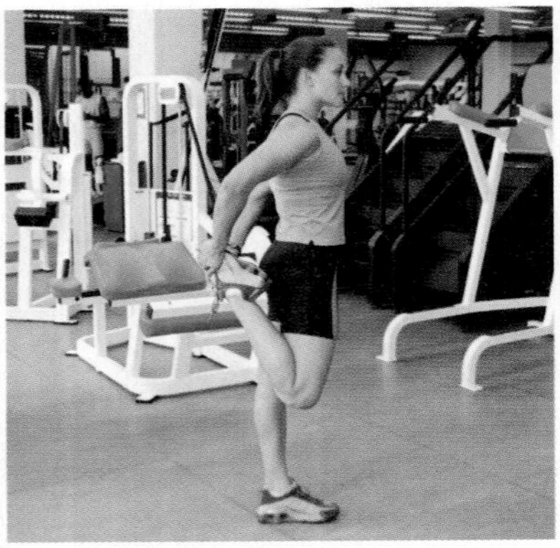

Front of Thigh

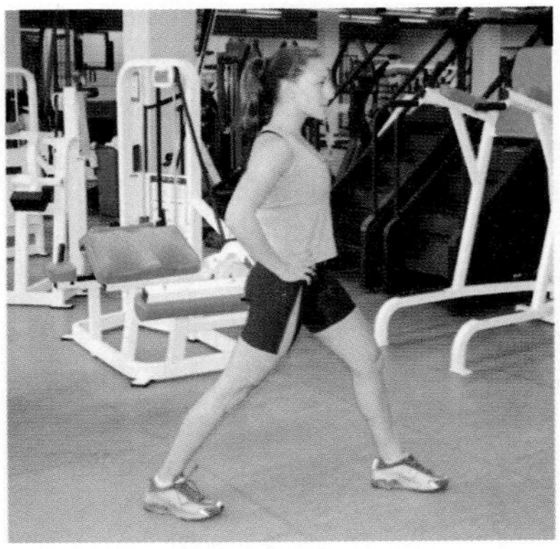

Ankle and Front of Hip

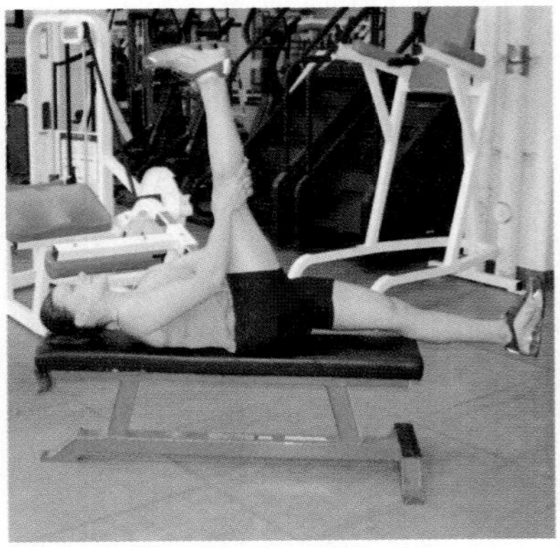

Back of Thigh

Photos Kristin Dilworth

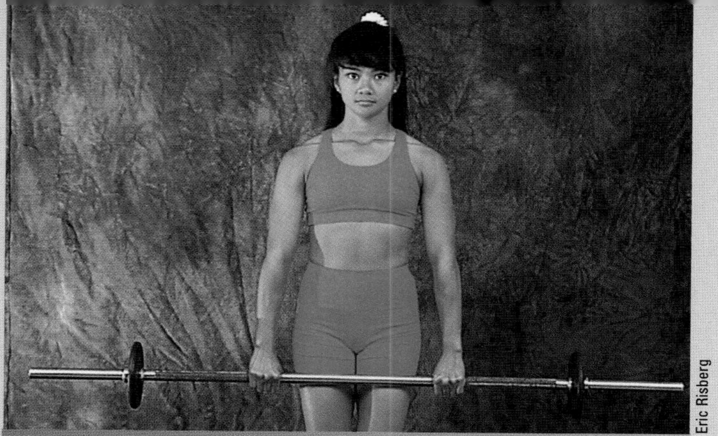

5

Safe and Effective Weight Training

Weight training involves a number of safety considerations. First, medical clearance is advised before you begin to participate in weight training. Then, as you begin weight training, you should learn the correct postures, the exercises that are right for you, and the proper way to execute them, as well as suggested clothing for weight training. Weight training also involves correct form, breathing, and often a training partner and spotting, among other safety features.

Medical Clearance

Experts recommend that you have a complete physical examination before you start any new exercise program. You should inform your physician that you want to start a weight training program and ask if there is any reason you should not do so. Medical clearance becomes more important as you get older, if you are overweight, or if you have not participated in a physical training program for a long time.

Clothing

Clothing for weight training should be comfortable and allow freedom of movement during all exercises through a complete range of motion. Figure 5.1 illustrates appropriate clothing for weight training. In warm environments, you should wear clothing to keep you cool. In cold environments, you should dress in clothing to keep you warm.

The clothing you select for weight training should be comfortable, durable, and keep your muscles warm during training. You should feel good about your appearance when you are weight training because if you don't feel good about yourself during an activity, the tendency is to quit participating. You should wear shoes when training with weights, as the weight room has many hard objects you might kick, drop, or step on.

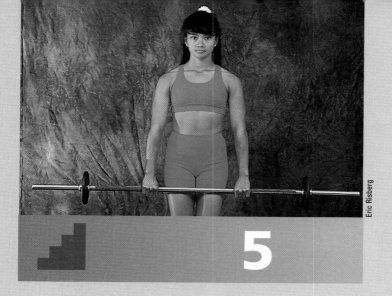

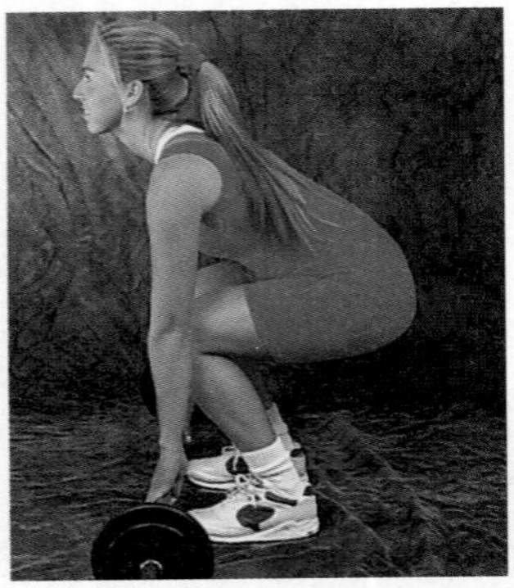
Eric Risberg

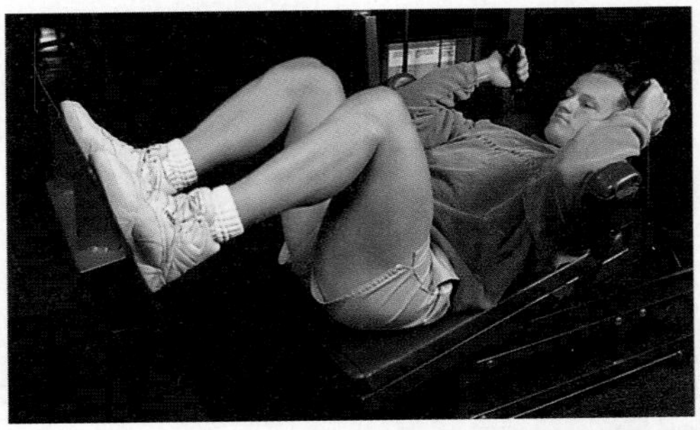
Eric Risberg

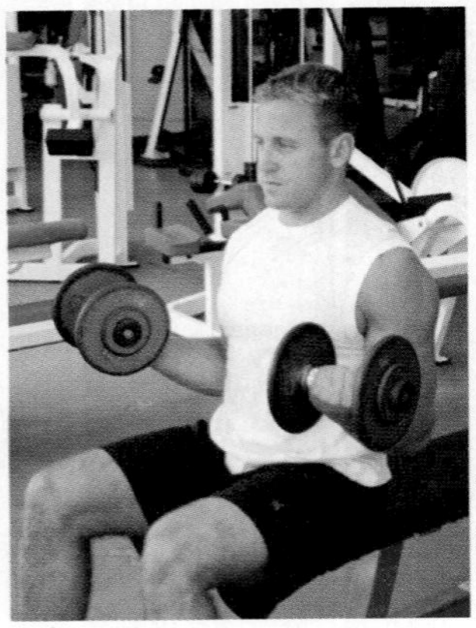
Kristin Dilworth

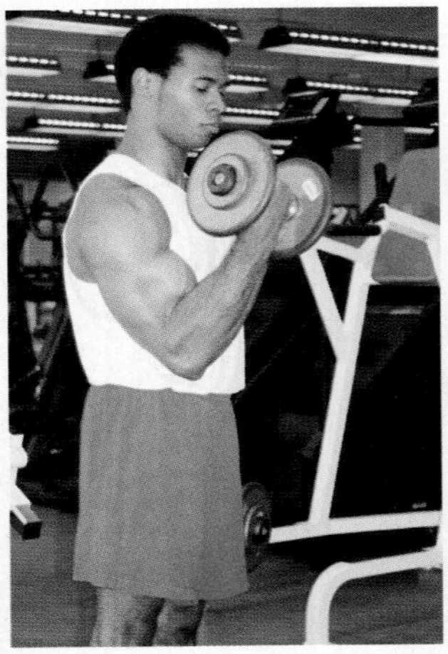
Kristin Dilworth

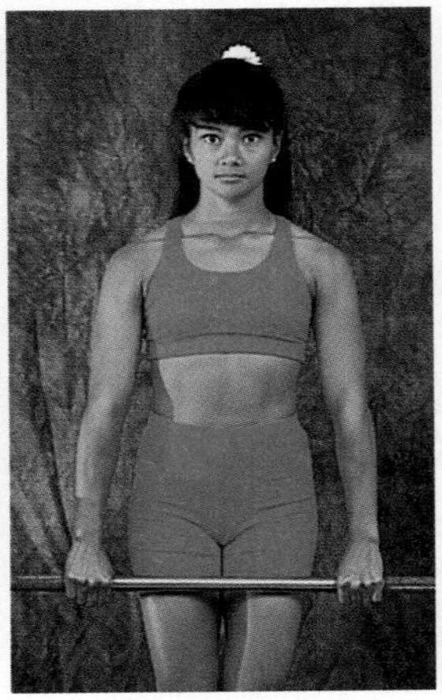
Eric Risberg

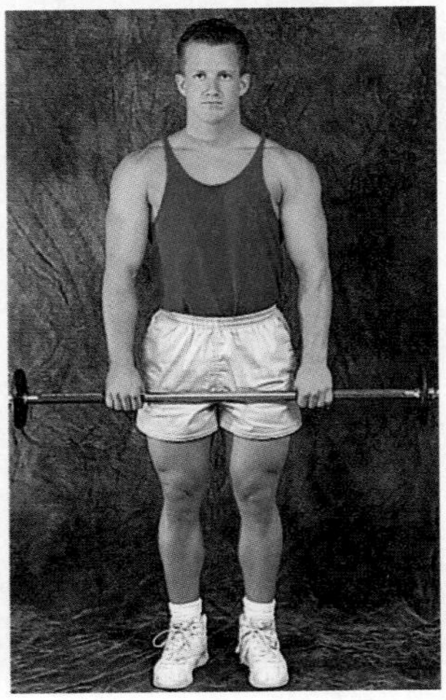
Eric Risberg

Figure 5.1 Appropriate clothing to wear while weight training.

Performing A Weight Training Exercise

The following are factors involved in performing a weight training exercise.

Strict Exercise Form

By maintaining strict exercise form (see Figure 5.2), you will keep the load on the muscles the exercise was designed to develop. When you do not maintain strict exercise form, you will reduce the load on the muscles you are trying to develop and increase your risk of injury.

Smooth Movement

Weight training exercises should be performed in a smooth, continuous movement rather than jerky motions. Some exercises are done faster than others, and some involve acceleration, but they should all be smooth. This allows the muscle to apply force to the resistance throughout the full range of motion. The purpose of weight training is to build healthy muscle tissue, not to tear it apart.

Full Range of Motion

Whenever possible, and when safe for the joints involved, a muscle should be exercised through a full range of motion (see Figure 5.3). This will result in strength gains throughout the complete range of motion of the muscle. It will also help to improve or maintain flexibility.

Phases of Exercise

Weight training exercises consist of a concentric phase and an eccentric phase.

Concentric Phase

In the *concentric phase* of an exercise, the muscle contraction overcomes the resistance. This causes the muscle to shorten as the weight is lifted. For most exercises this concentric phase should take about 2 seconds.

Eccentric Phase

During the *eccentric phase* of an exercise, the same muscles that lifted the weight will now lower the weight. In this phase the weight is allowed to overcome the force of muscle contraction. Therefore, even though the muscle is contracting and trying to shorten, it is being lengthened by the pull of the resistance. Eccentric contractions allow you to lower objects in a smooth, controlled manner. Weights should be lowered smoothly and continuously. The eccentric phase of an exercise should take at least as long as the concentric phase (at least 2 seconds), and sometimes up to twice as long (2 to 4 seconds).

Among those who gain the least from a weight training exercise are those who throw the weight upward using poor exercise form, incorrect muscle groups, and momentum. Then, once the weight has been lifted, they allow it to drop back to the starting position. Although they may move more weight, their muscles receive less benefit from the exercise and they have a much greater risk of injury.

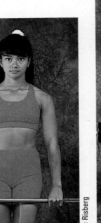

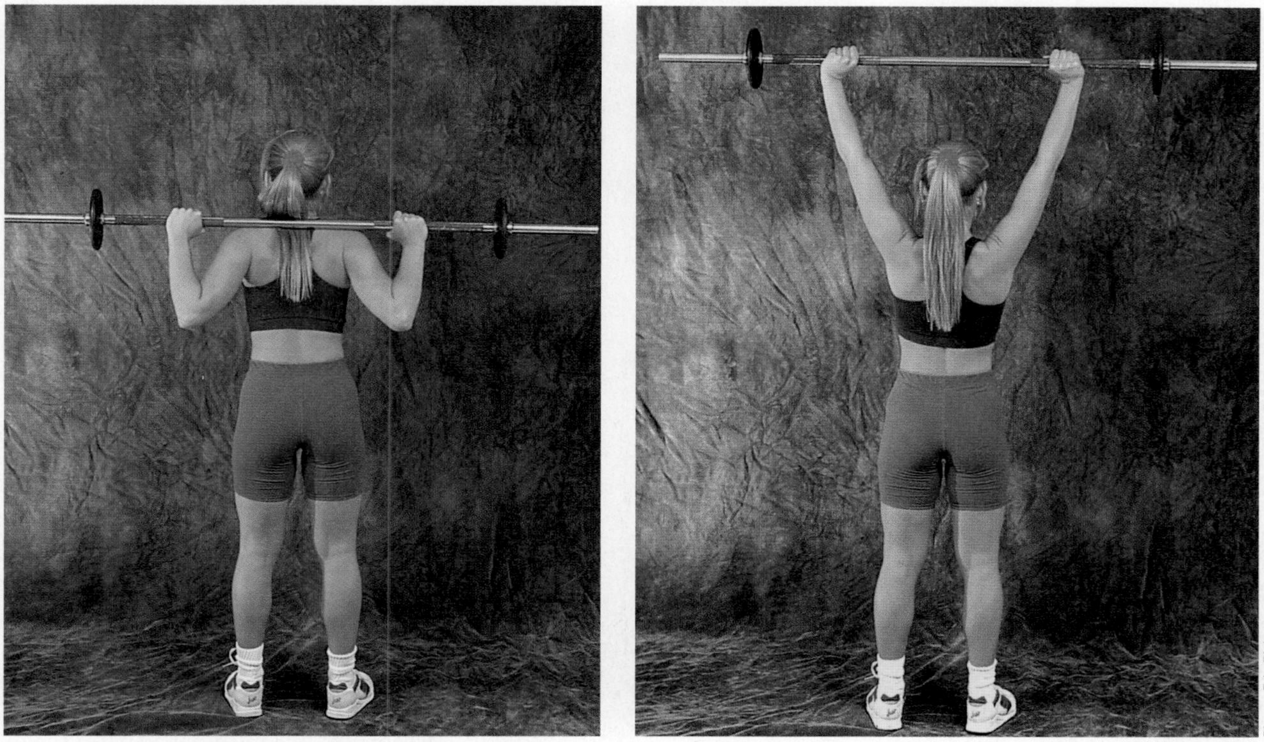

Photos Eric Risberg

Figure 5.2 Proper exercise form when lifting weights.

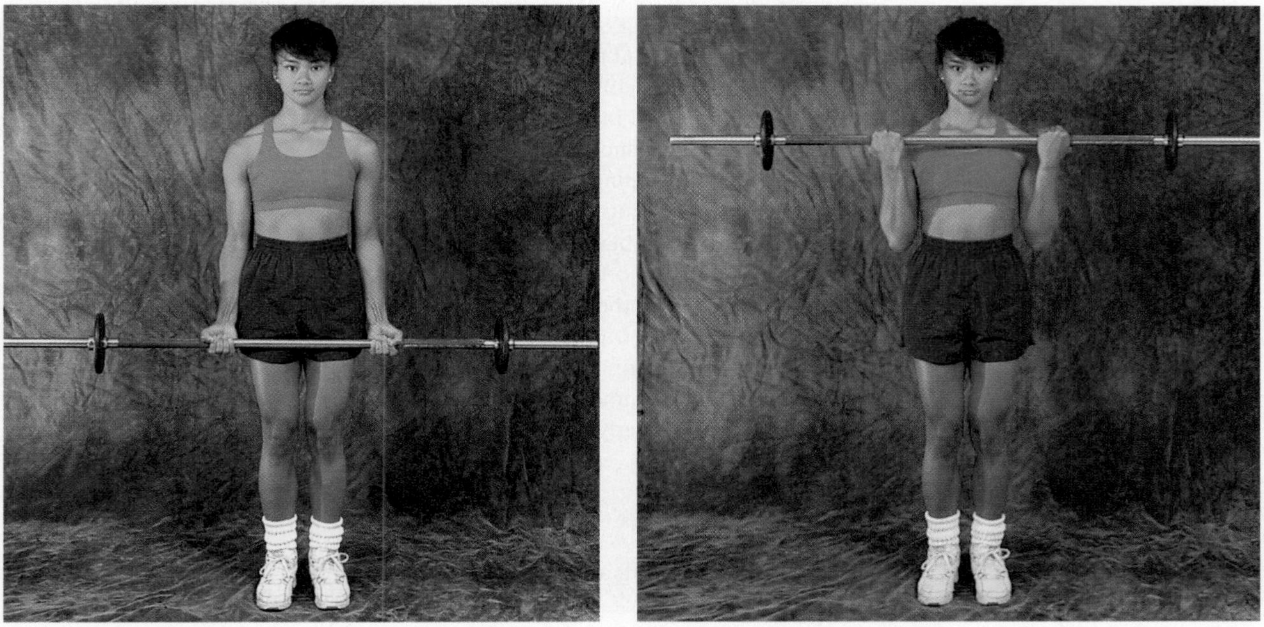

Photos Eric Risberg

Figure 5.3 Exercise muscles from full extension to full contraction and back to full extension.

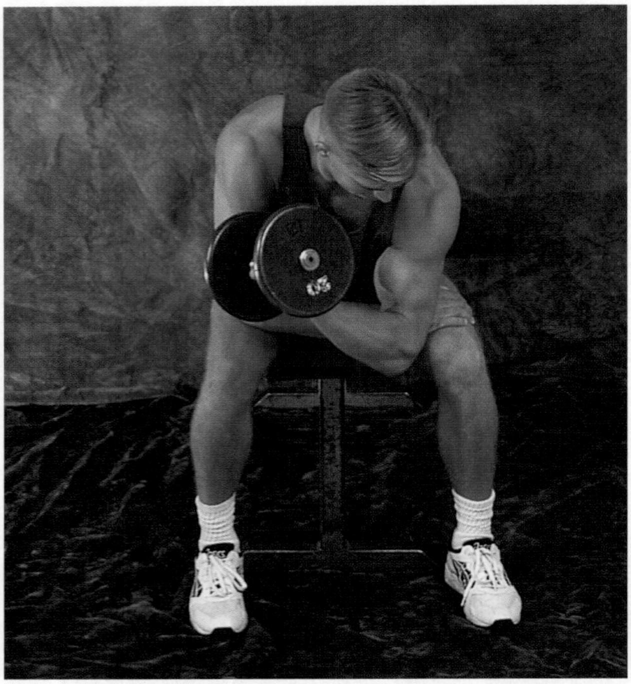

Figure 5.4 Focusing full attention on muscles moving the weight.

Breathing

A good general rule for breathing during weight training exercises is to exhale during the greatest exertion—usually the lifting phase of the exercise (concentric phase)—and inhale when lowering the weight (eccentric phase). One exception to this rule may be when performing overhead pressing movements. Some weight trainers are more comfortable inhaling as they press the weight overhead and exhaling as they lower it.

Proper breathing is an important part of correct exercise technique. You should practice proper breathing with lighter weights while you are learning new exercises. With each exercise, you should learn a breathing pattern. There is some room for individual differences and preferences.

If you hold your breath and strain while attempting to lift a heavy weight, this produces a great deal of pressure inside the chest cavity and the abdominal cavity, making it difficult, or even impossible, for the blood in the veins to return to the heart. The sudden high pressure caused by straining to lift a heavy weight while holding your breath could cause dizziness, a blackout, a stroke, a heart attack, or a hernia. Although events such as these are extremely rare in weight trainers, the possibility of their occurring should serve to emphasize the importance of learning to breathe properly during the exercises.

Concentration

You should focus your full attention on the muscles that are moving the weight (Figure 5.4). You should maintain this concentration on every repetition, and throughout every set, to gain the maximum benefit from the exercise. Weight trainers should not let their mind wander while performing a weight training exercise.

Isolated Intensity

Closely related to concentration and getting the greatest benefit from weight training in the least amount of exercise time is the concept of *isolated intensity*. This means focusing on a muscle, or group of muscles, that you wish to develop and forcing the muscle to work very hard. As you advance in your muscle training, you will learn how to force a muscle to work to temporary failure. This is beyond the point where you would like to quit and to the point where the muscle cannot perform the task. It is very intense exercise for an isolated group of muscles and is much more effective in producing gains than easier sets that are stopped when they begin to get difficult.

Caution: Working muscles to the point of temporary muscular failure increases the risk of injury and can result in extreme muscle soreness. Progress gradually and carefully to this level of intensity.

Additional Considerations for Machine Exercises

All of the guidelines for performing a weight training exercise apply to the use of weight training machines as well. A few additional considerations will make the use of weight machines safe and effective.

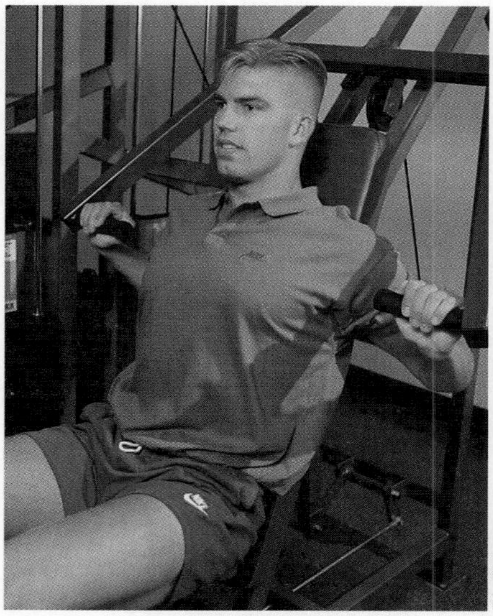

Figure 5.5 Correct body position on machines.

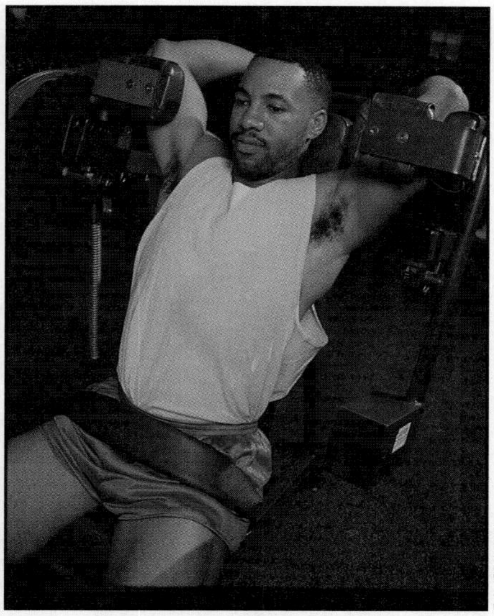

Figure 5.6 Seat belts on training machine.

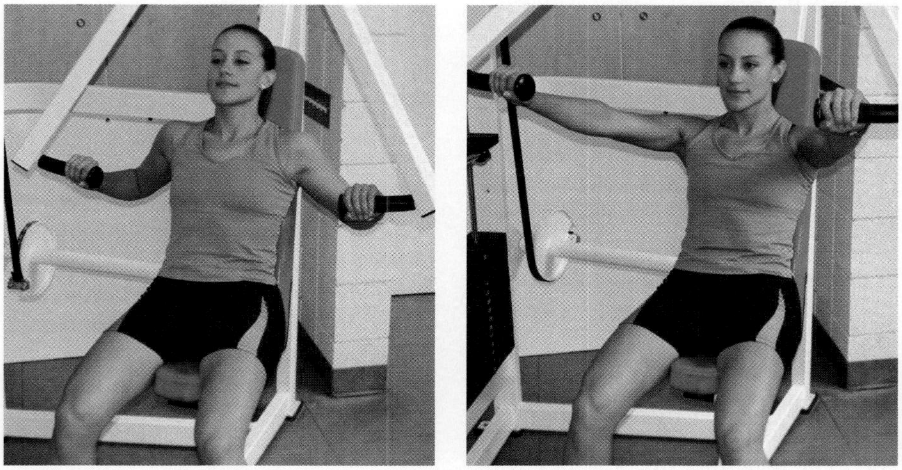

Figure 5.7 Using full range of motion.

Correct Body Position

You should position yourself on the machine so the pivot point of your body—the correct joint for the exercise movement—is lined up with the pivot point of the machine (see Figure 5.5 and Figure 5.6). For example, if you are on an arm curl machine, your elbow joint should be lined up with the pivot point of the arm curl machine. Most machines are designed to fit a wide range of body sizes. The adjustments are usually for height. Before you attempt to lift, make sure that you have adjusted the machine for correct body position and that all adjustments are locked in place.

Seat Belts

Several weight training machines have a seat belt to hold you on the machine and in the correct body position (Figure 5.6). Be sure to use the seat belt. It will make the exercise more effective and safer.

Speed of Movement

Most machines are not designed for speed and power training. Speed and momentum can cause problems for you and the machine. First, you are more likely to injure yourself if you use a fast, jerky motion to lift. Second, you are more likely to damage the machine if you lift too fast. Many machines have weight stacks, pulleys, cables, and chains. If you lift the weight stack too quickly, it will gain momentum and could continue upward at the end of the lift, causing the weight stack to bang against the top of the machine. This also may cause the cable or chain to jump off the pulley. At the very least, it will drop with a jerk, dramatically increasing the load on your muscles, tendons, ligaments, and joints.

The weight should be raised and lowered in a smooth, controlled manner. If you allow the weight to drop after lifting it, you may break a plate in the weight stack, the cable, the chain, or one of the pulleys. You can control the speed of movement on weight machines. Lifting the weight usually should take about 2 seconds, and lowering the weight should take 2 to 4 seconds. The weights should return to the weight stack gently and quietly. If you cannot control the speed of the weight, it is too heavy for you at this time. If you decrease the weight and perform the exercise correctly, you will get more benefit and achieve faster gains. Also, your machine will last much longer.

Full Range of Motion

Most weight machines are designed to allow you to lift through the full range of joint motion. If you lift through the full range of motion, you will develop strength, get better muscle development, and maintain a reasonable amount of flexibility. (See Figure 5.7.)

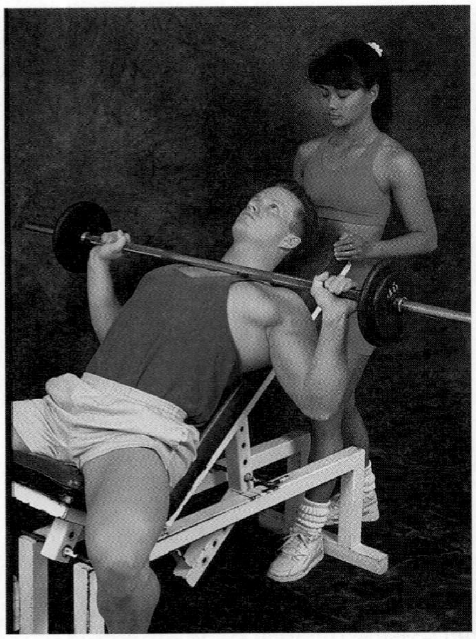

Eric Risberg

Figure 5.8 Training partner.

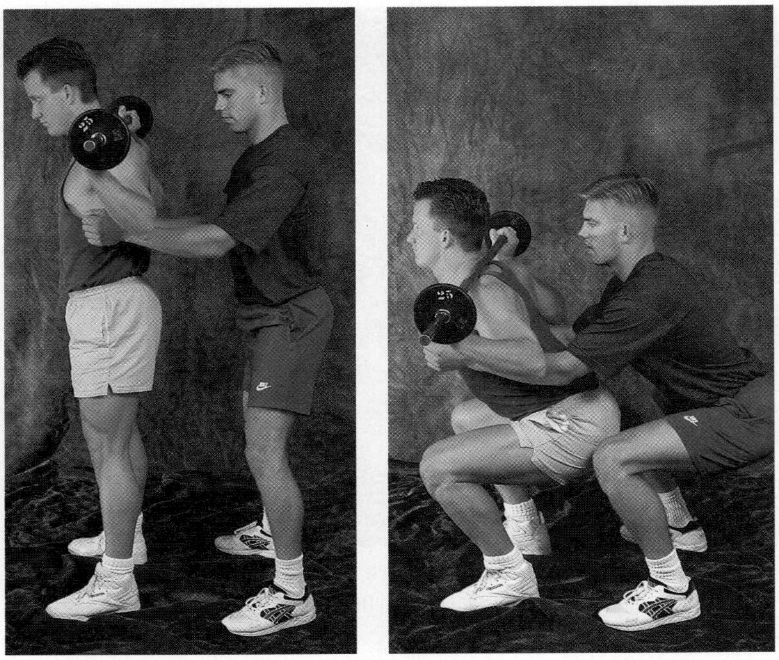

Photos Eric Risberg

Figure 5.9 Spotting.

Immediate Repairs

Like all machines, exercise machines have to be maintained properly. If you start to use a machine and find something that has to be tightened or adjusted, do it, or report it immediately. Usually it takes only a few turns of a screwdriver or wrench and a few seconds to make it right. But if you ignore it and something breaks, it probably will be much more costly in terms of time and money to get it repaired. Don't misuse weight machines. If you do your part to keep them working properly, they will give you years of good lifting.

Cleaning Machines

If many people use the same machines, it is courteous and thoughtful to carry a towel with you during your workout and wipe your perspiration off the machine when you are finished with the exercise. This takes only a second or two and makes it much nicer for the next lifter.

Moving Parts

You should maintain a safe distance from an exercise machine that someone else is using. Keep your hands and fingers away from moving weight stacks, cables, chains, levers, and pulleys.

Training Partner

A good training partner can be your greatest asset (see Figure 5.8.), and a bad training partner can be your greatest liability. A good training partner makes training safer by being alert on hazardous exercises so you can train to the limit of your capacity without fear of injury. A good training partner is always ready to help you load weights, change weights, and move equipment. A bad training partner lets you do all the work of setting up for exercises. A good training partner offers positive motivation and encouragement. A bad training partner maintains a negative attitude that dampens your enthusiasm. A good training partner is on time for every training session. A bad training partner frequently skips workouts or arrives late.

Even though you can make your best weight training progress with a good training partner, you can make excellent progress training alone. A bad training partner can hinder your weight training progress. If your partner is unwilling or unable to change, you should train alone or find a new training partner. You also should be prepared to listen—you may hear about some of your own faults as a training partner.

Spotting

When lifting weights, especially free weights, you could get pinned under a weight in some exercises if you could not complete the exercise movement. For safety, and to get the maximum benefit from the exercise, you should be spotted on these lifts. A *spotter* is a person who is in a position to help you complete the lift if it becomes necessary (see Figures 5.9 and 5.10).

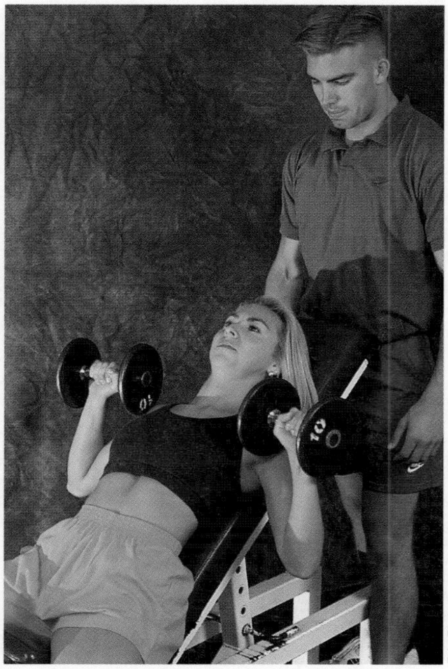

Figure 5.10 Stay alert! Give your full attention to spotting.

Communication

Effective communication is the key to effective spotting. Before the lift, the lifter and the spotter should talk briefly. Both the lifter and the spotter should know what exercise will be performed, how many repetitions will be attempted, how much help the lifter expects, if there will be any forced reps or negative reps at the end of the set, if the lifter expects help getting the weight into position (lift-off), and if the lifter expects help guiding the weight back onto a rack at the end of the set. This communication before the lift takes only a few seconds and is time well spent. It significantly increases safety and reduces misunderstandings.

General Guidelines for Spotters

1. Be sure you are strong enough to help with the weight being attempted. If not, tell the lifter and try to find more help.

2. Know how the lifter expects to be spotted. If you are not sure, ask the lifter before the lift is attempted.

3. Know what signs or signals the lifter will use to communicate during the lift. Know what words and gestures the lifter will use to let you know what to do.

4. Stay alert! Give your full attention to spotting the lift. Do not look away from the lifter. Do not be distracted. Do not carry on a conversation with someone else during the lift.

5. Do not touch the bar during the exercise if the lifter can complete the lift without your help. By doing so, you may decrease the overload stimulus the lifter needs to make the desired gains.

6. Before the lift, check the bar for balanced loading and secure collars.

7. Move weight plates or anything else near your feet that might cause you to trip or lose your balance.

8. Stay in a proper spotting and lifting position throughout the attempt so you are ready immediately if help is needed.

9. Do not jerk the bar away from the lifter or throw it off balance. Gently provide the least amount of help needed to complete the lift.

10. Be a responsible spotter. The lifter is depending on you to do the job right.

General Guidelines for Lifters Being Spotted

1. Make sure the spotter knows what you expect. Don't assume that the spotter can read your mind. If the spotter did not do what you were expecting, it was your fault for getting under the bar without communicating clearly before the lift.

2. Don't quit on a repetition. Even if you cannot complete the repetition by yourself, keep trying, and it should take very little lifting by the spotter to help you complete the lift. *Never* let go of the bar or quit on a lift when the spotter touches the bar.

3. Thank your spotter after each set.

Safety

The following are guidelines for safe weight training.

1. Move carefully and slowly in the weight room. The weight lifting area is not a good place for sudden, unexpected movements. Always be alert for movement around you. Do not back up without checking first. Look where you are going.

2. Stay clear of other lifters and spotters. Avoid collisions with people and equipment.

3. Stay clear of weight machines when someone is lifting or is in position to lift.

4. Fix broken equipment immediately, or set it aside, or put a sign on it. Do not attempt to use broken equipment.

5. Make sure you are in a stable position before you attempt a lift.

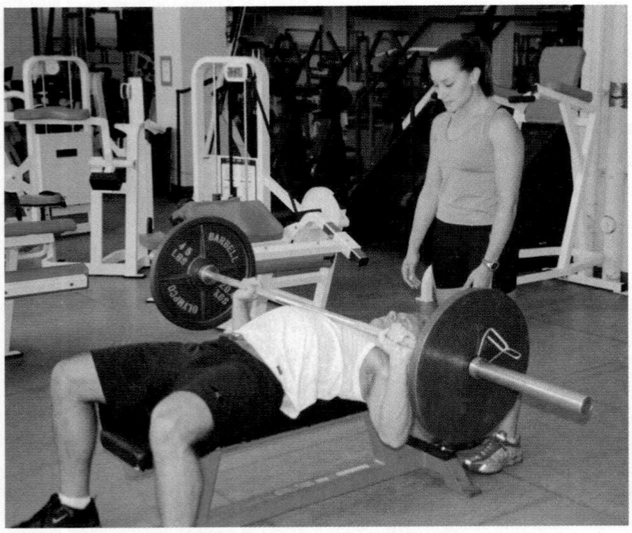

Figure 5.11 Do not perform a lift where you could be trapped under the weight unless you have a spotter.

6. Use collars on all plate-loading equipment such as barbells and dumbbells.

7. Perform all lifts using strict exercise form.

8. Do not hold your breath and strain to lift a weight.

9. Warm up before lifting.

10. Don't lift when you are sick. You are not likely to make much progress, and you expose everyone in the weight room to the same illness.

11. Don't fool around in the weight room. The weight lifting area is no place for practical jokes or wild behavior. Serious injuries can result from thoughtless and foolish behavior during weight training.

12. Do not twist your body, arch your back, or arch your neck while attempting to complete a lift.

13. Lift within your ability. Do not try to lift more weight than you can handle safely.

14. Adjust each machine to put you in the correct lifting position before starting a set.

15. Do not bounce weights off your body or off a weight stack. If you must bounce a weight to lift it, the weight is too heavy.

16. Be careful when loading and unloading barbells that are resting on a rack. If you get too much weight on one end of a barbell, it will flip off the rack. This is a dangerous but common mistake by beginning lifters. Add and remove weight from each end of the bar as evenly as possible, keeping the bar balanced on the rack.

17. Store all weight training equipment properly. Do not leave it lying around on the floor. All dumbbells, barbells, and weight plates should have storage racks where the lifter will put them after completing the exercise.

18. Always control the speed and direction of the lift. If you cannot control the lift, the weight is too heavy. Reduce the weight and perform the lift correctly.

19. Do not perform lifts where you could be trapped under the weight without spotters who know what to do. (See Figure 5.11.)

20. Always be polite, courteous, and helpful in the weight room. This will create a safer and more pleasant training environment for everyone.

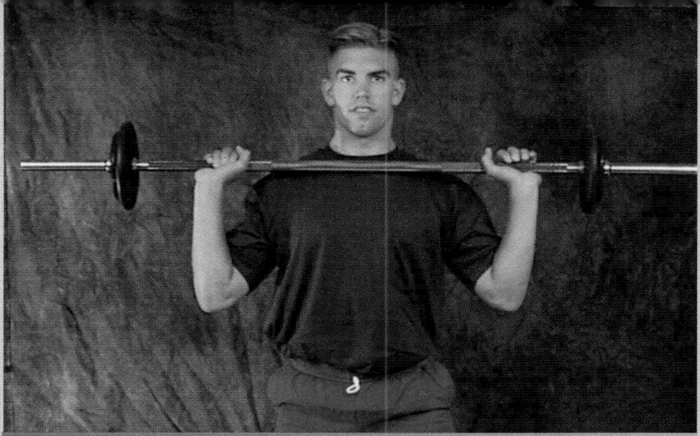

Eric Risberg

6

A Beginning Weight Training Program

This chapter presents and illustrates one beginning training program to get you started. Basic exercises are given for free weights and machines. You will need to choose which you will use based on your preference and what is available.

Free Weights or Machines?

Beginners often ask which is better, free weights or machines. The answer depends on several factors. The following are some of the factors to consider as you decide what is better for you.

Advantages of machines are:

1. Machines tend to be safer because you shouldn't be able to get trapped under a heavy weight. This is a real advantage if you will be training alone.

2. You can change from one weight to another more rapidly because you only need to move a selector pin to the new weight. This is a great advantage if you choose to spend less time exercising.

3. You can learn the exercise movements easier and faster because the machine controls the direction of the movement.

Advantages of free weights (barbells and dumbbells) are:

1. Free weights offer more variety of exercise movements than machines do because free weights are free to move in any direction.

2. Free weights are generally available at a much lower total cost than most exercise machines.

3. Free weights are easier to move from one location to another.

4. Adjustable barbells and dumbbells are the right size for almost everyone. Some machines are not.

5. You automatically use additional stabilizing and assisting muscles to hold your body in the correct exercise position, keep the weight moving along the correct path, and balance the weight.

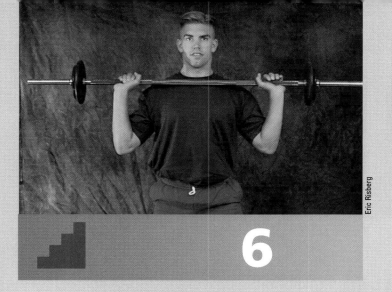

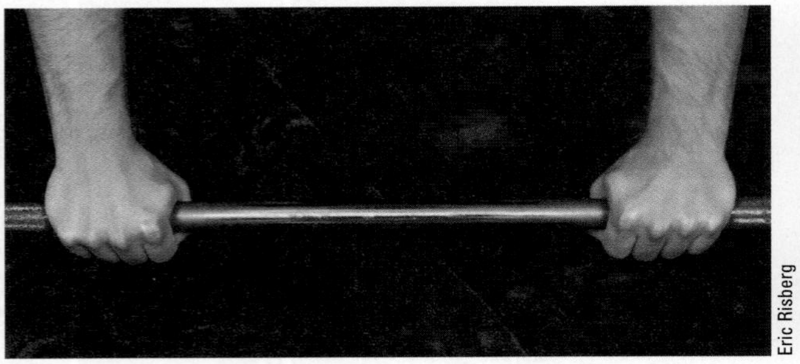

Figure 6.1 Pronated grip (overgrip).

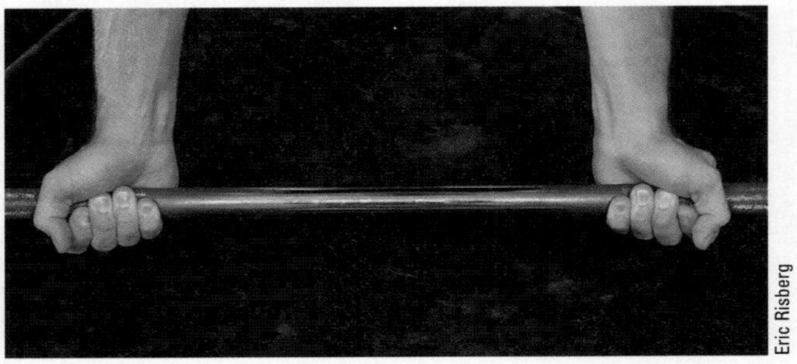

Figure 6.2 Supinated grip (undergrip).

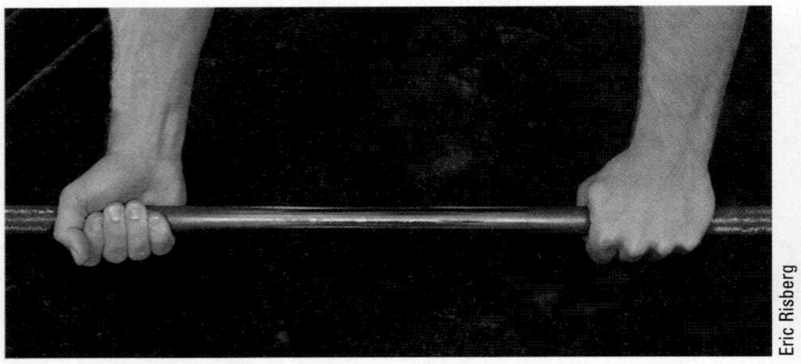

Figure 6.3 Mixed grip.

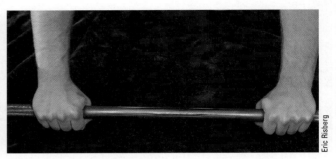

Figure 6.4 Shoulder-width grip.

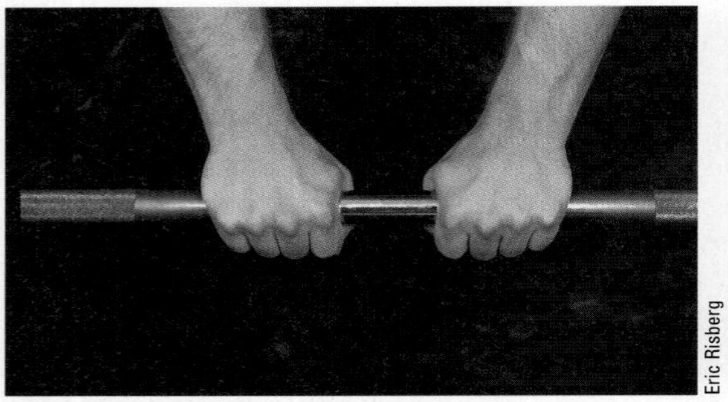

Figure 6.5 Narrow grip.

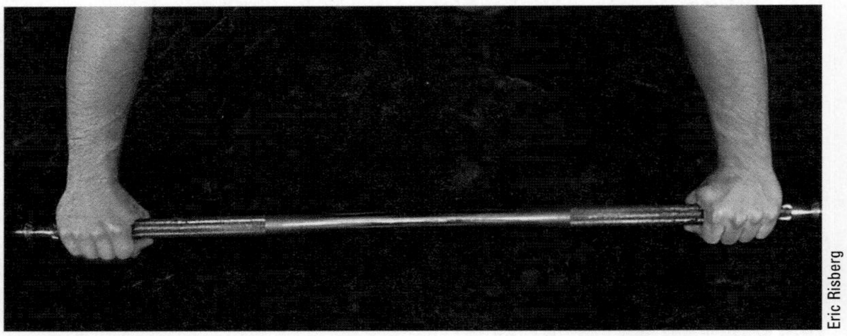

Figure 6.6 Wide grip.

Grips

Your grip on the barbell or exercise machine involves the position of your hands on the bar and the spacing between your hands.

Hand Position

The three basic hand positions are:

1. *Pronated grip* (thumbs toward each other), also referred to as the overhand grip, overgrip, overgrasp, and regular grip. (See Figure 6.1.)

2. *Supinated grip* (thumbs away from each other), also referred to as the underhand grip, undergrip, undergrasp, and reverse grip. (See Figure 6.2.)

3. *Mixed grip* (one thumb toward the other hand and one thumb away from the other hand), also referred to as the combined grip, alternate grip, and dead lift grip. (See Figure 6.3.)

You should always wrap your thumb around the bar for safety. Performing lifts in which the bar is over your body and your thumbs are not around the bar is risky and is not recommended. Locking your thumb around the bar and under your fingers places your thumb in a position that invites injury.

Hand Spacing

The three common distances for hand spacing on the bar are:

1. Regular or normal hand spacing, in which your hands are placed on the bar approximately shoulder-width apart. (See Figure 6.4.)

2. Narrow grip, which is recommended for some exercises. The hands are closer together than shoulder width, normally 4 to 8 inches apart. (See Figure 6.5.)

3. Wide grip, in which the hands are placed on the bar at a distance wider than shoulder-width. (See Figure 6.6.)

Dead Lift

Muscles developed: Erector spinae, gluteus maximus, quadriceps, trapezius, rhomboids.

Starting position: Bend over and assume a mixed grip on a barbell that is lying on the floor; bend your knees and hips so your hips are approximately knee level; keep your back flat.

Concentric phase (lifting the weight): Keep your neck and back straight while extending the trunk, hips, and knees to arrive at a standing position.

Eccentric phase (lowering the weight): Keep your neck and back straight as you slowly lower the weight back to the floor by bending your knees and hips.

Caution: Always use correct lifting technique. Do not try to lift a weight that is too heavy. Improper lifting technique may result in injury.

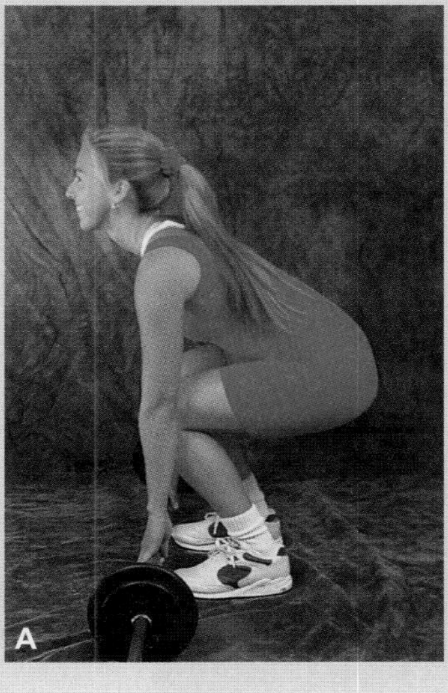
A

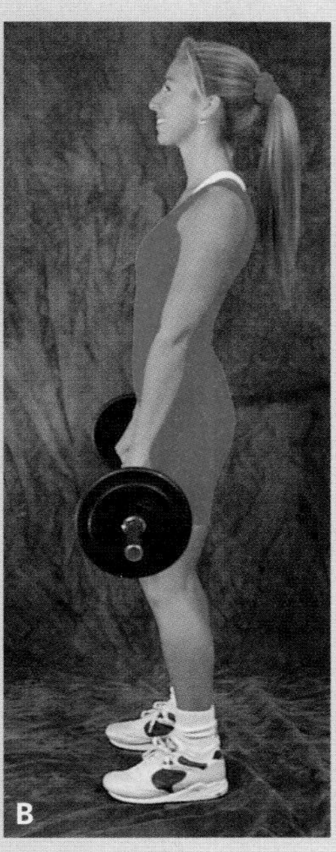
B

Photos Eric Risberg

When you are learning a new exercise, first try the hand spacing that is recommended or illustrated in the exercise portion of this book. Later, when you have more knowledge and experience, use a lighter weight and experiment with different hand spacing to find the most comfortable and effective hand spacing for you.

Getting in Position

If you lift with barbells and dumbbells, you often will need to lift the bar from the floor to assume the starting position for the exercise. There is a safe and correct way to do this. Every time you lift a weight from the floor, use the correct form, no matter how light the weight. You can injure your lower back by lifting improperly, and the low back does not tend to recover quickly or completely from injury. Therefore, it is important to avoid injury to your back in the first place. Ask anyone you know who has had a back injury!

Dead Lift

When you are lifting a barbell or dumbbells from the floor to the front of your thighs, use the proper grip for the exercise to be performed. For example, if you are picking up the bar to perform barbell arm curls, grasp the bar with a supinated grip and perform the dead lift as described to get into the starting position for the exercise.

Clean

When you are lifting a barbell or dumbbells to the front of your shoulders, use a lift called the *clean.* For some free weight exercises, such as the overhead press, you will have to get the weight to shoulder level to start the exercise. If a shoulder-height rack is available, you can lift the weight from the rack. If a rack is not available, you will have to lift the weight from the floor to your shoulders.

To clean a weight, keep your back flat and lift with your legs. The proper body position for the pull on the clean is the same as the pull on the dead lift. Keep your back flat and lift with your legs. More advanced lifters use the clean as an exercise. It is not generally recommended for beginners as an exercise without supervision and excellent instruction.

Cleans

Muscles developed: Trapezius, erector spinae, gluteus maximus, quadriceps.

Starting position: Bend over and grasp a barbell that is on the floor, with your hands approximately shoulder-width apart and in a pronated (thumbs in) grip; bend your knees and hips, keeping your head in line with your body and your neck and back flat.

Concentric phase (lifting the weight): Inhale as you lift the bar from the floor and accelerate the bar upward, gaining speed as it rises to the highest position to which you can pull it. The pull should continue upward to the level of your chest or shoulders. As the bar nears its highest point, quickly rotate your arms under the bar and bend your knees, catching the bar on your shoulders. Straighten your legs to a standing position and exhale.

Eccentric phase (lowering the weight): Inhale and quickly rotate your arms from under the bar. Bend your arms, legs, and hips to decelerate the bar to a hang position with the bar resting against the upper thighs. Then slowly bend the knees and hips to lower the bar back to the floor. Exhale.

Caution: Keep your back straight. Lift with your legs. Do not jerk the weight from the floor, but lift and accelerate the weight.

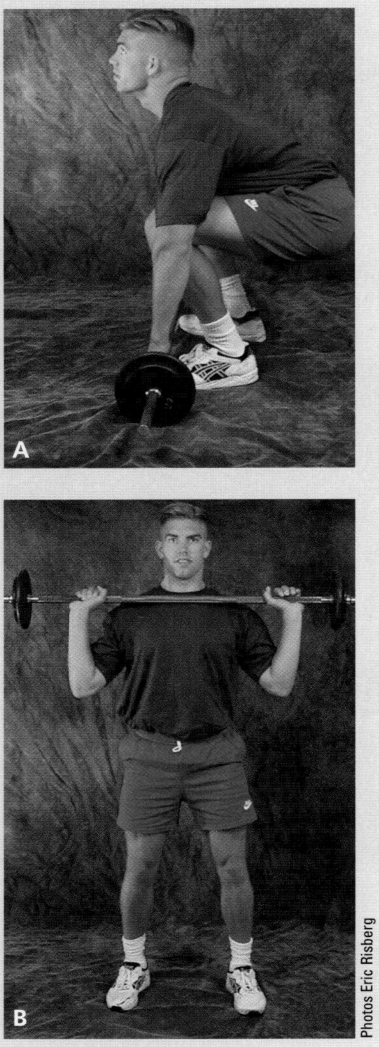

Basic Exercises

All of the exercises for the beginning program are basic exercises described in the exercise portion of this book. One exercise for each major muscle group or joint action is recommended for beginning weight trainers. Those who are weight training to develop physical fitness usually do not need more than one exercise per body part; however, it is a good idea to occasionally change the exercise you are performing to develop that body part.

Frequency and Resistance

The exercises in Table 6.1 should be performed three times each week with at least 48 hours of rest between training sessions. Start light, and progress slowly. If you are just starting a weight training program, you should begin with very light weight and learn to do each exercise with correct technique before you add resistance. Then, gradually add weight, but never at the cost of losing correct lifting technique. Ask your training partner or instructor to watch you perform each lift, and compare your technique with the photographs and descriptions in the exercise sections of this book. Have someone videotape your lifts so you can critique them yourself. Some weight training instructors grade students on correct lifting technique.

Weight training can be one of the most intense forms of exercise you will ever perform. Muscles can be isolated and worked extremely hard within a minute or two without experiencing total body fatigue. Therefore, beginners tend to *overtrain* and develop extreme delayed-onset muscle soreness during the first few days. This tendency to overtrain is also a product of the false belief that "If a little is good, more must be better." This is not always the case with weight training. Beginners can

Exercise Description	Free Weights	Machines
Chest (Chapter 8)	Barbell Bench Press	Prone or Seated Chest Press
Back (Chapter 9)	One Dumbbell Rowing	Seated or Low Pulley Rowing
Shoulders (Chapter 10)	Military Press	Seated Shoulder Press
Arms (Chapter 11)	Barbell Curl	Arm Curl
Thighs (Chapter 12)	Squat	Leg Press
Calves (Chapter 12)	One Dumbbell Calf Raise	Calf Raise or Calf Press
Abdominals (Chapter 13)	Abdominal Crunches	Ab Machine Crunches
Back Extension (Chapter 13)	Back Extension	Back Extension

Table 6.1 Recommended Exercises for Beginners

easily overtrain the muscles to the point that they cannot recover before the next training session. The result is a decrease in performance and no gain.

The program suggested in this chapter is recommended for healthy young people of high school and college age (approximately 15 to 22 years old) who are near their peak of physical growth and who have been physically active. If you are older, or if you have been inactive for a long time, you should progress more slowly. Weight training is a lifetime activity. If you progress slowly and safely, you can avoid the injuries and extreme soreness that result from doing too much too soon.

The First Six Weeks

Safety and correct exercise technique are the most important things to learn during the first few weeks of a weight training program. Start with light weights and learn to perform each exercise in your program correctly. Learn the breathing pattern that works best, and develop a habit of breathing correctly during your exercises.

Allow your body to gradually adapt to this new demand. Progress slowly to keep muscle soreness to a minimum. Learn to concentrate on the muscles being developed during each repetition of each exercise.

Weeks 1 and 2 (1 × 20)

For the first 2 weeks (6 exercise sessions), perform each exercise once (one set), completing 20 exercise movements (20 repetitions) in that set. *Example:* Bench Press: 1 set of 20 repetitions (1 × 20).

If you complete all 20 repetitions while maintaining correct exercise technique, you may increase the resistance for the next training session. If a weight feels very light and the repetitions are extremely easy, you could make a large increase in the weight for the next training session. If a weight feels moderately difficult, you should make a small increase for the next training session. By the end of 2 weeks (6 training sessions), you should be training with a weight that makes it difficult for you to complete 20 repetitions while maintaining correct lifting technique.

If you complete at least 15 repetitions, but fewer than 20, use the same resistance for your next training session and try to increase the number of repetitions you complete. If you complete fewer than 15 repetitions, reduce the resistance for your next training session. Any time you begin to use incorrect lifting technique to move the weight, stop, use a lighter weight, and repeat the set or schedule a lighter weight for the next training session.

Don't sacrifice proper exercise form to complete repetitions. When you can no longer perform repetitions correctly, stop the set and record the number of repetitions you performed correctly. See the progress log at the end of this chapter.

Weeks 3 and 4 (1 × 20) (1 × 10)

During the next 2 weeks (6 training sessions) perform 1 set of 20 repetitions (1 × 20), followed by 1 set of 10 repetitions (1 × 10). Keep trying to find the heaviest weight you can lift 20 times on the first set.

After resting 1 or 2 minutes, perform 1 set of 10 repetitions. Each time you complete 10 repetitions in the second set, schedule a heavier weight for the next training session. Following this procedure, gradually work toward the heaviest weight you can lift 20 times in the first set and the heaviest weight you can lift 10 times in the second set while maintaining strict exercise form. If you cannot complete at least 8 repetitions in the second set, reduce the resistance for the next training session.

Weeks 5 and 6 (1 × 20) (1 × 10) (1 × 5)

During weeks 5 and 6 (the next 6 workouts), perform 1 set of 20 repetitions (1 × 20) first, 1 set of 10 repetitions (1 × 10) second, and 1 set of 5 (1 × 5) third. Continue to search *safely* for the heaviest weight you can handle in each set. If you complete 5 good repetitions in the third set, schedule a heavier weight for the next training session. If you complete at least 3 repetitions in the third set, keep the weight and try to increase your reps. If you cannot complete at least 3 good repetitions, reduce the weight for the next training session.

Guidelines for Productive Training

After this first 6 weeks of training, you should have had time to develop a good foundation of total body strength and time to finish reading this book so you are able to plan your own weight training programs based on goals you have set for yourself. You also should be able to plan a method of record keeping and measuring your progress toward your goals. Some overall guidelines are:

1. Perform each repetition with correct technique and complete concentration.

2. Make gradual but consistent increases in resistance as you are able.

3. Complete each scheduled training session. Form the habit of never missing a scheduled training session.

4. Maintain a positive attitude. Enjoy each training session. Have fun. Make this the most fun part of your day.

5. Eat right. Healthy eating is critical to optimal weight training progress.

6. Get enough rest. Weight training serves only as a stimulus for positive changes to take place in your body. The changes are biological adaptations that actually take place between exercise sessions. Without adequate nutrition and rest, it is difficult for these positive changes to take place.

7. Stay healthy. You may not normally think of this as a choice, but it is. Your health is closely related to your lifestyle. Make healthy choices.

Strength and Muscular Endurance Progress Log

Name																				
Date																				
Exercise	Wt	Rep	Wt	Rep	Wt	Rep	Wt	Rep	Wt	Rep	Wt	Rep	Wt	Rep	Wt	Rep	Wt	Rep	Wt	Rep

Strength and Muscular Endurance Progress Log

Name

Date																								
Exercise	Wt	Rep	Wt	Rep	Wt	Rep	Wt	Rep	Wt	Rep	Wt	Rep	Wt	Rep	Wt	Rep	Wt	Rep	Wt	Rep	Wt	Rep	Wt	Rep

Strength and Muscular Endurance Progress Log

Name																				
Date																				
Exercise	Wt	Rep	Wt	Rep	Wt	Rep	Wt	Rep	Wt	Rep	Wt	Rep	Wt	Rep	Wt	Rep	Wt	Rep	Wt	Rep

Strength and Muscular Endurance Progress Log

Name																								
Date																								
Exercise	Wt	Rep	Wt	Rep	Wt	Rep	Wt	Rep	Wt	Rep	Wt	Rep	Wt	Rep	Wt	Rep	Wt	Rep	Wt	Rep	Wt	Rep	Wt	Rep

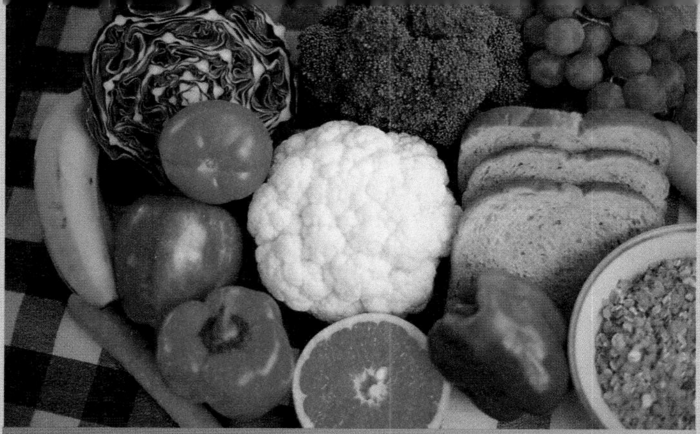

7

Nutrition, Rest, and Drugs

Good nutrition and rest are necessary accompaniments to any weight training program, In addition, this chapter addresses the use of drugs—anabolic steroids, alcohol, and tobacco.

Nutrition

The average American will spend approximately 6 years of his or her life eating. That will include about 70,000 meals and 60 tons of food. Sound dietary practices will help you maintain a high level of health throughout your life. The nutrients your body needs to function properly have been classified into six categories:

1. Water
2. Minerals
3. Vitamins
4. Carbohydrates
5. Fats
6. Proteins

Carbohydrates, fats, and proteins supply energy, which is measured in *calories.* Water, minerals, and vitamins do not supply energy, but they are necessary for the release of energy and other aspects of metabolism. The nutrients in these six categories provide most of the chemicals necessary for your body to:

- produce energy
- grow and develop new tissue
- repair damaged tissue
- conduct nerve impulses
- reproduce
- regulate physiological processes.

Water

Water contains no calories or vitamins, yet it is essential in relatively large quantities for your body to function properly. Although most people seldom think about the importance of adequate water intake, approximately 60% of a person's body weight consists of water. Water molecules make up a large portion of the blood, muscle, and brain. You can survive for weeks without food, but only days without water.

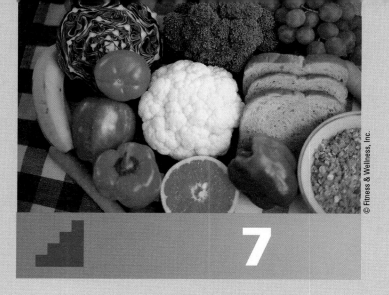

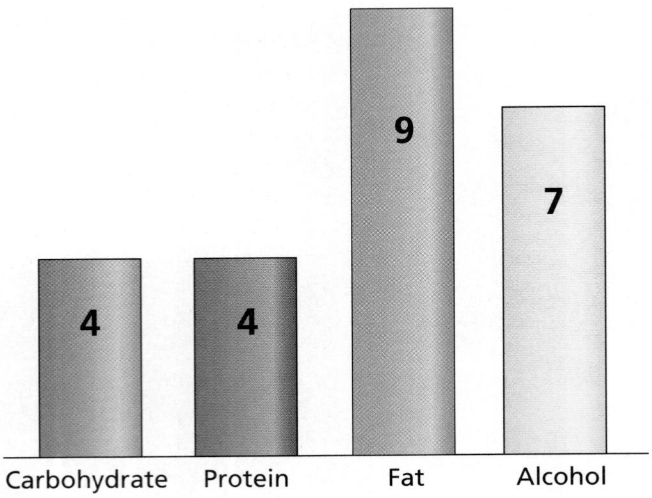

Source: *Principles and Labs For Fitness & Wellness* by Werner W. K. Hoeger and Sharon A. Hoeger. Wadsworth/Thomson Learning, 2002, pg. 60.

Figure 7.1 Caloric value of food.

When you are thirsty, your body is asking for water (H_2O), but thirst is not always an accurate indicator of your need for water. You should drink at least 8 to 10 glasses of water a day. You also get some water from the foods you eat. For example, some fruits, such as melons, are as much as 80% water. Factors including your size, activity level, environment, and diet affect your need for water intake.

What should you give your body when you are thirsty? Not all fluids contribute to your water needs. Some beverages (coffee, tea, and alcohol) actually dehydrate your body and increase your need for additional water.

It would be difficult for you to drink too much water. If you do happen to take in more than your body needs, you get rid of any excess easily. You lose water every day in urine, feces, sweat, and evaporation from your lungs. If you do not take in enough water, your body cannot continue to function normally. Your health and performance will suffer.

Minerals

Minerals are inorganic substances necessary for some of the chemical activity that goes on in your body. If your body does not have the appropriate minerals, certain chemical changes cannot take place. Minerals are essential in regulating body functions such as muscle contraction, protein synthesis, and heart function.

The *major minerals* that your body needs include calcium, phosphorus, magnesium, sodium, potassium, and chloride. Because they are found in a variety of foods, mineral deficiencies are not common in people who are eating a balanced diet. The one exception is calcium. In a National Academy of Sciences study, 80% of the women over age 18 who were surveyed consumed too little calcium. Adequate calcium intake during childhood and adolescence is vital for strong, healthy bones. A calcium deficiency can cause osteoporosis (a thinning of the bones).

Bones respond to physical activity by becoming more dense and stronger. If you use your arms regularly to lift weights, then, the bones in your arms will become stronger.

Trace minerals—those you need in small amounts—include minerals such as iron, zinc, copper, fluoride, and selenium. Even though the body requires trace minerals in only small amounts, they are still essential for your health. Some women do not get enough iron. A survey by the U. S. Department of Agriculture discovered that many women between ages 19 and 50 get only about 60% of the iron they need each day. This can lead to too few red blood cells in the bloodstream, a condition known as iron-deficiency anemia. Eating a balanced diet is the safest way to prevent mineral deficiencies.

Vitamins

Vitamins are organic substances that are necessary for some of the chemical activity that goes on in the body. Vitamins do not contain calories and therefore do not directly supply energy. Nevertheless, they are essential to release the energy stored in carbohydrates, fats, and proteins. They also are necessary for building tissue and controlling the body's use of food.

The body needs 13 vitamins. The two major categories of vitamins are:

1. *Fat-soluble* vitamins (A, D, E, K)
2. *Water-soluble* vitamins (C and the eight B-complex vitamins).

Excess water-soluble vitamins normally are excreted in the urine. Because the body can store fat-soluble vitamins, you can take in too much of these. A toxic effect can result when certain vitamins are taken in excessive amounts. Getting your vitamins from a balanced diet instead of vitamin supplements is generally healthier.

The body needs adequate amounts of water, minerals, and vitamins. A deficiency will decrease optimal bodily function and performance. The findings of independent research to date, however, indicate that more than the required amount does not improve performance or progress. A good guideline to follow is to eat a balanced diet from a variety of good foods and to drink at least 8 to 10 glasses of water a day.

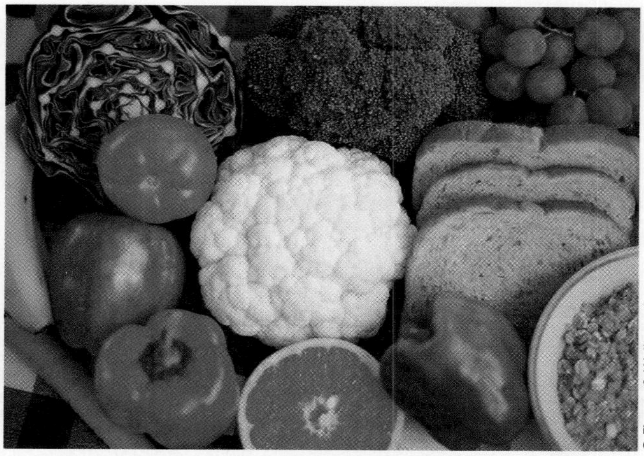

A balanced diet is essential for maintaining good health.

Carbohydrates

Calories (body fuel) are contained in carbohydrates, fats, and proteins (see Figure 7.1). Carbohydrates are a major source of energy for the body, particularly during high-intensity exercise. Each gram of carbohydrate contains approximately 4 calories.

Simple carbohydrates, sometimes referred to as simple sugars, tend to have little nutritive value. Foods such as cookies, soft drinks, and candy are high in simple sugars. People are often attracted to these instead of more nutritious foods.

Complex carbohydrates provide your body with many of the valuable nutrients needed to keep you healthy. They are the foundation of a healthy diet. These complex carbohydrates are found primarily in foods from plant sources such as breads, fruits, vegetables, rice, pasta, and cereals. The exception is milk, which is the only significant animal source of complex carbohydrates.

Fiber, another complex carbohydrate, is the indigestible material in food. Nutritionists urge people to add fiber to their diets because of proven health benefits such as lower blood cholesterol and proper digestion and elimination.

Fats

Dietary fats, or *lipids*, are the most concentrated source of energy at 9 calories per gram. That is more than twice the calories in a gram of carbohydrates or proteins. Fats have a higher energy value than carbohydrates and provide up to 70% of the body's energy needs in a resting state or during low-level physical activity. Fats also are an essential component of cell walls and nerve fibers. They are involved in absorbing and transporting fat-soluble vitamins, supporting and cushioning organs, and insulating the body.

Although fats have useful functions in the body, it is possible to have too much of a good thing. Excess fat in the diet contributes to high blood pressure, heart disease, diabetes, and other diseases. Too much body fat is a risk factor for heart disease and has been associated with certain cancers (colon, breast, prostate, and uterus).

The correct amount of fat is good and too much is bad, so what you need is the right amount of fat in your diet. The American Heart Association and the U.S. Department of Health and Human Services recommend that less than 30% of your daily calories come from fats. Fats should not be cut out of your diet completely, nor should you eat too many fats. Either extreme can be detrimental.

Of the different categories of fats, *saturated fats* require special mention because of their associated risk for cardiovascular disease. Saturated fats contribute to an increase in blood cholesterol levels. Cholesterol level in the body is affected more by the percent of fat in your diet than by the cholesterol you eat. Elevated blood cholesterol is a major risk factor for heart disease. Less than 10% of your total daily caloric intake should come from saturated fats. Figure 7.2 shows the fat content of selected foods.

Fat Content of Selected Foods

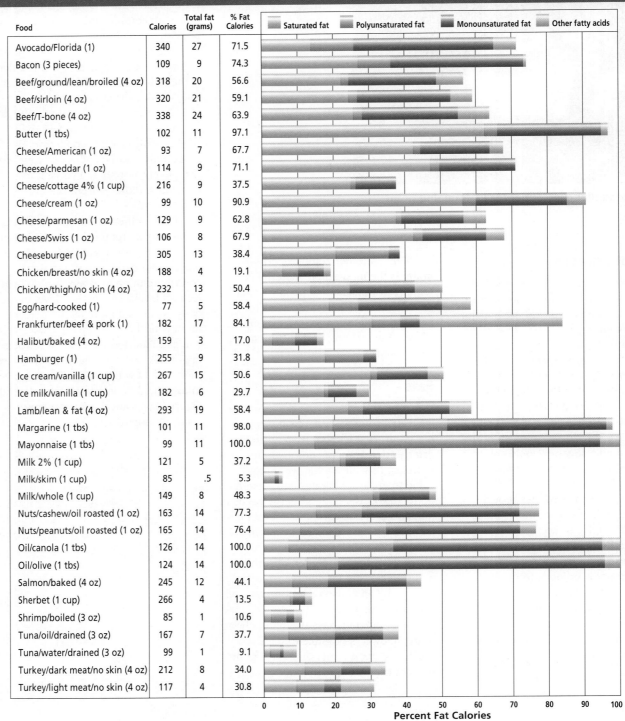

Food	Calories	Total fat (grams)	% Fat Calories
Avocado/Florida (1)	340	27	71.5
Bacon (3 pieces)	109	9	74.3
Beef/ground/lean/broiled (4 oz)	318	20	56.6
Beef/sirloin (4 oz)	320	21	59.1
Beef/T-bone (4 oz)	338	24	63.9
Butter (1 tbs)	102	11	97.1
Cheese/American (1 oz)	93	7	67.7
Cheese/cheddar (1 oz)	114	9	71.1
Cheese/cottage 4% (1 cup)	216	9	37.5
Cheese/cream (1 oz)	99	10	90.9
Cheese/parmesan (1 oz)	129	9	62.8
Cheese/Swiss (1 oz)	106	8	67.9
Cheeseburger (1)	305	13	38.4
Chicken/breast/no skin (4 oz)	188	4	19.1
Chicken/thigh/no skin (4 oz)	232	13	50.4
Egg/hard-cooked (1)	77	5	58.4
Frankfurter/beef & pork (1)	182	17	84.1
Halibut/baked (4 oz)	159	3	17.0
Hamburger (1)	255	9	31.8
Ice cream/vanilla (1 cup)	267	15	50.6
Ice milk/vanilla (1 cup)	182	6	29.7
Lamb/lean & fat (4 oz)	293	19	58.4
Margarine (1 tbs)	101	11	98.0
Mayonnaise (1 tbs)	99	11	100.0
Milk 2% (1 cup)	121	5	37.2
Milk/skim (1 cup)	85	.5	5.3
Milk/whole (1 cup)	149	8	48.3
Nuts/cashew/oil roasted (1 oz)	163	14	77.3
Nuts/peanuts/oil roasted (1 oz)	165	14	76.4
Oil/canola (1 tbs)	126	14	100.0
Oil/olive (1 tbs)	124	14	100.0
Salmon/baked (4 oz)	245	12	44.1
Sherbet (1 cup)	266	4	13.5
Shrimp/boiled (3 oz)	85	1	10.6
Tuna/oil/drained (3 oz)	167	7	37.7
Tuna/water/drained (3 oz)	99	1	9.1
Turkey/dark meat/no skin (4 oz)	212	8	34.0
Turkey/light meat/no skin (4 oz)	117	4	30.8

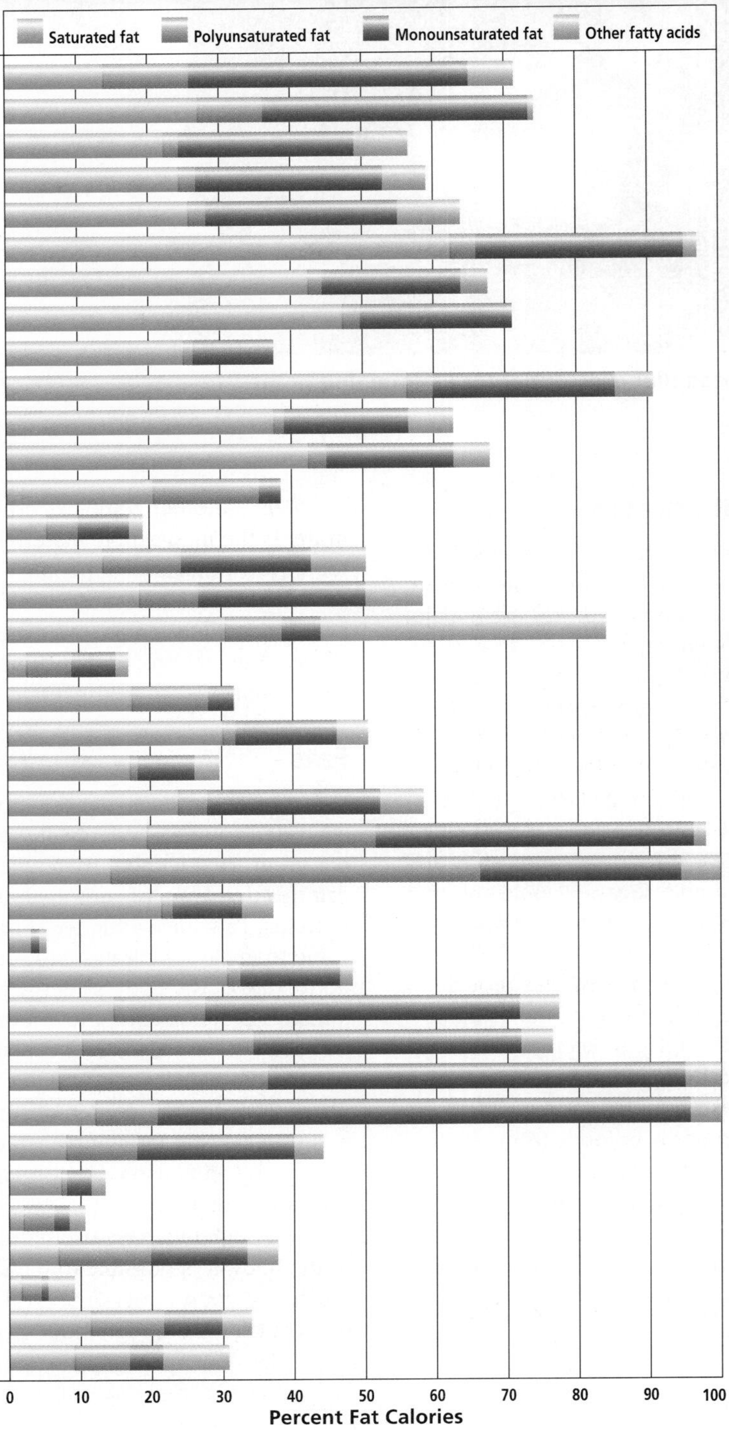

Figure 7.2 Saturated fat, polyunsaturated fat, and monounsaturated fat content of selected foods.

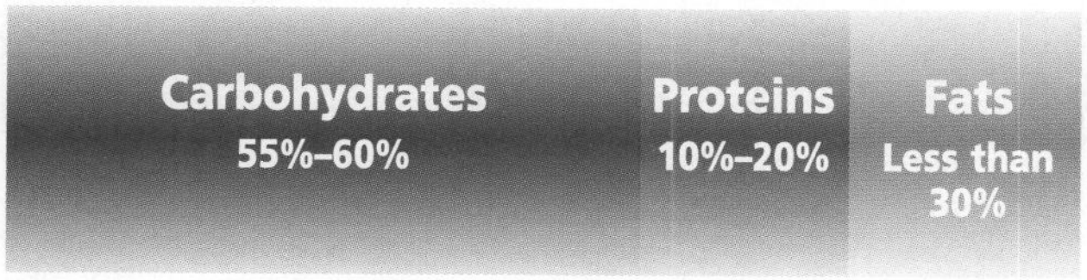
Carbohydrates
55%–60%
Proteins
10%–20%
Fats
Less than 30%

Figure 7.3 A balanced diet.

Proteins

Proteins are complex organic compounds made up of *amino acids*. This nutrient is essential for growth and repair of body tissues. Proteins are a potential source of energy but are not normally used for fuel when carbohydrates and fats are available.

Of the 20 amino acids that have been identified, nine are essential in the human diet. A food that contains all nine essential amino acids is called a *complete protein* food. Foods from animal sources such as fish, poultry, meat, eggs, and dairy products provide complete proteins. Incomplete proteins come from plant sources such as beans, peas, grains, and nuts. Combining selected incomplete proteins, such as beans and rice, ensures that the body gets sufficient protein.

Carbohydrates, fats, and proteins are all necessary in your daily food intake. In each case, a deficiency creates a problem, an adequate amount is optimal, and more is not better. The suggested caloric intake balance for adults as shown in Figure 7.3 is:

- 55% to 60% from carbohydrates
- Less than 30% from fats
- 10% to 20% from proteins.

The "Secret" Weight Training Diet

Many weight trainers and athletes are looking for the "secret" or "magic" diet that will make them successful and produce miraculous results. The truth is that no one food or special diet will do that. The "secret" diet is a balanced diet that includes all of the nutrients your body needs in the correct amounts.

The only major difference between the diet that is best for the average sedentary adult and the diet that is best for the active athlete or weight trainer is the total number of calories consumed. Athletes and weight trainers use more total calories because they expend more energy.

Fundamental principles of the "secret" weight training diet are moderation, variety, and balance. The diet should consist of a wide variety of good quality food in the proper amounts. You must eat right to gain healthy muscle tissue and remove excess stored body fat. Choose foods that are high in nutrients compared to their calories—those with *high nutrient density*. Foods that have few nutrients and are high in calories are called "junk foods." Carbonated drinks and chips will not produce quality muscle tissue but certainly can be stored as fat. Remove the junk food from your diet and eat high quality foods. Learn to tell the difference. One of the top body builders in the world has claimed that his body building success was 80% nutrition and 20% training.

Food Guide Pyramid

One relatively easy way to balance all of your complex nutritional requirements is to follow the U. S. Department of Agriculture's Food Guide Pyramid (Figure 7.4). The pyramid translates nutrient recommendations into a food group plan. This plan guides you to a balanced intake of essential nutrients, based on a recommended number of servings from five food groups (Table 7.1). The tip of the pyramid is not considered to be a major food group because the foods found there provide extra calories but little in the way of nutrients.

1. 6 to 11 servings daily from the bread, cereal, rice, and pasta group.

2. 3 to 5 servings daily from the vegetable group.

3. 2 to 4 servings daily from the fruit group.

4. 2 to 3 servings daily from the milk, yogurt, and cheese group.

5. 2 to 3 servings daily from the meat, poultry, fish, dry beans, eggs, and nuts group.

6. Sparingly (use very little) from the fats, oils, and sweets group.

The Food Guide Pyramid is a general guide, not an exact prescription, to healthy eating. Nevertheless, knowing the recommendations from the Pyramid should help you in making healthy food choices for a diet that is right for you. Also refer to Figure 7.4 to assist in making healthy food choices.

The Food Guide Pyramid

Key
● Fat (naturally occurring and added)
▲ Sugars (added)
These symbols show fats, oils, and added sugars in foods.

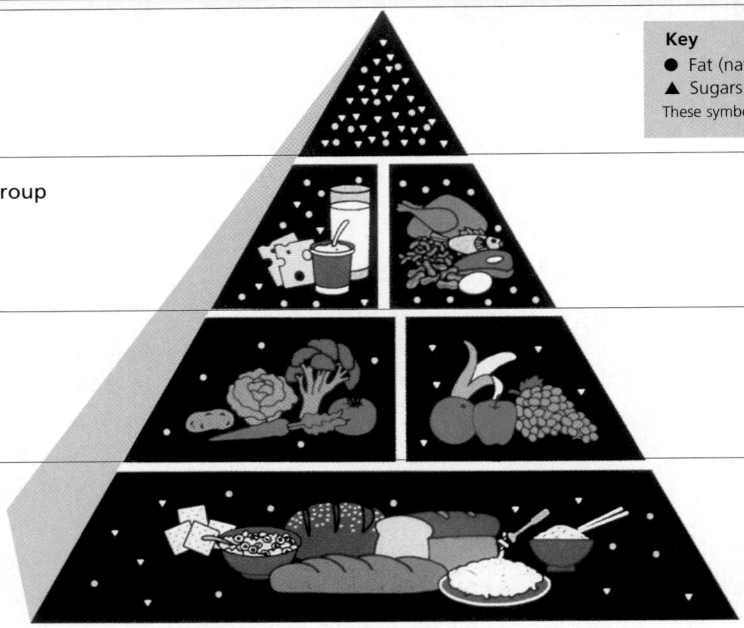

Fats, Oils, and Sweets
USE SPARINGLY

Milk, Yogurt, and Cheese Group
2–3 SERVINGS

Milk, Poultry, Fish, Dry Beans, Eggs, and Nuts Group
2–3 SERVINGS

Vegetable Group
3–5 SERVINGS

Fruit Group
2–4 SERVINGS

Bread, Cereal, Rice, and Pasta Group
6–11 SERVINGS

What counts as one serving?

Breads, Cereals, Rice, and Pasta
1 slice of bread
1/2 cup of cooked rice or pasta
1/2 cup of cooked cereal
1 ounce of ready-to-eat cereal

Vegetables
1/2 cup of chopped raw or cooked vegetables
1 cup of leafy raw vegetables

Fruits
1 piece of fruit or melon wedge
3/4 cup of juice
1/2 cup of canned fruit
1/4 cup of dried fruit

Milk, Yogurt, and Cheese
1 cup of milk or yogurt
1½ to 2 ounces of cheese

Meat, Poultry, Fish, Dry Beans, Eggs, and Nuts
2½ to 3 ounces of cooked lean meat, poultry, or fish
Count 1/2 cup of cooked beans, or 1 egg, or 2 tablespoons of peanut butter as 1 ounce of lean meat (about 1/3 serving)

Fats, Oils, and Sweets
LIMIT CALORIES FROM THESE

The amount you eat may be more than one serving. For example, a dinner portion of spaghetti would count as two or three servings of pasta.

How many servings do you need each day?

	Women and some older adults	Children, teen girls, active women, most men	Teen boys and active men
Calorie level*	about 1,600	about 2,200	about 2,800
Bread group	6	9	11
Vegetable group	3	4	5
Fruit group	2	3	4
Milk group	2–3**	2–3**	2–3**
Meat group	2, for a total of 5 ounces	2, for a total of 6 ounces	3, for a total of 7 ounces

* These are the calorie levels if you choose lowfat, lean foods from the 5 major food groups and use foods from the fats, oils, and sweets group sparingly.

** Women who are pregnant or breastfeeding, teenagers, and young adults to age 24 need 3 servings.

A Closer Look at Fat and Added Sugars

The small tip of the Pyramid shows fats, oils, and sweets. These are foods such as salad dressings, cream, butter, margarine, sugars, soft drinks, candies, and sweet desserts. Alcoholic beverages are also part of this group. These foods provide calories but few vitamins and minerals. Most people should go easy on foods from this group.

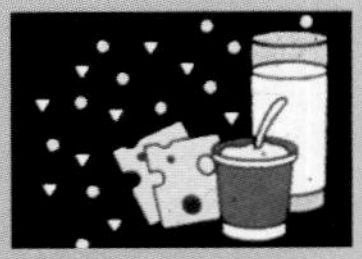

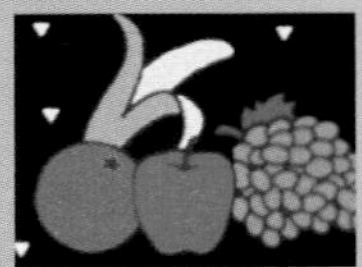

Some fat or sugar symbols are shown in the other food groups. That's to remind you that some foods in these groups can also be high in fat and added sugars—such as cheese or ice cream from the milk group or french fries from the vegetable group. When choosing foods for a healthful diet, consider the fat and added sugars in your choices from all the food groups, not just fats, oils, and sweets from the Pyramid tip.

Source: Developed by the U. S. Department of Agriculture to promote a healthy diet for people in the United States.

Figure 7.4 Food Guide Pyramid.

	Functions	Sources
Water	Carries nutrients and removes waste; dissolves amino acids, glucose, and minerals; cleans body by removing toxins; regulates body temperature	Liquids, fruits, and vegetables
Proteins	Help build new tissue to keep hair, skin, and eyesight healthy; build antibodies, enzymes, hormones, and other compounds; provide fuel for body	Meat, poultry, fish, eggs, beans, nuts, cheese, vegetables, some fruits, pastas, breads, cereal, tofu, and rice
Carbohydrates	Provide energy	Grains, cereal, pasta, some fruits and vegetables, nuts, milk, and sugars
Fats		
Saturated Fats	Provide energy; trigger production of cholesterol and LDL	Red meat, dairy products, egg yolks, and coconut and palm oils
Unsaturated fats	Also provide energy, but trigger more HDL production and less cholesterol and LDL production	Some fish; avocados; olive, canola, and peanut oils; shortening; stick margarine; baked goods
Vitamins	Facilitate use of other nutrients; involved in regulating growth, maintaining tissue, and manufacturing blood cells, hormones, and other body components	Fruits, vegetables, grains, some meat and dairy products
Minerals	Help build bones and teeth; aid in muscle function and nervous system activity; assist in various body functions including growth and energy production	Many foods

Table 7.1 Essential Nutrients

Dietary Guidelines for Americans, 2000

Among the most widely used of the guidelines for healthy eating are the Dietary Guidelines for Americans, developed jointly by the U. S. Departments of Agriculture and Health and Human Services (Table 7.2). The 10 dietary guidelines are:

1. Aim for a healthy weight.

2. Be physically active each day.

3. Let the Pyramid guide your food choices.

4. Choose a variety of grains daily, especially whole grains.

5. Choose a variety of fruits and vegetables daily.

6. Keep foods safe to eat.

7. Choose a diet that is low in saturated fat and cholesterol and moderate in total fat.

8. Choose beverages and foods that limit your intake of sugars.

9. Choose and prepare foods with less salt.

10. If you drink alcoholic beverages, do so in moderation.

Use the food logs at the end of this chapter to keep track of what you eat for 3 days. Compare your diet to the recommendations on the Food Guide Pyramid and the Dietary Guidelines for Americans. *A balanced diet should include plenty of fruits and vegetables.*

Nutrient Supplementation

If you are eating according to the recommendations of the U. S. Department of Agriculture (USDA) Food Guide Pyramid, you will be consuming a balanced diet of high-quality foods that should meet all of your nutritional needs. Independent researchers (those who do not sell food supplements) have found no benefit from the use of supplements when the subjects were on a healthy diet that was meeting all of their nutritional needs.

If you have dietary deficiencies, supplements might be beneficial, but you should improve your diet before resorting to "quick fix" supplements to

The following ten Dietary Guidelines point the way to good health using three basic messages—the ABCs for health:

Aim for fitness. These two guidelines will help keep you healthy and fit.

- Aim for a healthy weight.
- Be physically active each day.

Build a healthy base. These four guidelines build a base for healthy eating.

- Let the Pyramid guide your food choices.
- Choose a variety of grains daily, especially whole grains.
- Choose a variety of fruits and vegetables daily.
- Keep food safe to eat.

Choose sensibly. These four guidelines help you make sensible choices that promote health.

- Choose a diet that is low in saturated fat and cholesterol and moderate in total fat.
- Choose beverages and foods that limit your intake of sugars.
- Choose and prepare foods with less salt.
- If you drink alcoholic beverages, do so in moderation.

Tips for Following the Dietary Guidelines

Aim for a healthy weight.	Choose a lifestyle that combines sensible eating with regular physical activity. Evaluate your current weight. If you are overweight, first aim to prevent further weight gain, and then lose weight to improve your health. Choose a healthy assortment of foods that includes vegetables, fruits, whole grains, fat-free milk, and fish, lean meat, poultry, or legumes.
Be physically active each day.	Physical activity and nutrition work together for better health. Engage in 30 minutes or more of moderate physical activity on most, preferably all, days of the week. A moderate physical activity is any activity that requires about as much energy as walking 2 miles in 30 minutes. Choose activities that you enjoy and that you can do regularly.
Let the Pyramid guide your food choices.	To get all the nutrients and other beneficial substances you need for health, use the Food Guide Pyramid to help you make healthy food choices. Build your eating pattern on a variety of plant foods, including whole grains, fruits, and vegetables. Also choose moderate amounts of low-fat dairy products and low-fat foods from the meat, poultry, fish, dry beans, eggs, and nuts group each day. Go easy on foods high in fat or sugars.
Chose a variety of grains daily, especially whole grains.	Eat six or more servings of grain products daily (whole-grain and enriched breads, cereals, pasta, and rice). Include several servings of a variety of whole-grain foods—such as whole wheat, brown rice, oats, and whole corn—every day. Prepare or choose grain products with little added saturated fat and low amounts of added sugars.
Choose a variety of fruits and vegetables daily.	To promote your health, eat a variety of fruits and vegetables—at least two servings of fruits and three servings of vegetables—each day (see Figure 7.4 for serving sizes). Choose fresh, frozen, dried, or canned forms and a variety of colors and kinds. Choose dark-green leafy vegetables, bright orange and red fruits and vegetables, and cooked dried peas and beans often. Enjoy fruits as a naturally sweet end to a meal.
Keep food safe to eat.	Keep things clean: Wash hands and surfaces often. Don't cross-contaminate: Keep raw meat, poultry, eggs, fish, and shellfish away from contact with other foods, surfaces, utensils, or serving plates. Keep hot foods hot (above 140°F). Cook and reheat foods to a safe temperature. Choose pasteurized milk and juices. The risk of contamination is high from rare hamburger, raw eggs, fish (including sushi), clams, and oysters. Keep cold foods cold (below 40°F): refrigerate perishable foods promptly.
Choose a diet that is low in saturated fat and cholesterol and moderate in total fat.	Limit use of animal fats, hard margarines, and partially hydrogenated shortenings. Choose fat-free or low-fat dairy products, legumes, fish, and lean meats and skinless poultry. Trim fats from meats. Use egg yolks and whole eggs in moderation (use egg whites and egg substitutes freely). Limit breaded and deep-fried foods, and foods with creamy sauces.
Choose beverages and foods that limit your intake of sugars.	Use less sugar, syrup, and honey. Use fewer concentrated sweets such as candy, soft drinks, cakes, cookies, and fruit drinks. Read food labels for sugar content. Don't let soft drinks, or other sweets crowd out other foods you need to maintain health, such as low-fat milk or other good sources of calcium.
Choose and prepare foods with less salt.	Use herbs, spices, and fruits to flavor foods. Add little or no salt at the table. Limit salty foods. Read the Nutrition Facts label to compare and help identify foods lower in sodium. Go easy on condiments such as soy sauce, ketchup, mustard, pickles, and olives—they can add a lot of salt to your food.
If you drink alcoholic beverages, do so in moderation.	Limit alcoholic beverages to one drink per day for women or two drinks per day for men, and take with meals to slow absorption, "One drink" means 12 oz of beer, 5 oz of wine, or 1½ oz of distilled spirits. Pregnant women should not use alcohol. If you drink, do not drive.

*These guidelines are intended for healthy children (ages 2 years and older) and adults of any age.

Source: U. S. Department of Agriculture, U. S. Department of Health and Human Services, *Dietary Guidelines for Americans*, 5th ed., 2000.

Table 7.2 Dietary Guidelines for Americans, 2000*

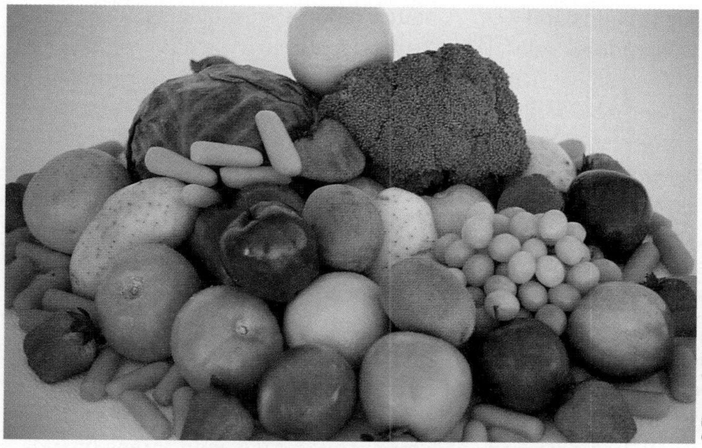

A balanced diet should include plenty of fruits and vegetables.

make up for your poor eating habits. If you suspect that you have dietary deficiencies, consult with a nutrition expert such as a dietician. *Weight training for life* encourages a lifelong pattern of healthy, balanced exercise supported by healthy, balanced eating.

Sports Drinks

Most people who exercise for an hour or less in moderate temperatures need only water to replace fluids. The electrolytes lost will be replaced by a balanced diet. For longer periods of exertion or exercise in hot and humid conditions, however, the American Dietetic Association suggests a sports beverage as part of the hydration-replacement process. Sports drinks are not a substitute for water. They should be consumed in addition to water. Sports drinks replace fluid and electrolytes that are lost in sweat and provide energy to working muscles.

Protein Supplementation

Contrary to a common myth, most individuals and even athletes do not need more protein. The exception may be those who are engaged in intense strength training. Most Americans consume in excess of the RDA for protein and do not need more protein. For adult men and women the recommended dietary allowance (RDA) for protein is 0.8 grams of protein per kilogram of body weight. Heavy, intense, high-volume strength training can increase this requirement to 1.7 grams of protein per kilogram of body weight.

Muscle requires the right kind and amount of exercise to stimulate growth and enough protein in the diet to build it. Claims that building muscle boosts the need for certain amino acids (the building blocks of protein) are not proven. A balanced diet can provide all the protein needed. If your diet is low in protein, you can get what you need without turning to expensive drinks and bars. Protein beyond what is needed is burned for energy or stored as fat.

Weight Gain

To gain muscular body weight, perform brief heavy weight training workouts. Work the largest muscles in your body, and eat a balanced diet of high-quality foods. Increase your total caloric intake by 500 to 1,000 calories per day. Eat smaller meals and more frequently. Get plenty of rest. Slow down, stay calm, and decrease your other activities. Set a healthy goal to gain muscle and not just total body weight. Watch your body fat level. Any diet in which caloric intake exceeds caloric need can lead to fat storage and unhealthy weight gain.

Weight Loss

Concerns about losing weight are increasing for many Americans, and these concerns may be justified. According to the National Center for Health Statistics, 58 million people—one in every three men and women—are *obese*, weighing at least 20% more than they should. Starting at age 25, the typical American gains 1 pound of weight per year.

At any given time, 33% to 40% of women and 20% to 24% of men are trying to lose weight. Another 28% of all adults are trying to maintain a weight loss—usually without success. The simple and well-documented truth is that diets are not an effective weight-loss strategy. Only about 10% of the people who begin a diet without exercise are able to lose the desired weight. Only one in 200 is able to maintain the weight loss for any significant amount of time. Diets don't work.

So what is the key to weight management? The formula is to maintain a moderate level of total calories, minimize fat calories, and get regular exercise. A well-rounded exercise program including aerobic exercise, weight training, and flexibility activities is best for weight management and overall fitness.

Continuous, rhythmic activities that use large muscle groups are good for high-caloric expenditure. Examples of good fat-loss activities are walking, cycling, and jogging. Combining these aerobic exercises with strength training exercises produces even better results.

How does weight training fit into a fat-loss program? When you start a weight training program, you will gain muscle and lose fat. Therefore, you may not see an immediate loss of total body weight. To lose excess body fat, you should perform longer training sessions consisting of more sets, repetitions, and exercises, which will use more total calories. You cannot "spot reduce" body fat. For example, sit-ups do not "spot reduce" fat from the abdominal area.

Weight training increases *lean body mass*. Because of the high energy needs of muscle tissue, more calories are required just to maintain muscle tissue.

Each additional pound of muscle tissue can raise the basal metabolic rate by as much as 35 calories per day. Lean body mass has such an important role in *metabolism* that maintaining muscle tissue causes increased caloric expenditure even when you are not exercising. Weight training increases lean body mass (muscle), which in turn increases metabolic rate. This results in greater caloric expenditure.

Because weight training increases muscle mass (calorie-burning cells), it is also beneficial for people who are at their recommended body weight but have a higher than recommended percentage of body fat.

An added benefit of weight training is the firm and fit appearance that results from regular training. Muscle tissue is more dense than fat tissue, so increasing muscle tissue and decreasing fat tissue results in a trim, healthy, toned appearance.

The secret to healthy weight loss is found in the following guidelines:

1. Eat a balanced diet of good quality food.

2. Do not skip meals or omit any food group. Did you know that the fewer meals people eat, the greater is their tendency toward obesity?

3. Decrease your total caloric intake by about 500 to 1,000 calories per day. This should translate into a safe 1- to 2-pound fat loss per week.

4. Increase your level of physical activity.

5. Select activities where food is not easily available.

6. Decrease the amount of rest and sleep you get. Your metabolic rate and caloric expenditure are higher when you are awake and moving.

7. Eat more slowly. Your brain needs about 20 minutes to register that you are full.

Rest

Although weight training exercise is the stimulus, the positive changes in the muscular system as a result of weight training take place between exercise sessions as your body rebuilds and adapts to the exercise overload. Adequate rest and nutrition are necessary for these positive changes to occur.

Weight training progress is best when a muscle receives 2 to 4 days of rest between exercise sessions. Fewer than 2 days of rest or more than 4 days of rest between workouts results in slower progress.

An average amount of sleep is 8 hours per night. Sleep requirements, however, vary from one person to another, and for the same person based upon changes in activity levels. At first, beginning weight trainers may find that they need more sleep to recover from this new demand. As they become accustomed to the increased physical activity and their bodies begin to function more efficiently, they often return to normal sleep patterns.

"Hard gainers"—individuals who have a hard time gaining muscle—sometimes need as many as 10 hours of sleep each night. Some "easy gainers" gain weight on 7 hours of sleep per night. Not getting adequate rest can be one of the greatest obstacles to weight training progress for young adults. Many high school students, college students, and young adults train hard with weights but do not get enough sleep to recover completely from their training sessions.

Weight training is intense and demanding. Too many other physical activities will slow your weight training progress. If you want to maximize your weight training gains, you should cut down on other physically strenuous activities. Young adults (ages 16 to 30) often wear themselves out with a large number of activities. This combination of too much activity and not enough rest can cancel out all the hard work you put into your weight training exercises. Some experienced weight trainers believe that they progress better if they train hard for 6 to 8 weeks, take one week off, and then start a new training program.

As you get older, some of your bodily functions will naturally begin to slow down. You should not view this as a totally negative experience. Many older adults report that they need less sleep, less food, and less exercise to stay healthy and physically fit. Beyond an approximate age of 40 or 50, two weight training workouts per week might be sufficient to maintain the muscular system in excellent condition. This depends on your weight training goals and your personal ability to recover from your workouts.

Some days you will feel better than others. On some days you likely will not feel like doing your normal workout. On those days you probably should train anyway but reduce your intensity and your total workload. You should not skip workouts completely on those days. You should maintain the frequency of workouts. Once you skip a training session, it becomes easier to skip another and another until soon you have no training schedule at all. It is easy to stop training completely and difficult to get started again. Many people begin weight training, but few have what it takes to continue for the rest of their lives. Persistence is a common word but a rare human quality.

The only time you should not train is when you are sick or injured. If you are truly physically sick, you should not work out, because it will further stress your body. You cannot "sweat out" a cold or any other illness. Instead, you should follow your doctor's advice and rest completely so you can get well in the shortest possible time. If you keep training, an illness can drag on for weeks, and you probably will not experience any progress in spite of your training efforts.

Weight training should contribute to your health. When you are not well, you should stop training and get well, then start again. If you are sick more than two or three times a year, you should examine your lifestyle.

If you feel exhausted when you wake up and are sleepy all day long, even during activities you normally enjoy, you may not be getting enough rest. If you are sleeping about 8 hours each night but are still feeling tired, you may be overtraining. In that case, try reducing the total number of sets in your weight training program and see if

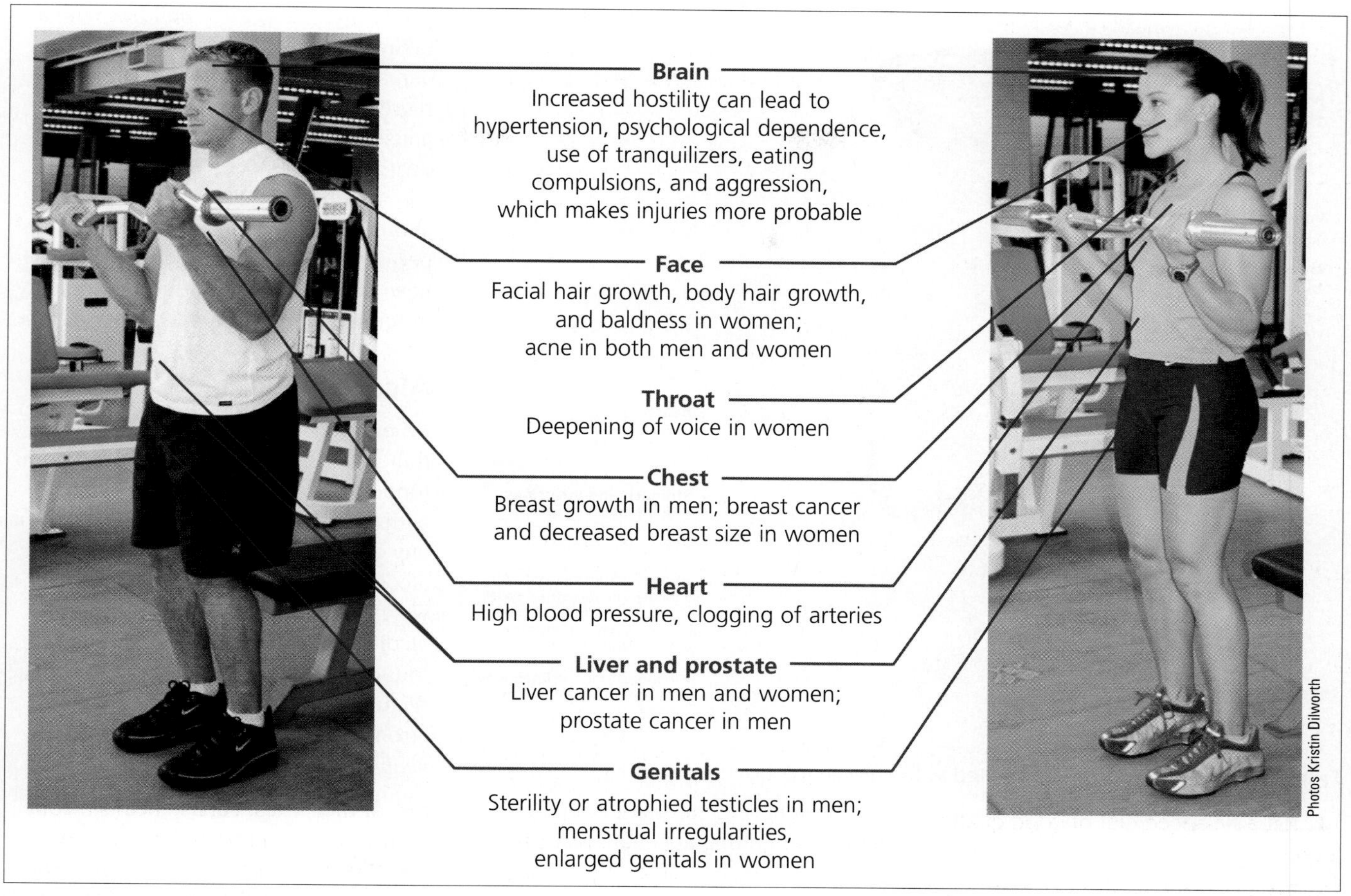
Brain
Increased hostility can lead to hypertension, psychological dependence, use of tranquilizers, eating compulsions, and aggression, which makes injuries more probable
Face
Facial hair growth, body hair growth, and baldness in women; acne in both men and women
Throat
Deepening of voice in women
Chest
Breast growth in men; breast cancer and decreased breast size in women
Heart
High blood pressure, clogging of arteries
Liver and prostate
Liver cancer in men and women; prostate cancer in men
Genitals
Sterility or atrophied testicles in men; menstrual irregularities, enlarged genitals in women
Photos Kristin Dilworth

Figure 7.5 Adverse effects of steroids on parts of the body.

you feel better. Adequate rest and recovery time are essential to your weight training progress.

Drugs

The drugs discussed here are anabolic steroids, alcohol, and tobacco. Although the topic of drugs is much broader, these are the ones that are most prominent in weight trainers.

Anabolic Steroids

One drug problem in weight training is the use of *anabolic steroids,* synthetic compounds that are like the natural hormones the body produces. Most of the steroids that weight trainers and athletes use to gain muscle mass are similar to the hormone testosterone.

Anabolic steroids are thought to promote muscle growth. They have been difficult to study because they also produce highly undesirable and dangerous side effects. Therefore, they can be studied only at safe (low) levels. Athletes who claim that steroids work take massive doses—sometimes 10 to 20 times greater than the safe dose an ethical physician would allow in a research study with human subjects.

Steroid use is dangerous because it can produce serious, life-threatening side effects and adverse reactions (see Figure 7.5). The side effects for women are just as dangerous as they are for men. Some of the undesirable side effects that users have reported and doctors have observed include endocrine disturbances, atrophy of the testicles, male impotency, liver damage, liver cancer, psychological disturbances, and coronary artery disease. The effects on specific parts of the body are given in Figure 7.5.

Steroid users agree that steroids work only when accompanied by extremely hard weight training. Therefore, steroids are not "easy gain" muscle drugs that replace hard work. Intense workouts are still necessary to gain muscle. This is another reason that steroid effects are hard to study. It is difficult to determine how much of the improvement is a result of training and how much can be attributed to the steroid effect.

Many steroid users have reported an increase in aggressiveness. This can result in more intense weight training workouts, which might produce greater gains. Because anabolic steroids do not produce scientifically proven and predictable benefits, and they do have documented and dangerous side effects, their use is not recommended. Some

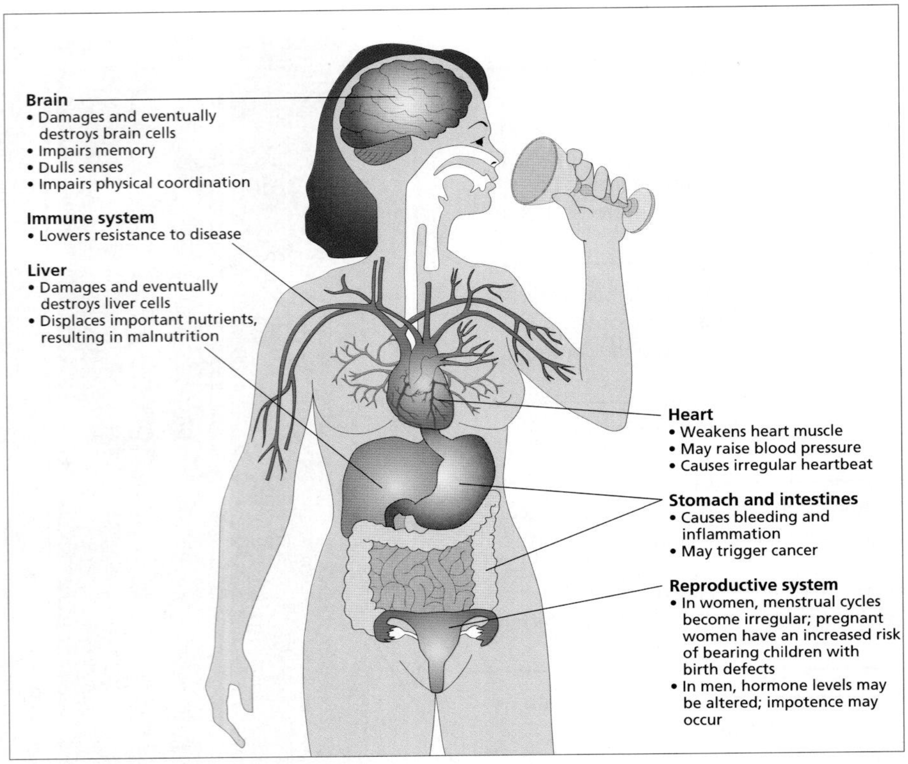

Brain
• Damages and eventually destroys brain cells
• Impairs memory
• Dulls senses
• Impairs physical coordination
Immune system
• Lowers resistance to disease
Liver
• Damages and eventually destroys liver cells
• Displaces important nutrients, resulting in malnutrition
Heart
• Weakens heart muscle
• May raise blood pressure
• Causes irregular heartbeat
Stomach and intestines
• Causes bleeding and inflammation
• May trigger cancer
Reproductive system
• In women, menstrual cycles become irregular; pregnant women have an increased risk of bearing children with birth defects
• In men, hormone levels may be altered; impotence may occur

Figure 7.6 Long-term risks associated with chronic alcohol use.

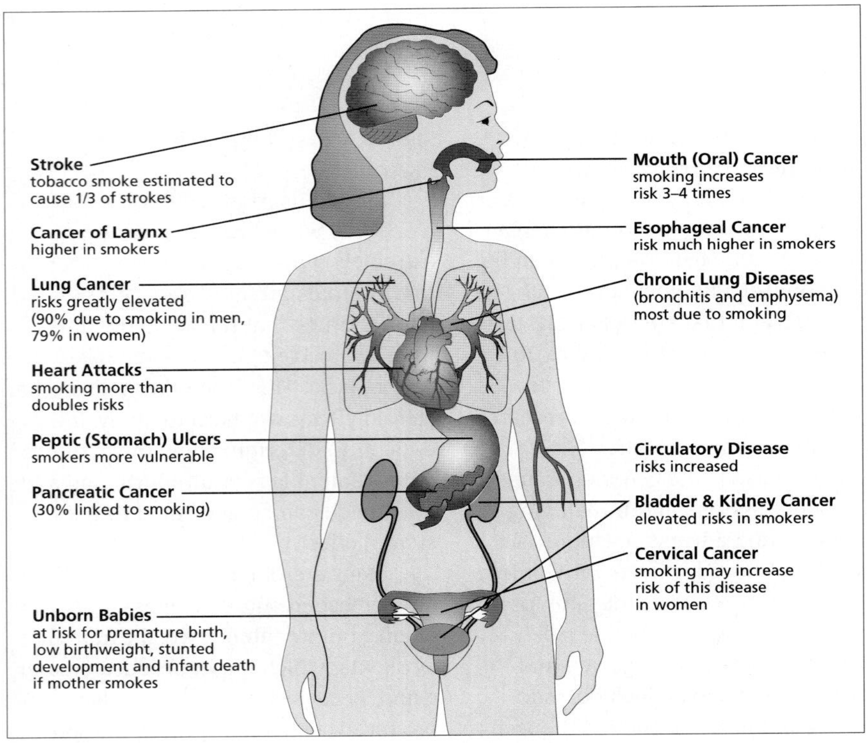

Figure 7.7 Adverse health effects of smoking.

young lifters and body builders who are taking steroids are causing lifelong damage to their bodies that they will regret when they get older. Steroid abuse has also caused a number of deaths.

Weight training is an activity that should improve your health and natural performance level. Drug use and abuse have no place in a health development program such as *weight training for life*.

Alcohol

No evidence is available to suggest that a low level of alcohol consumption (one drink per day or less) interferes with weight training progress. Neither is any evidence available indicating that alcohol has any beneficial effect on weight training progress. But heavy alcohol consumption does have profound detrimental effects on your body (Figure 7.6). If your desire is to have a strong and healthy body, you need to keep your alcohol consumption to a minimum or eliminate it completely.

Tobacco

Smoking or chewing tobacco has no known beneficial effects, but smoking does harm the respiratory and circulatory systems (Figure 7.7). It decreases performance and training capacity. Smoking reduces the ability to finish demanding weight training workouts and interferes with the ability to recover from workouts. Smoking and chewing tobacco both have been proven to cause cancer and other diseases, and neither will help you reach your weight training goals.

FOOD DIARY

	Name			Date		Total Caloric Intake							
	Time	Place	Associated Activity	Reason/Mood	Food and Amount	Food Groups							
						Dairy	Meat	Grain	Vegs	Fruits	Fats	Misc.	Water
Breakfast													
Snack													
Lunch													
Snack													
Dinner													
Snack													
Exercise													

FOOD DIARY

	Name			Date		Total Caloric Intake							
	Time	Place	Associated Activity	Reason/Mood	Food and Amount	Food Groups							
						Dairy	Meat	Grain	Vegs	Fruits	Fats	Misc.	Water
Breakfast													
Snack													
Lunch													
Snack													
Dinner													
Snack													
Exercise													

FOOD DIARY

	Name			Date		Total Caloric Intake							
	Time	Place	Associated Activity	Reason/Mood	Food and Amount	Food Groups							
						Dairy	Meat	Grain	Vegs	Fruits	Fats	Misc.	Water
Breakfast													
Snack													
Lunch													
Snack													
Dinner													
Snack													
Exercise													

FOOD DIARY

	Name			Date		Total Caloric Intake							
	Time	Place	Associated Activity	Reason/Mood	Food and Amount	Food Groups							
						Dairy	Meat	Grain	Vegs	Fruits	Fats	Misc.	Water
Breakfast													
Snack													
Lunch													
Snack													
Dinner													
Snack													
Exercise													

FOOD DIARY

	Name			Date		Total Caloric Intake							
	Time	Place	Associated Activity	Reason/Mood	Food and Amount	Food Groups							
						Dairy	Meat	Grain	Vegs	Fruits	Fats	Misc.	Water
Breakfast													
Snack													
Lunch													
Snack													
Dinner													
Snack													
Exercise													

FOOD DIARY

Name | Date | Total Caloric Intake

	Time	Place	Associated Activity	Reason/Mood	Food and Amount	Food Groups							
						Dairy	Meat	Grain	Vegs	Fruits	Fats	Misc.	Water
Breakfast													
Snack													
Lunch													
Snack													
Dinner													
Snack													
Exercise													

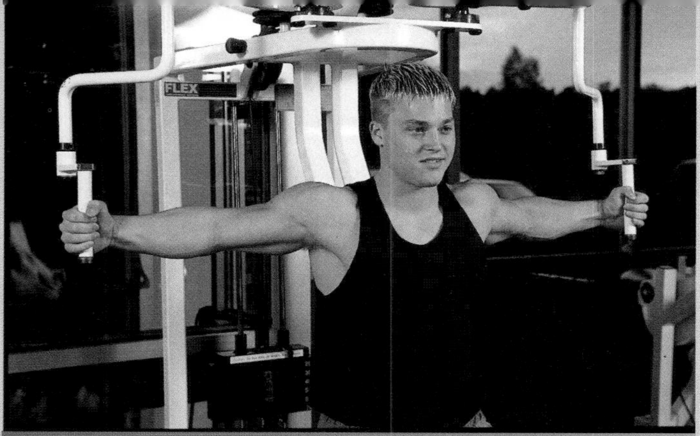

Jon Kelley

Part II: Learning More Weight Training Exercises

The weight training exercises in this book are arranged into the following chapters.

Chapter 8: Chest Exercises
Chapter 9: Back Exercises
Chapter 10: Shoulder Exercises
Chapter 11: Arm Exercises
Chapter 12: Leg Exercises
Chapter 13: Trunk Flexion and Extension Exercises

The exercise descriptions in this book are consistent with the exercise technique recommendations of the National Strength and Conditioning Association (NSCA). The general pattern in these chapters is to present a basic barbell and dumbbell exercise on the left page along with a description of the exercise and an illustration of the major muscles used to perform the exercise. Then, on the right page directly across from it are common exercise machine positions for the same exercise.

Various exercise machines have been used here because of the many good ones on the market. The idea is for you to recognize that you can either perform the basic barbell or dumbbell exercise or perform the same exercise movement on the machines you have available, and realize you are working the same muscles. Some exercise machines use a cam or a pivot system to vary the resistance as you move through the range of motion. This is not really important for you to understand as a beginner as long as you provide your muscles with an appropriate overload stimulus.

The *concentric phase* of a weight training exercise is the portion of the exercise during which your muscular contractions overcome the resistance and the weight is lifted. The *eccentric phase* of a weight training exercise is the portion of the exercise during which the resistance overcomes your muscular contraction and the weight is lowered. The same muscles are working during both the concentric phase and the eccentric phase of a weight training exercise.

Almost any barbell exercise can be performed using dumbbells. In many dumbbell exercises the dumbbells may be moved together or in an alternating manner.

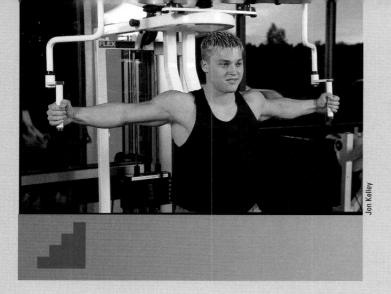

Major Muscles of the Human Body

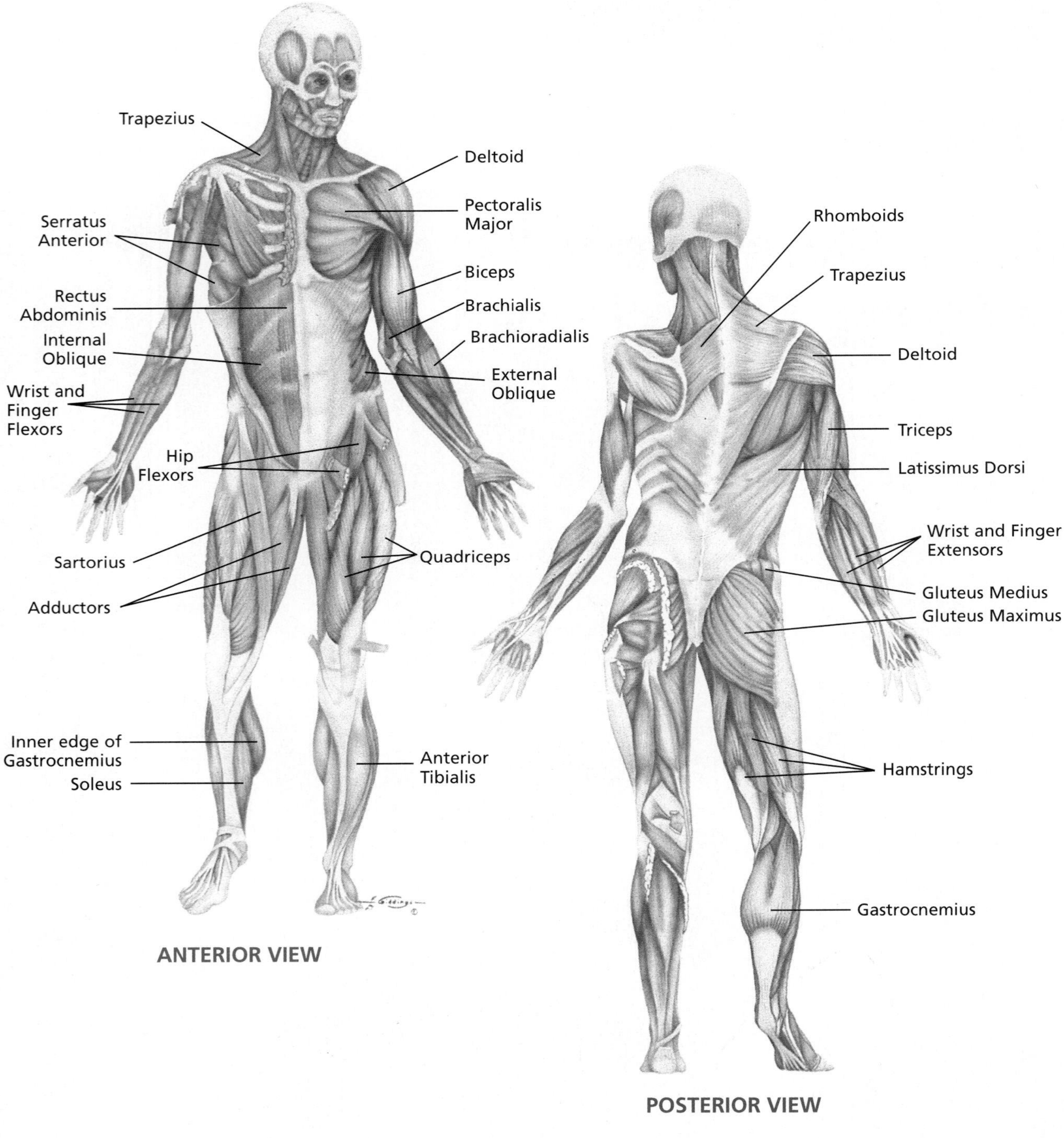
Trapezius
Deltoid
Pectoralis Major
Serratus Anterior
Biceps
Rectus Abdominis
Brachialis
Brachioradialis
Internal Oblique
External Oblique
Wrist and Finger Flexors
Hip Flexors
Sartorius
Quadriceps
Adductors
Inner edge of Gastrocnemius
Anterior Tibialis
Soleus
ANTERIOR VIEW
Rhomboids
Trapezius
Deltoid
Triceps
Latissimus Dorsi
Wrist and Finger Extensors
Gluteus Medius
Gluteus Maximus
Hamstrings
Gastrocnemius
POSTERIOR VIEW

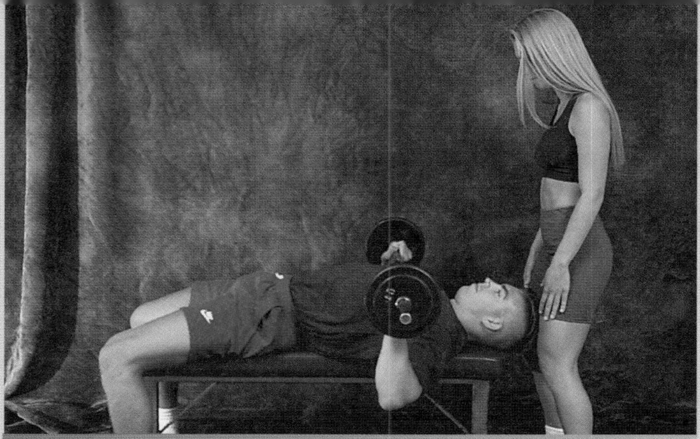

Eric Risberg

8

Chest Exercises

Chest (Pectoralis major)

Barbell Bench Press
Dumbbell Bench Press
Prone Bench Press Machine
Cybex Seated Chest Press Machine

Incline Barbell Bench Press
Incline Dumbbell Bench Press
Boss Incline Bench Press Machine
Cybex Incline Bench Press Machine

Bent-Arm Flyes
Body Master Bent-Arm Machine Flyes
Pec Deck Machine
Nautilus 10-Degree Chest Machine

Chest/Back (Pectoralis major and Latissimus dorsi)

Barbell Bent-Arm Pullover
Dumbbell Straight-Arm Pullover
Hammer Bent-Arm Pullover Machine
Nautilus Pullover Machine

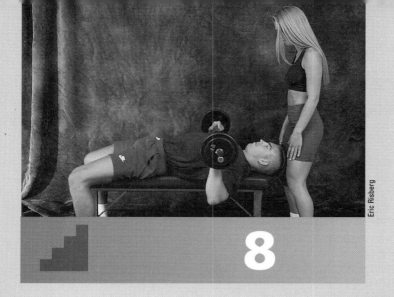

CHEST (PECTORALIS MAJOR)

Bench Press

Muscles developed: Pectoralis major, anterior deltoid, triceps.

Starting position: Start on your back on a flat bench; hold a barbell directly above your shoulders, arms straight, and both feet flat on the floor (A).

Eccentric phase: Inhale as you lower the bar to touch your chest (B).

Concentric phase: Exhale as you press the weight back up to the starting position.

Spotting: Have a spotter stand at the head end of the bench in case you cannot press the weight back to the starting position.

Variations: Change the angle of the bench and change the width of the hand spacing on the bar to achieve many variations of this basic chest exercise. You also may choose to perform this exercise with dumbbells.

Additional information: To make this exercise easier, use a rack to hold the weight above the bench. Some people prefer to place their feet on the bench to keep the lower back flat on the bench.

Caution: Do not arch your lower back during this lift. Use a spotter.

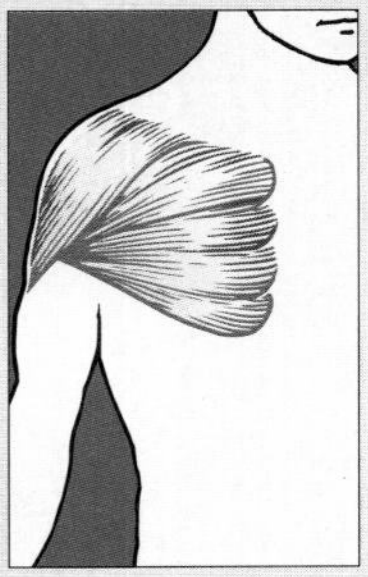
Front

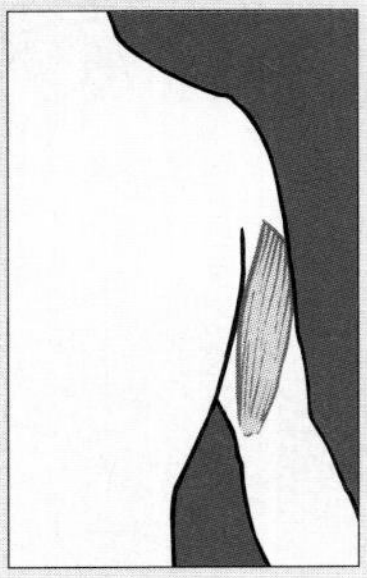
Back

Barbell

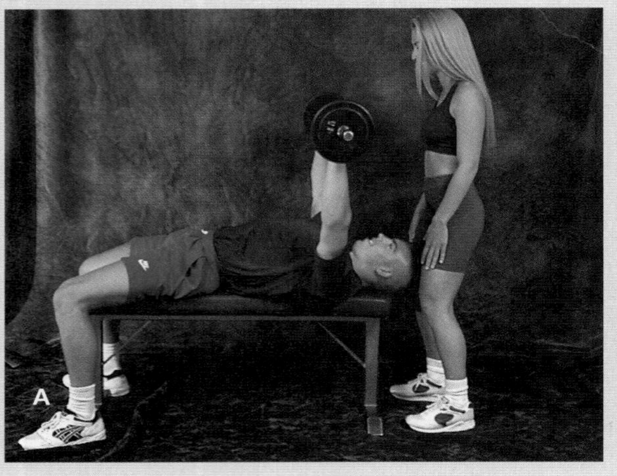

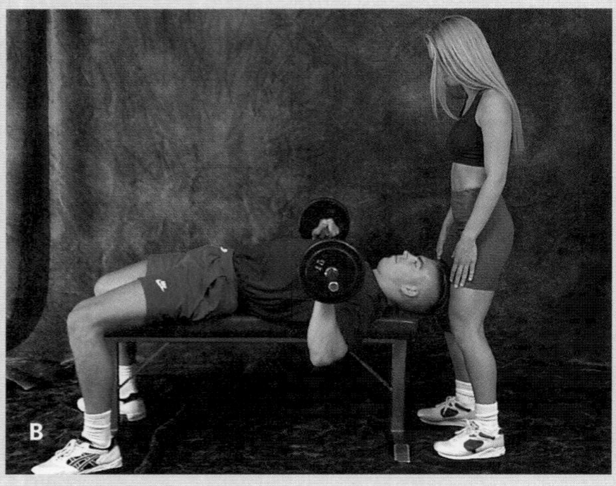

Photos Eric Risberg

Dumbbell

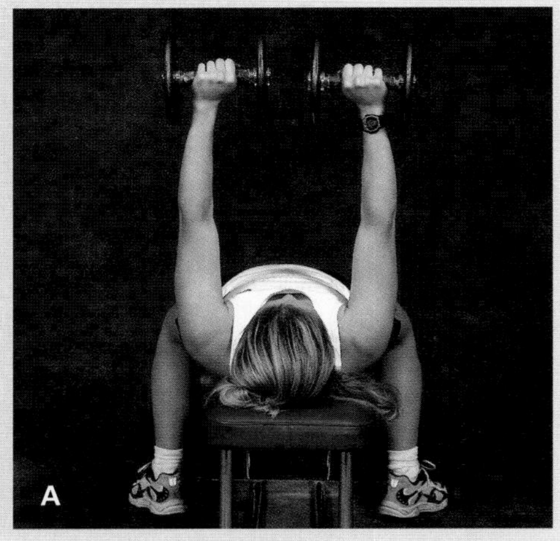

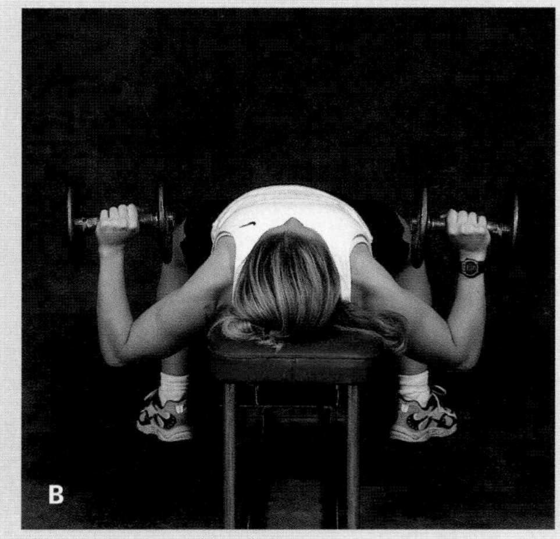

Photos Eric Risberg

Prone Bench Press Machine

Muscles developed: Pectoralis major, anterior deltoid, triceps.

Starting position: Start on your back on a flat bench; grasp the bar with your hands wider than shoulder-width and your elbows bent; place both feet flat on the floor or on the end of the bench (A).

Concentric phase: Exhale as you press the weight upward to a straight arm position (B).

Eccentric phase: Inhale as you lower the weight to the starting position.

Cautions:

1. Do not arch your lower back or lift your hips off the bench when you do this lift.

2. Keep your head a safe distance away from the weight stack and the selector pin.

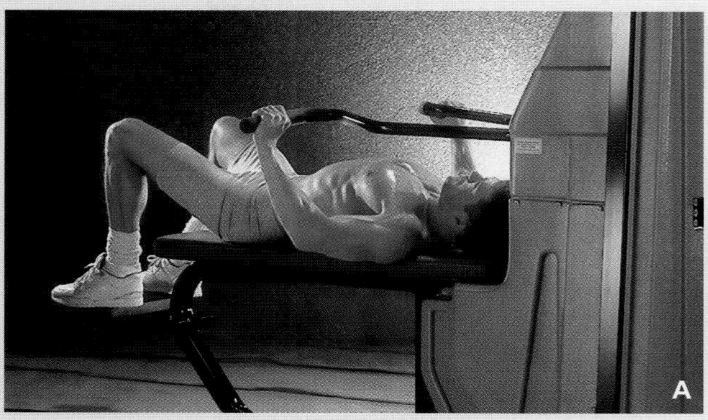

A

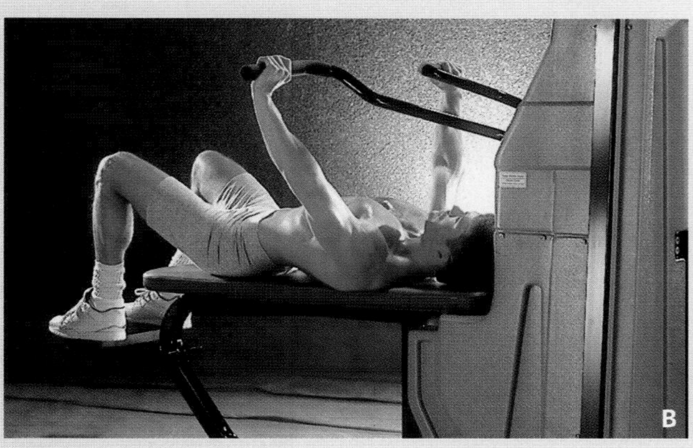

B

Photos © Nautilus Sports/Medical Industries, Inc.

Cybex Seated Chest Press Machine

Muscles developed: Pectoralis major, anterior deltoid, triceps.

Starting position: Adjust the machine so you start in a seated position with the exercise handles at chest level. Grasp the exercise handles with your hands wider than shoulder-width and your elbows bent (A).

Concentric phase: Exhale as you press forward to a straight arm position (B).

Eccentric phase: Inhale as you allow the weight to return to the starting position.

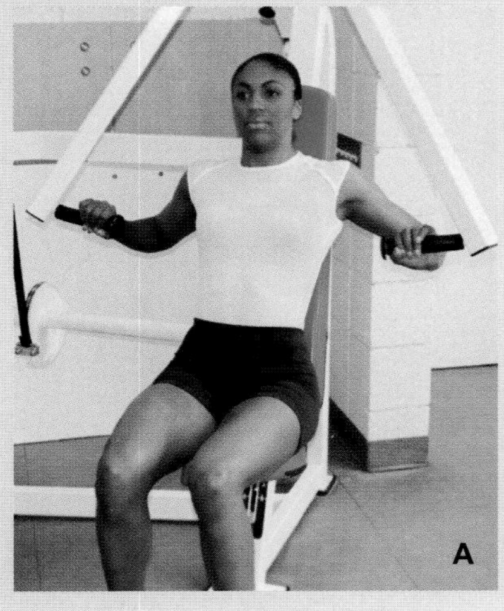

A

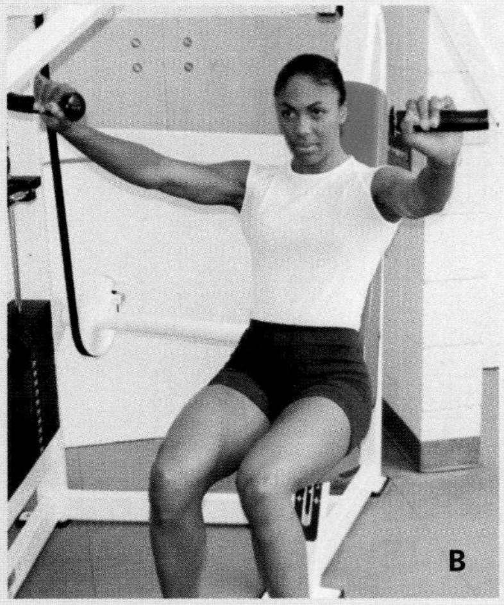

B

Photos Kristin Dilworth

Incline Bench Press

Muscles developed: Upper pectoralis major, anterior deltoid, triceps.

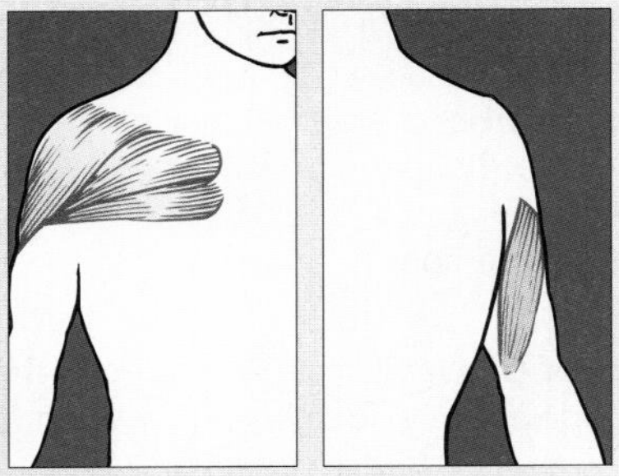

Starting position: Start on your back on an incline bench; hold a barbell directly above your shoulders with both arms straight and both feet flat on the floor (A).

Eccentric phase: Inhale as you lower the bar to touch your chest (B).

Concentric phase: Exhale as you press the weight back up to the starting position.

Spotting: Have a spotter stand behind the bench in case you cannot get the weight back to the starting position.

Variations:

1. Change the angle of the incline bench.
2. Change your hand spacing on the bar.
3. Use dumbbells instead of a barbell.

Additional information: To make this exercise easier to perform, use a weight rack to support the weight above the bench.

Caution: Dumbbells can be difficult to control because they are free to move in any direction. Begin with a light weight and master the movement before using heavier dumbbells. Have a spotter in position to help if you begin to lose control of the exercise movement.

Barbell

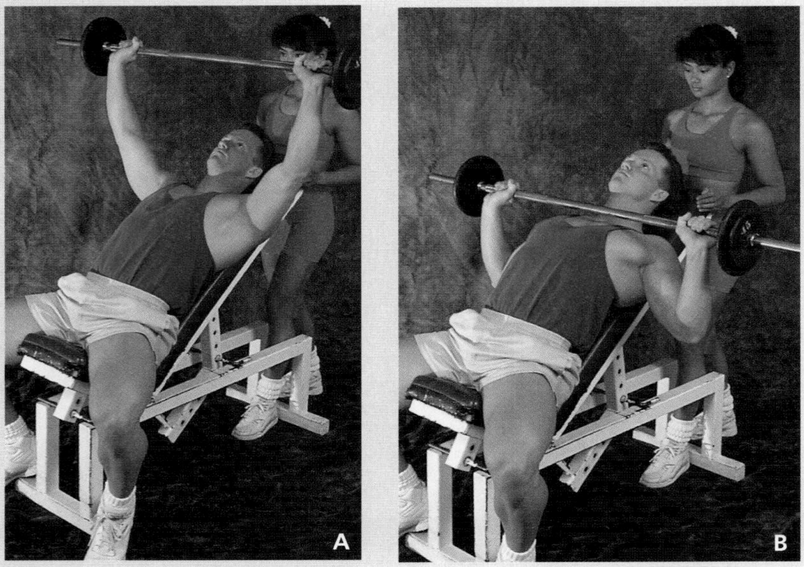

Photos Eric Risberg

Dumbbell

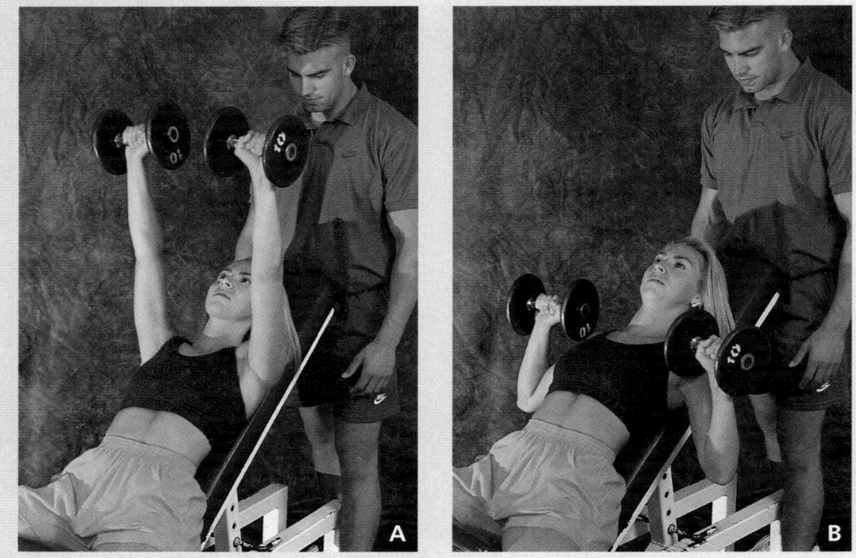

Photos Eric Risberg

Boss Incline Bench Press Machine

Muscles developed: Upper pectoralis major, anterior deltoid, triceps.

Starting position: Start in a seated position on an incline bench press machine (A).

Concentric phase: Exhale as you press the weight upward to a straight arm position (B).

Eccentric phase: Inhale as you slowly lower the weight to the starting position.

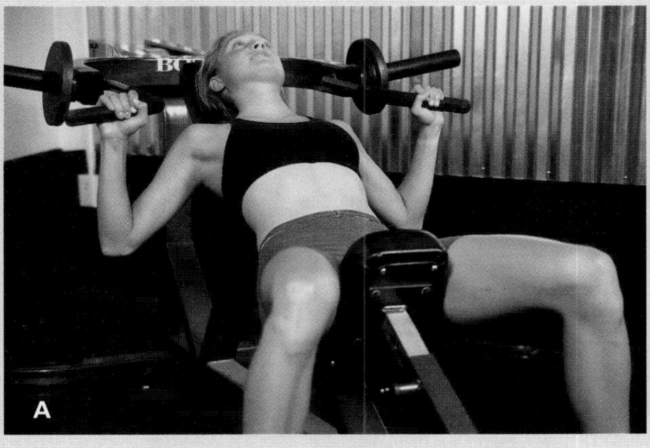

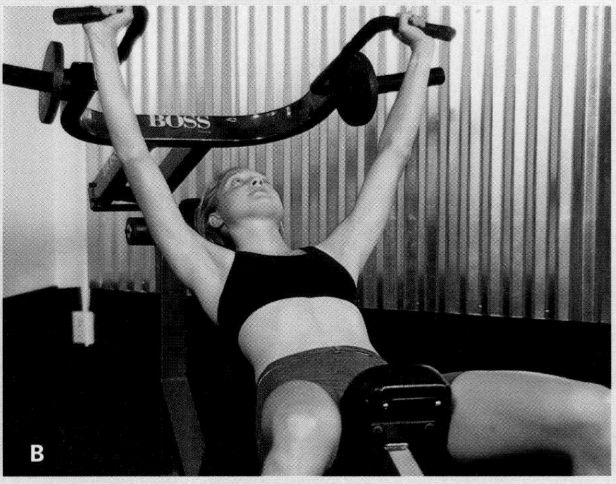

Photos Jon Kelley

Cybex Incline Bench Press Machine

Muscles developed: Upper pectoralis major, anterior deltoid, triceps.

Starting position: Start in a seated position on an incline bench press machine (A).

Concentric phase: Exhale as you press the weight upward to a straight arm position (B).

Eccentric phase: Inhale as you slowly lower the weight to the starting position.

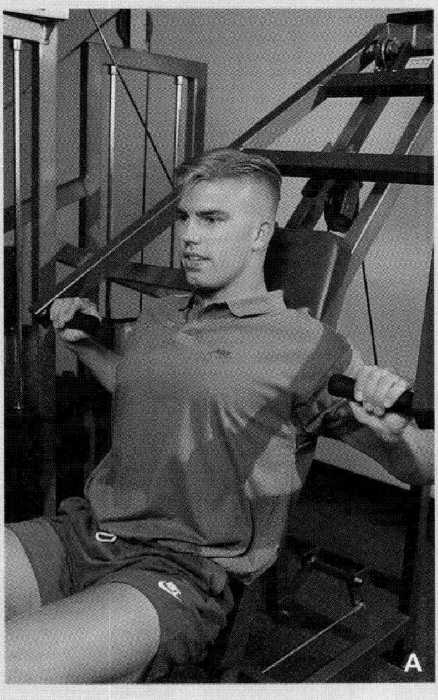

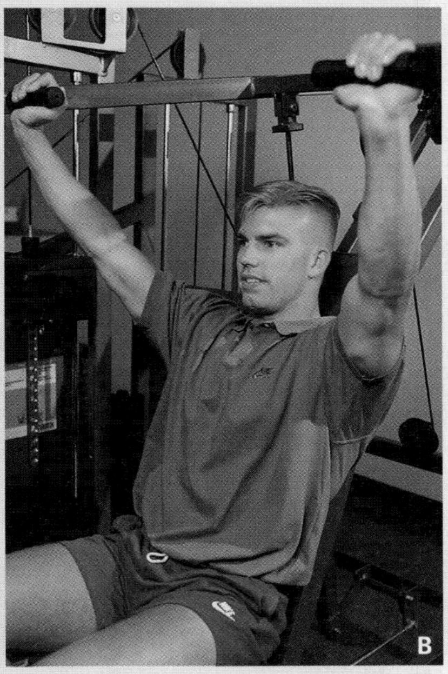

Photos Eric Risberg

Bent-Arm Flyes

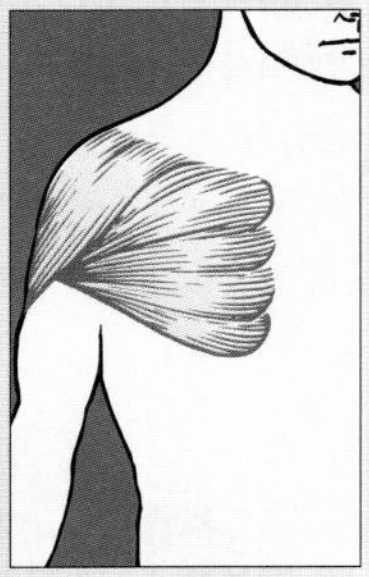

Front

Muscles developed: Pectoralis major, anterior deltoid.

Starting position: Start on your back on a flat exercise bench; hold one dumbbell in each hand above your shoulders, with your arms slightly bent (A).

Eccentric phase: Inhale as you move the dumbbells away from each other and lower them toward the floor (B).

Concentric phase: Exhale as you return the dumbbells to the starting position.

Variations: Perform this exercise on an incline or decline bench.

Caution: Keep your elbows slightly bent throughout this exercise to place the exercise stress on the pectoralis major muscle and relieve the stress on the elbow joint.

Dumbbell

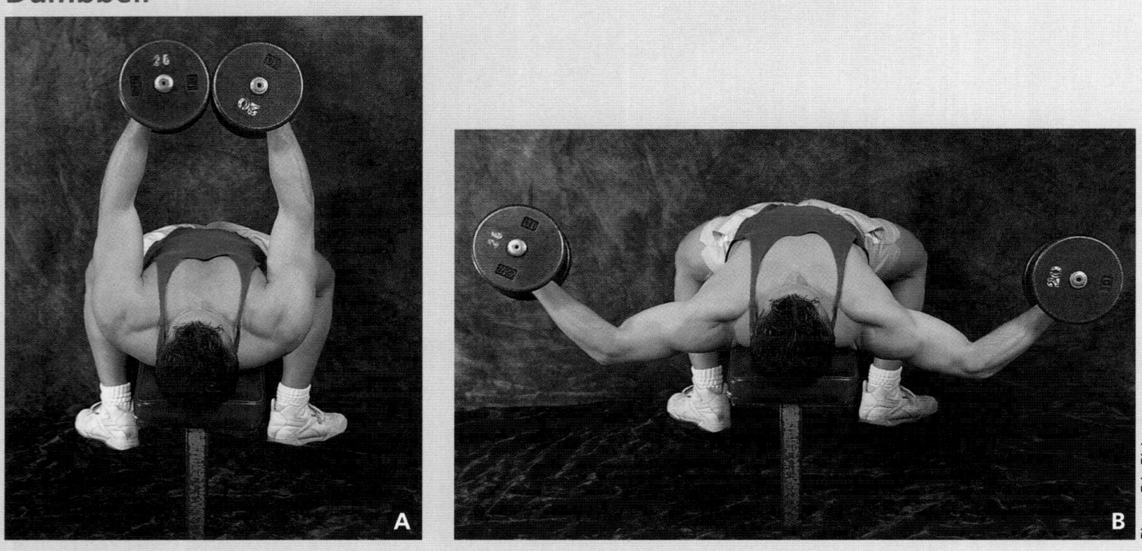

Photos Eric Risberg

Body Master Machine Flyes

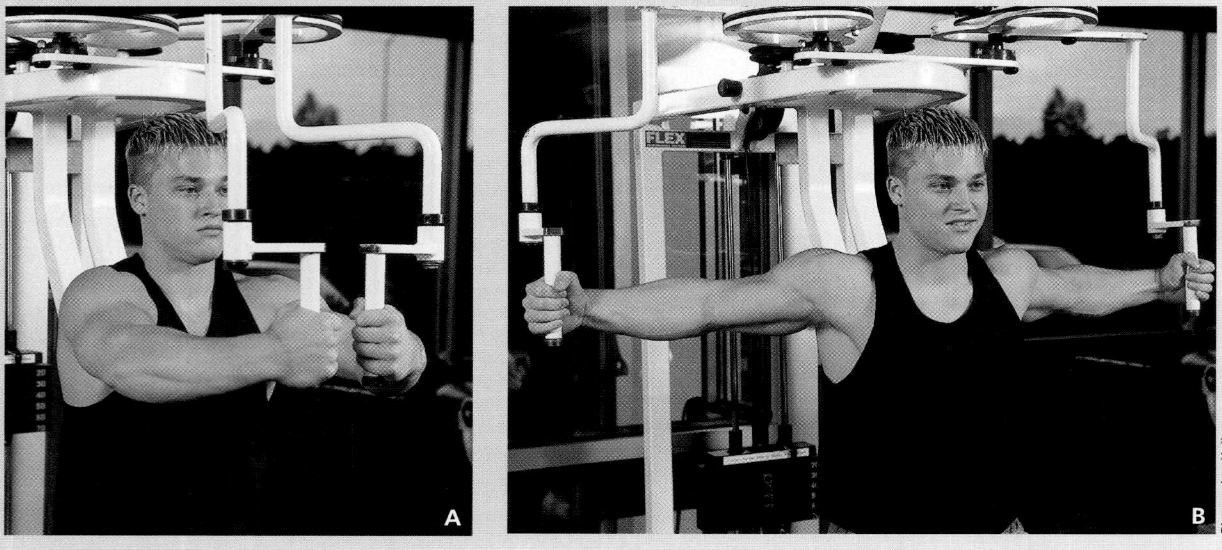

Photos Jon Kelley

Pec Deck Machine

Muscles developed: Pectoralis major, anterior deltoid.

Starting position: Start in a seated position with your elbows bent and your forearms on the padded exercise bars. Adjust the seat so that your elbows are shoulder height (A).

Concentric phase: Exhale as you pull your arms forward and toward each other. Keep pulling until the exercise bars gently touch each other (B).

Eccentric phase: Inhale as you slowly allow your arms to return to the starting position.

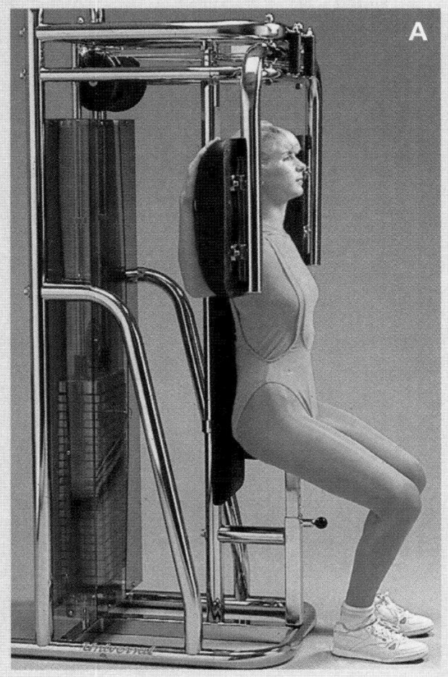

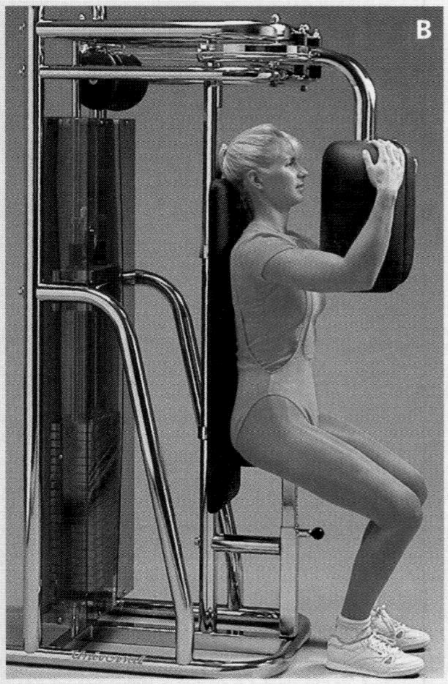

Photos © Universal Gym Equipment, Inc.

Nautilus 10-Degree Chest Machine

Muscles developed: Pectoralis major, anterior deltoid.

Starting position: Start on your back on the bench and place your arms under the padded exercise bars. (See photo.)

Concentric phase: Exhale as you pull your bent arms upward and toward each other. Keep pulling until the exercise bars gently touch each other or come to the end of their travel. Pause briefly and try to squeeze your arms together.

Eccentric phase: Inhale as you slowly allow your arms to return to the starting position.

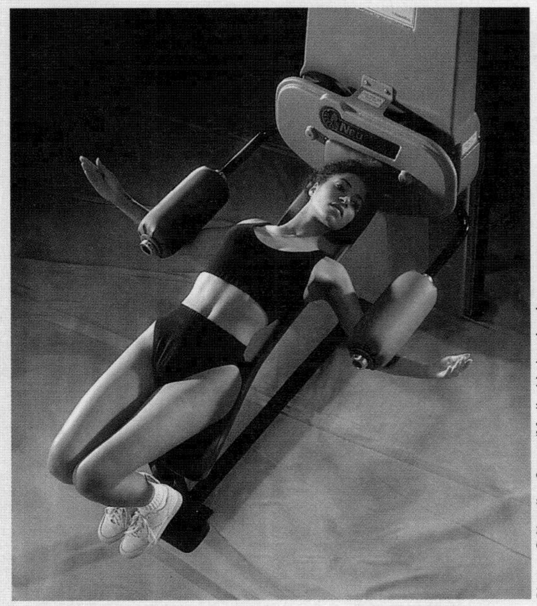

Photos © Nautilus Sports/Medical Industries, Inc.

CHEST / BACK

Barbell Bent-Arm Pullover

Muscles developed: Latissimus dorsi, pectoralis major.

Starting position: Start on your back on a flat bench; hold a barbell supported on your chest, hands 6 to 12 inches apart, elbows bent, and head beyond the end of the bench (A).

Eccentric phase: Inhale as you lower the weight past your face toward the floor (B).

Concentric phase: Exhale as you pull the weight back to the starting position.

Additional information: Keep your elbows bent and your arms in close to your head.

Caution: Keep your arms pressed inward toward each other to avoid placing too much strain on the medial side or inside of your elbow joints.

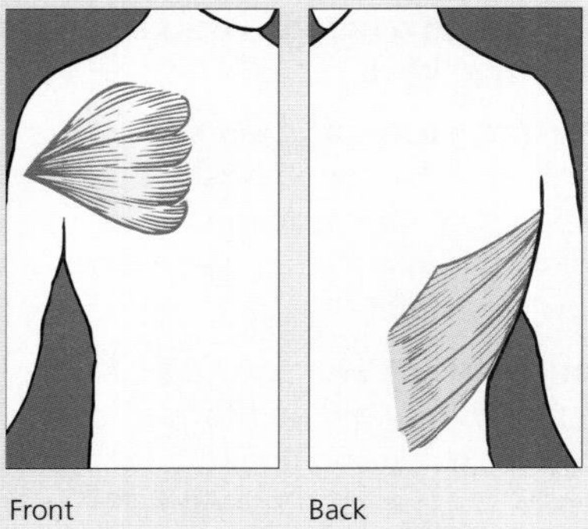

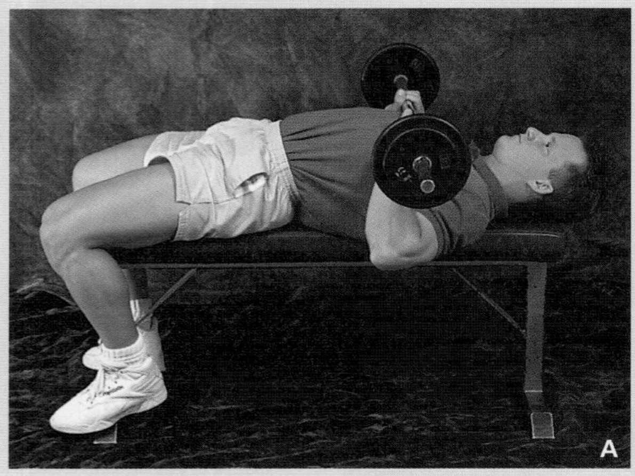

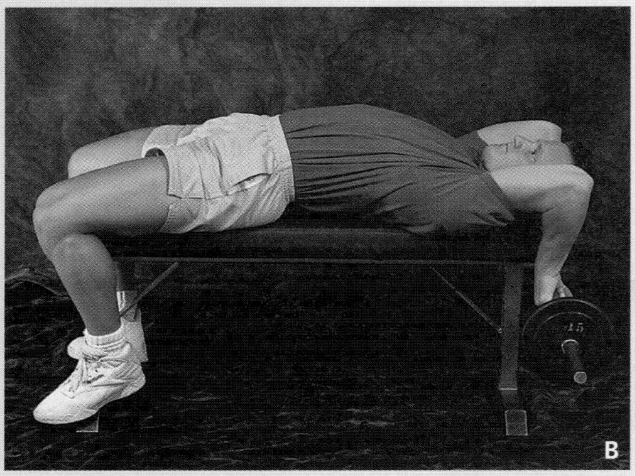

Photos Eric Risberg

Dumbbell Straight-Arm Pullover

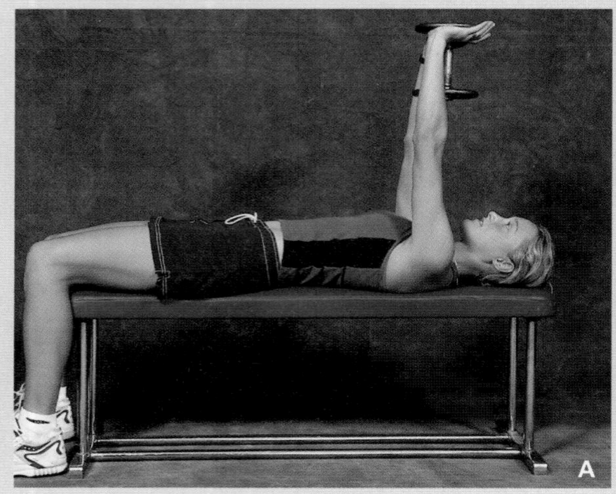

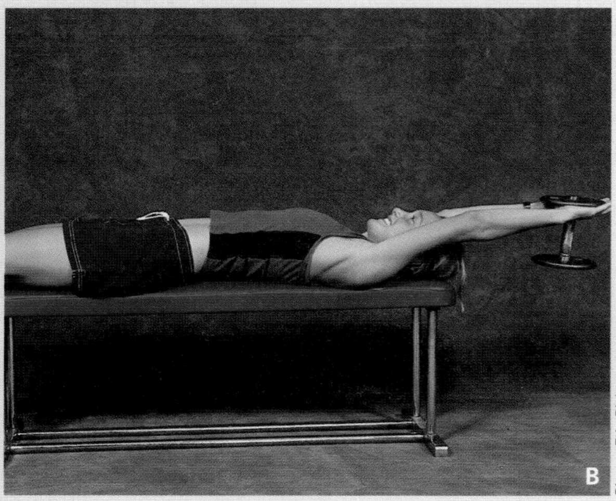

Photos Eric Risberg

Hammer Strength Bent-Arm Pullover Machine

Muscles developed: Pectoralis major, latissimus dorsi.

Starting position: Start in a seated position with your shoulder joints aligned with the pivot point of the machine. Fasten the seat belt to hold your hips in the correct position. Grasp the exercise bar behind your head with a palms-up grip (A).

Concentric phase: Exhale as you pull the exercise bar over your head and all the way to your abdomen (B).

Eccentric phase: Inhale as you slowly allow the bar to return to the starting position.

Caution: Push on the elbow pads more than pull with your hands.

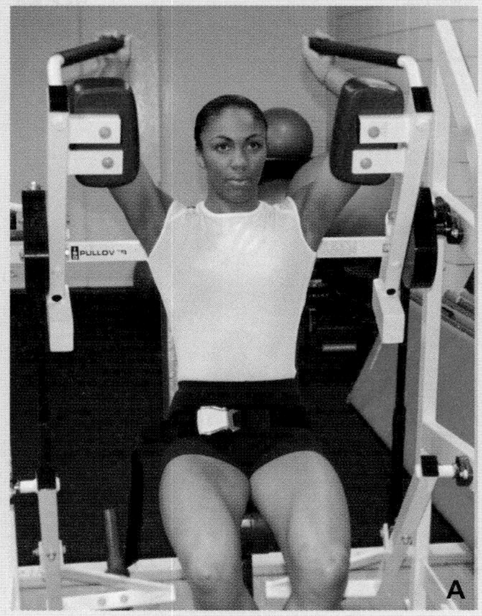
A

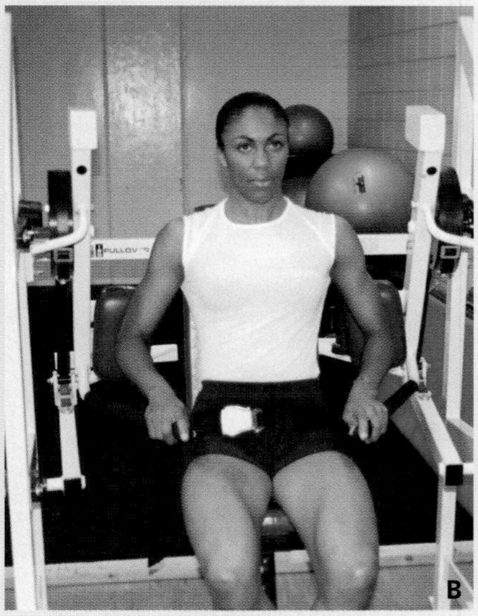
B

Photos Kristin Dilworth

Nautilus Pullover Machine

Muscles developed: Pectoralis major, Latissimus dorsi.

Starting position: Start in a seated position with your shoulder joints aligned with the pivot point of the pullover machine. Fasten the seat belt to hold your hips in the correct position. Push down on the foot bar to bring the exercise bar forward to a position where you can place your upper arms on the padded portion of the exercise bar as shown in the photograph (A). Allow the bar to gently pull your arms back to the starting position, then remove your feet from the foot bar.

Concentric phase: Exhale as you pull the exercise bar over your head and all the way to your abdomen (B).

Eccentric phase: Inhale as you slowly allow the exercise bar to return to the starting position.

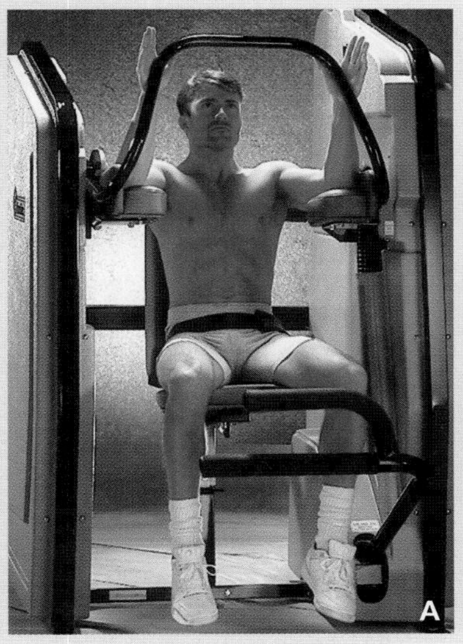
A

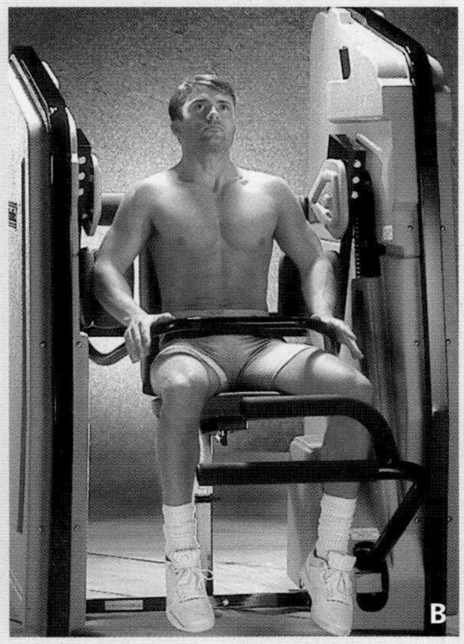
B

Photos © Nautilus Sports/Medical Industries, Inc.

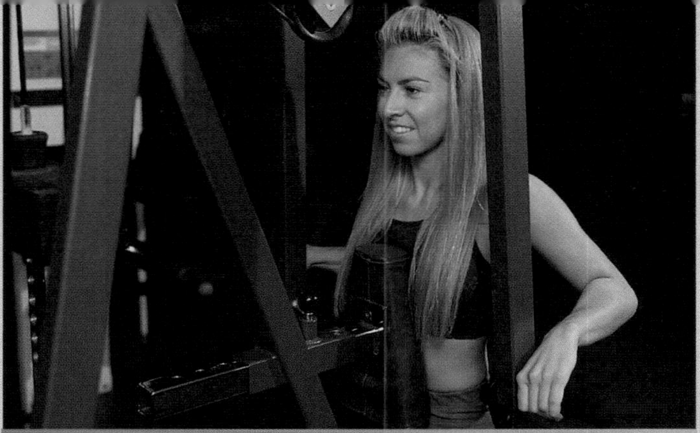

9

Back Exercises

Back (Latissimus dorsi)

Barbell Rowing
One-Dumbbell Rowing
Cybex Seated Rowing Machine
Nautilus Seated Rowing Machine

Pull-Ups
Chin-Ups
Lat Pulldown Machine
Cybex Weight-Assisted Pull-Up Machine

Upper Back (Trapezius)

Barbell Shoulder Shrug
Dumbbell Shoulder Shrug
Low Pulley Shoulder Shrug
Nautilus Shoulder Shrug Machine

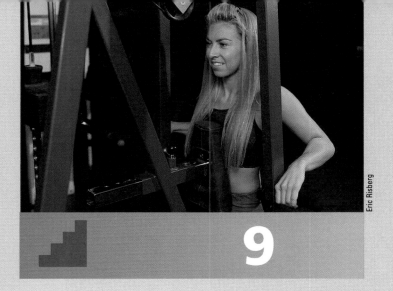

BACK (LATISSIMUS DORSI)

Rowing

Muscles developed: Latissimus dorsi, teres major, posterior deltoid, trapezius, rhomboids.

Starting position: Bend over with your knees slightly bent; hold a barbell in your hands with your arms straight so the barbell is hanging directly below your shoulders (A).

Concentric phase: Exhale as the weight is pulled upward (B) until the bar touches your chest. Pause briefly with the bar held against your chest.

Eccentric phase: Inhale as the weight is lowered slowly to the starting position.

Variations:

1. Stand on a bench or block to get more stretch in the starting position when larger plates are used.
2. Change the distance between your hands.
3. Pull the bar to your shoulders or chest or abdomen.
4. Perform this exercise with dumbbells, bringing both up at the same time or alternately.

Caution: Your lower back will be in a potentially dangerous position. To reduce the risk of injury to your lower back, keep your back flat, do not jerk or drop the weight, and keep your knees bent.

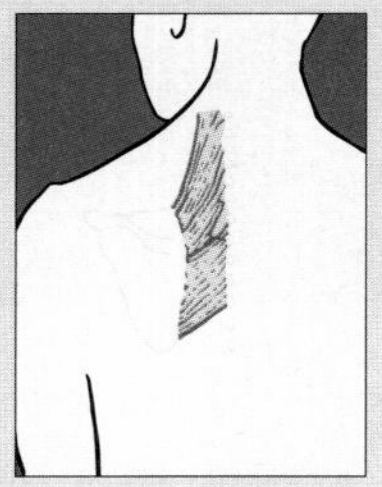

Back

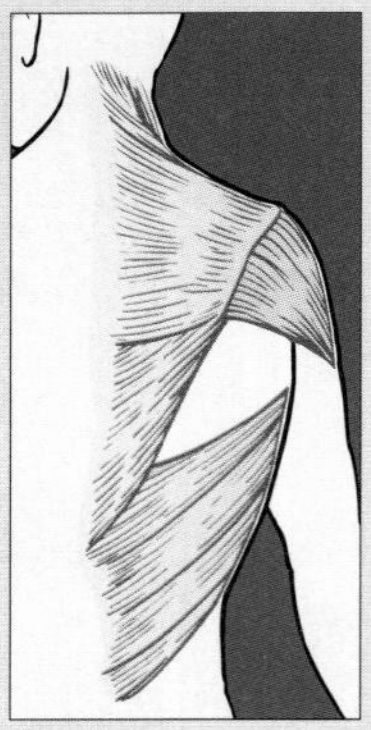

Back

Barbell

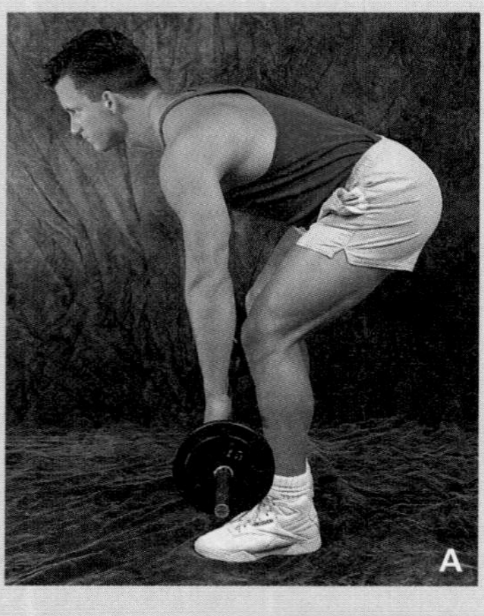

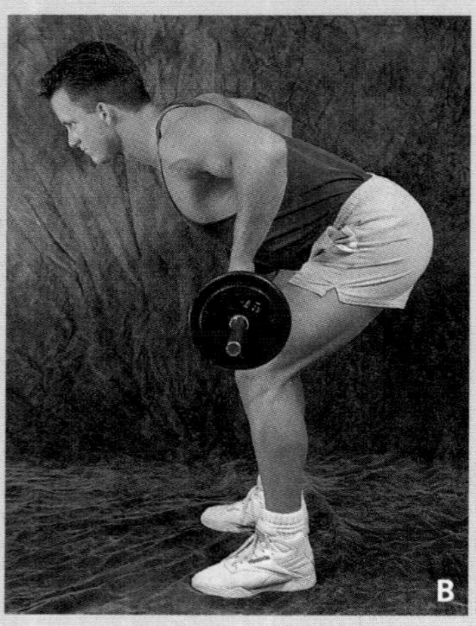

Photos Eric Risberg

One-Dumbbell

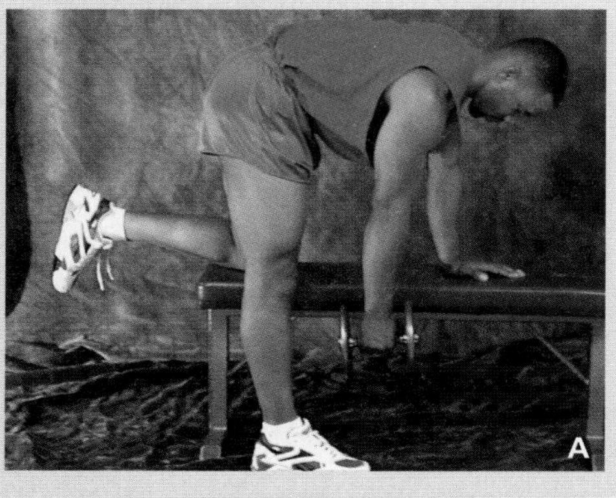

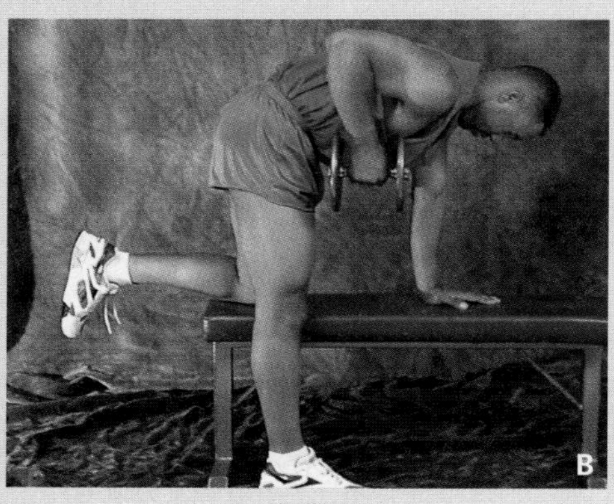

Photos Eric Risberg

Cybex Seated Rowing Machine

Muscles developed: Latissimus dorsi, teres major, posterior deltoid, trapezius, rhomboids.

Starting position: Adjust the chest pad so you can just reach the handles of the exercise bar with your arms fully extended (A).

Concentric phase: Exhale as you pull the exercise handles toward your chest (B). Pause briefly in the fully contracted position.

Eccentric phase: Inhale as you slowly allow the exercise handles to return to the starting position.

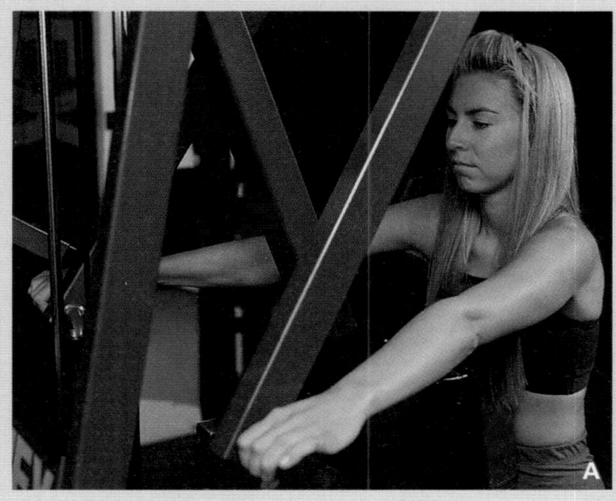

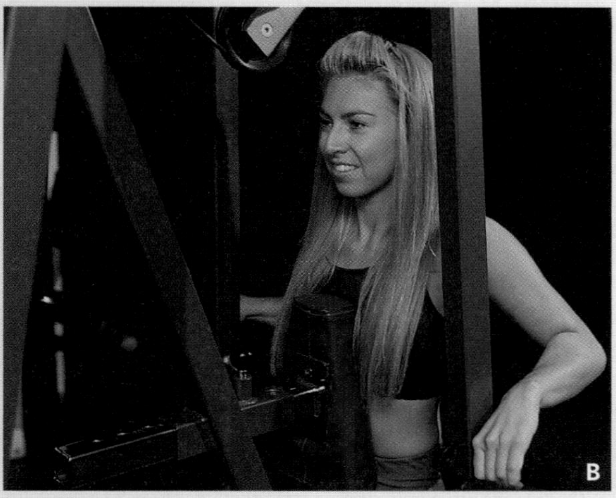

Photos Eric Risberg

Nautilus Seated Rowing Machine

Muscles developed: Latissimus dorsi, teres major, posterior deltoid, trapezius, rhomboids.

Starting position: Start facing the machine and grasp one exercise bar in each hand.

Concentric phase: Exhale as you pull the exercise bars toward your chest. Pause briefly in the fully contracted position and squeeze your shoulder blades together.

Eccentric phase: Inhale as you slowly allow the exercise bars to return to the starting position.

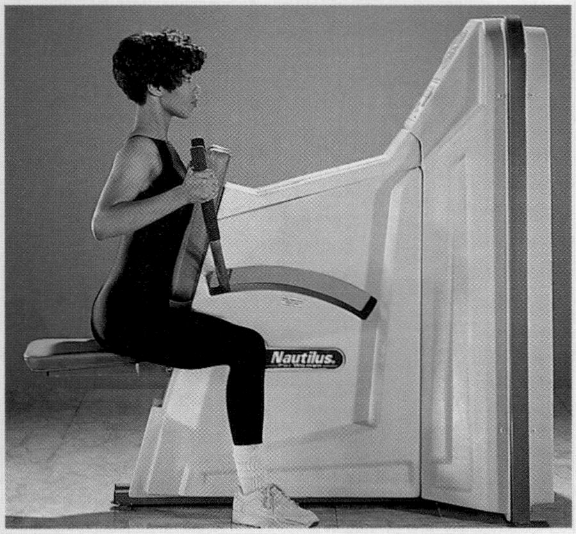

Photos © Nautilus Sports/Medical Industries, Inc.

Pull-Ups

Muscles developed: Latissimus dorsi, teres major, biceps brachii.

Starting position: Hang from a bar with a pronated grip (thumbs in) (A). For chin-ups use a supinated grip (thumbs out) (A).

Concentric phase: Exhale as you pull yourself upward to a position with your chin above the bar (B).

Eccentric phase: Inhale as you lower yourself slowly to the starting position.

Variations: Change grip direction and hand spacing for variations of this exercise.

Additional information: Start each pull-up from a full hang. Pause with your chin above the bar, then lower yourself slowly to the starting position. Add weight by suspending a dumbbell from a wide strap that passes around your lower back and placing the dumbbell between your thighs.

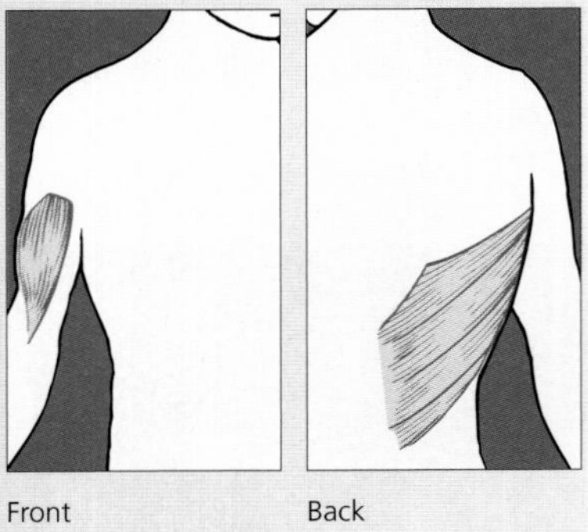

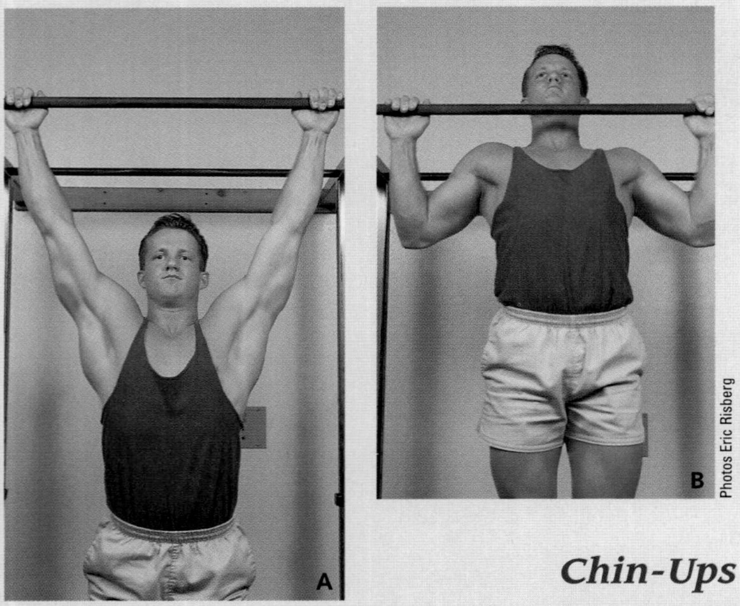

Chin-Ups

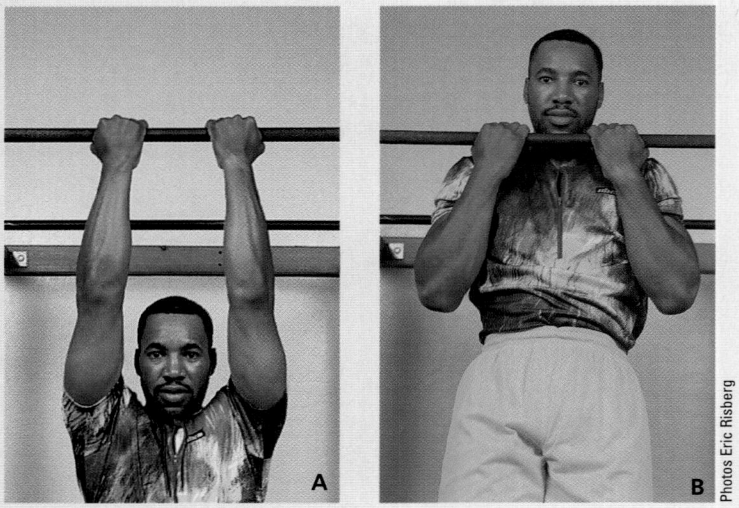

Lat Pulldown Machine

Muscles developed: Latissimus dorsi, teres major, biceps.

Starting position: Grasp the bar with a pronated grip and your hands wider than shoulder width. Assume a seated position with your arms straight (A).

Concentric phase: Inhale and pull the exercise bar down to your upper chest (B). Pause briefly in the fully contracted position and squeeze your shoulder blades together.

Eccentric phase: Exhale as you slowly allow the exercise bar to return to the starting position.

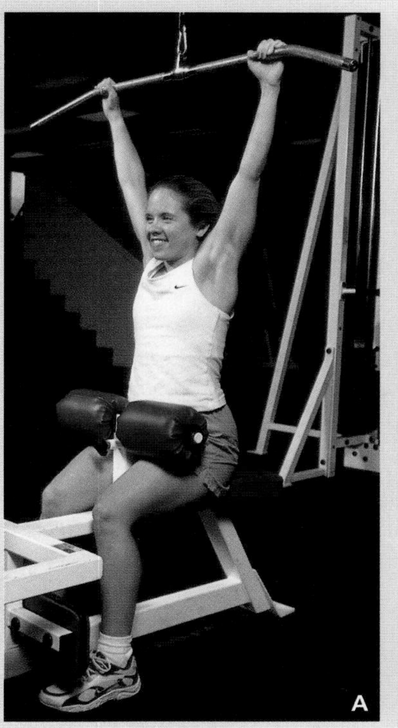

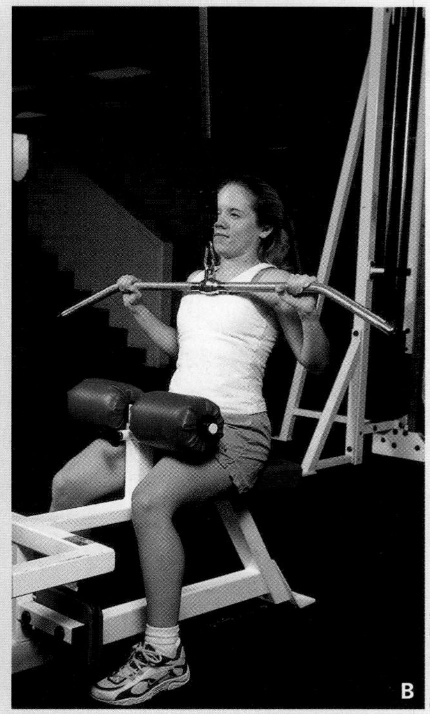

Photos Jon Kelley

Cybex Weight-Assisted Pull-Up Machine

Muscles developed: Latissimus dorsi, teres major, biceps.

Starting position: Set the weight for the amount of assistance you want from the machine. Grasp the overhead bar with a pronated grip. Step from the platform onto the weight-assist bar and lower yourself to the fully stretched starting position (A).

Concentric phase: Exhale as you pull yourself upward to a position with your chin above the bar (B). Pause briefly and squeeze your shoulder blades together.

Eccentric phase: Inhale as you lower yourself slowly to the starting position.

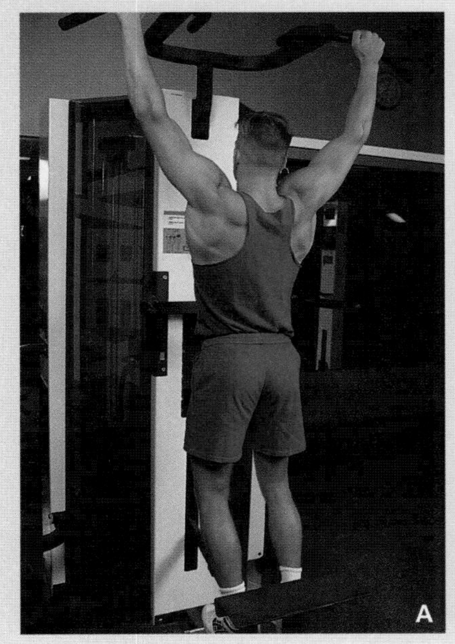

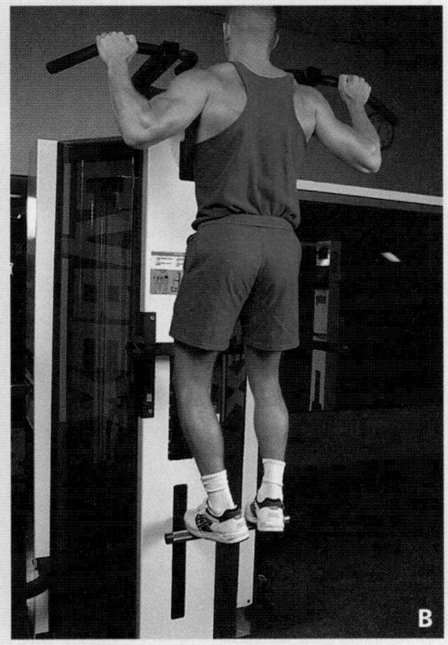

Photos Eric Risberg

UPPER BACK (TRAPEZIUS)

Shoulder Shrug

Muscles developed: Trapezius, levator scapulae.

Starting position: Start with a barbell hanging at arms length in front of your body; hold the bar with both hands in a pronated (thumbs in) grip (A).

Concentric phase: Inhale as you lift or shrug your shoulders to the highest possible position (B). Hold that position briefly.

Eccentric phase: Exhale as you slowly lower the bar to the starting position.

Variations:

1. Roll your shoulders forward and up, then back and down.

2. Roll your shoulders back and up, then forward and down.

Additional information: Do not bend your elbows or pull with your arm muscles. The hands and arms serve as hooks to hang the weight on during this exercise.

Caution: Do not jerk the weight upward or let it drop back to the starting position.

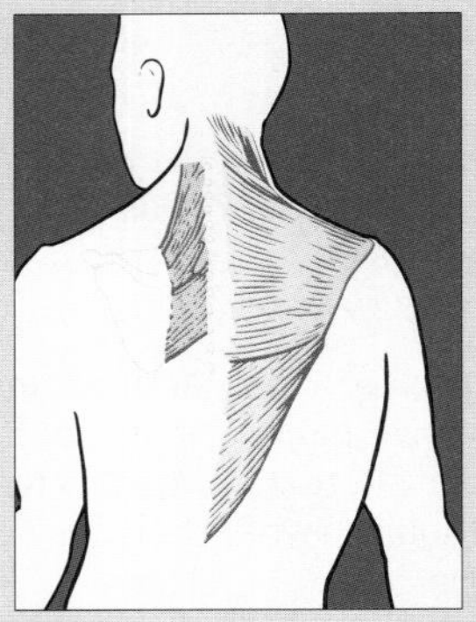

Back

Barbell

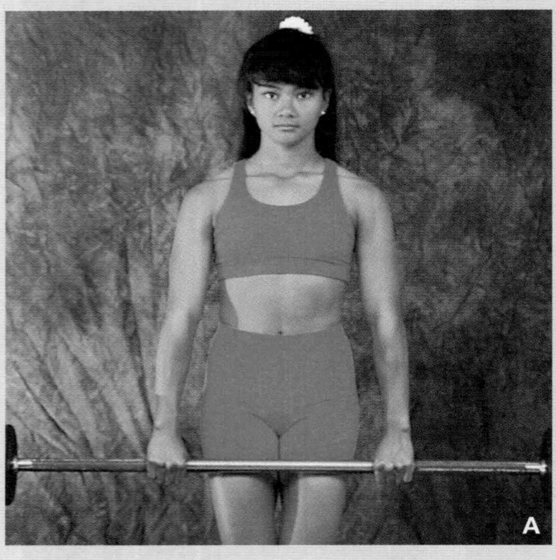

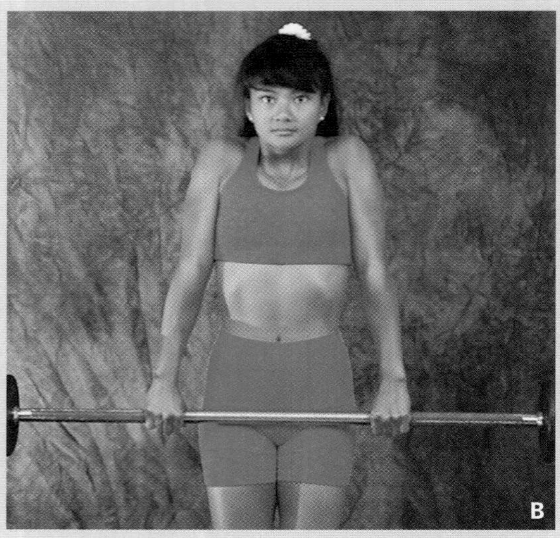

Photos Eric Risberg

Dumbbell

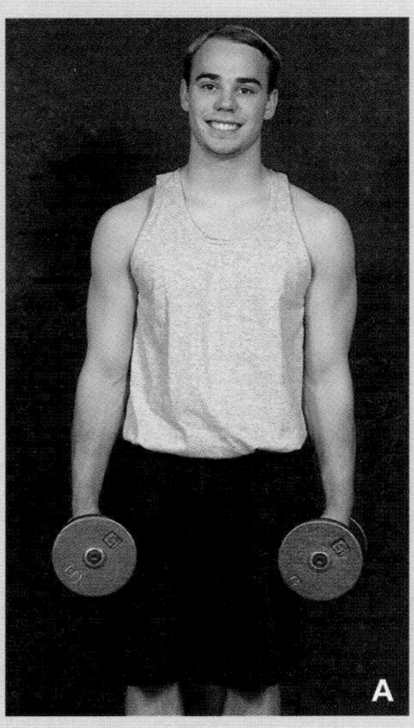

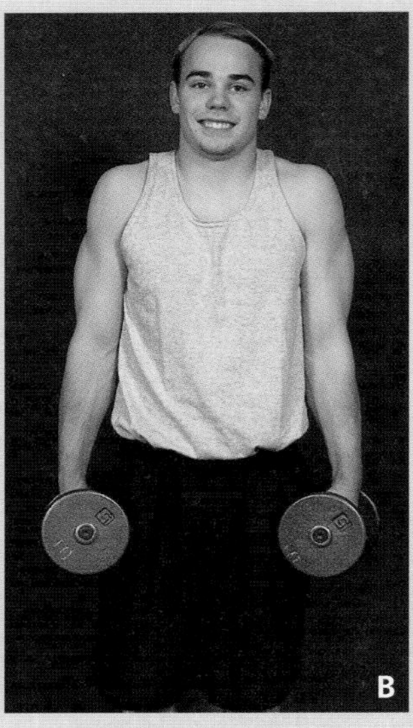

Photos Eric Risberg

Low Pulley Shoulder Shrug

Muscles developed: Trapezius, levator scapulae.

Starting position: Start in a standing position holding the low pulley handle with a pronated grip. With your arms straight, allow the weight to pull your shoulders down as far as possible (A).

Concentric phase: Inhale as you pull your shoulders upward as high as possible while keeping your arms straight (B). Pause briefly and hold this position.

Eccentric phase: Exhale as you slowly lower the weight to the starting position.

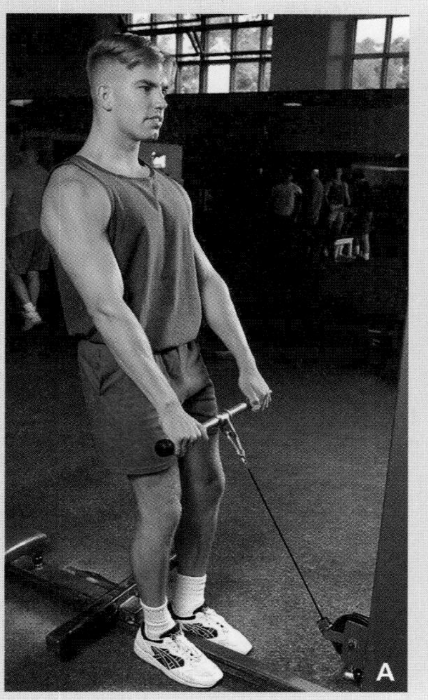
A

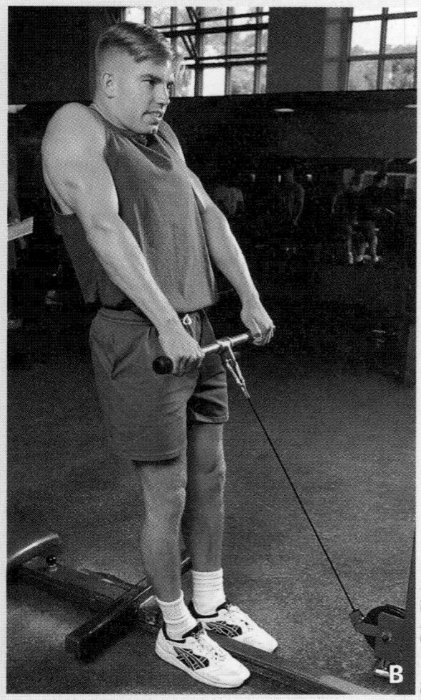
B

Photos Eric Risberg

Nautilus Shoulder Shrug Machine

Muscles developed: Trapezius, levator scapulae.

Starting position: Start in a seated position with your forearms between the padded exercise bars.

Concentric phase: Inhale as you pull your shoulders upward as high as possible. Pause briefly at the top of the pull and hold this position.

Eccentric phase: Exhale as you slowly lower the weight to the starting position.

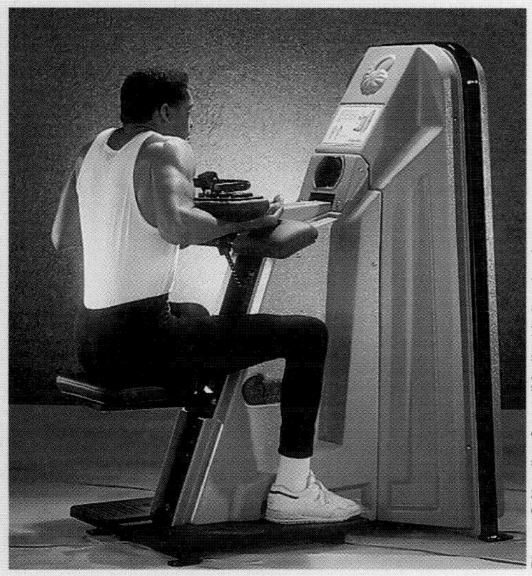

Photos © Nautilus Sports/Medical Industries, Inc.

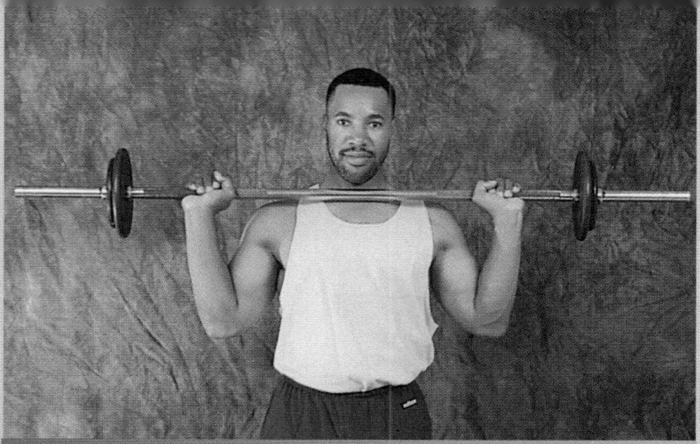
Eric Risberg

10

Shoulder Exercises

Shoulder (Deltoid)

Barbell Overhead Press or Military Press
Dumbbell Overhead Press
Hammer Strength Overhead Press Machine
Boss Overhead Press Machine

Barbell Upright Rowing
Dumbbell Upright Rowing
Low Pulley Upright Rowing (Curved Bar)
Low Pulley Upright Rowing (Straight Bar)

Dumbbell Lateral Raise
Cybex Seated Lateral Raise Machine
Dumbbell Front Raise
Dumbbell Bent-Over Lateral Raise

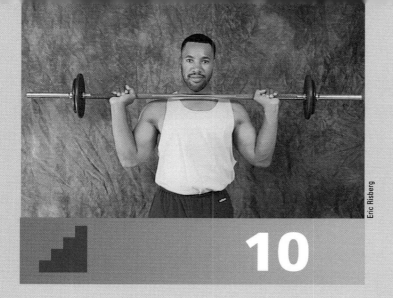

SHOULDER (DELTOID)

Overhead Press or Military Press

Muscles developed: Deltoid, triceps.

Starting position: Start with a barbell supported at shoulder-level in front of your body with your hands placed slightly wider apart than shoulder-width (A).

Concentric phase: Inhale while pressing the weight overhead to a straight arm position (B).

Eccentric phase: Exhale while lowering the weight to the starting position.

Variations: This overhead press has many variations. The exercise can be done standing or sitting, with a barbell from the shoulders in front of the head or behind the neck, with dumbbells together, or alternating.

Caution: Do not lean back or arch your back. Do not close your eyes.

Additional information: This exercise is called the military press because you stay in an erect posture (military posture) while forcing the muscles of the arms and shoulders to do all the work. Do not bend or sway the back to complete a repetition.

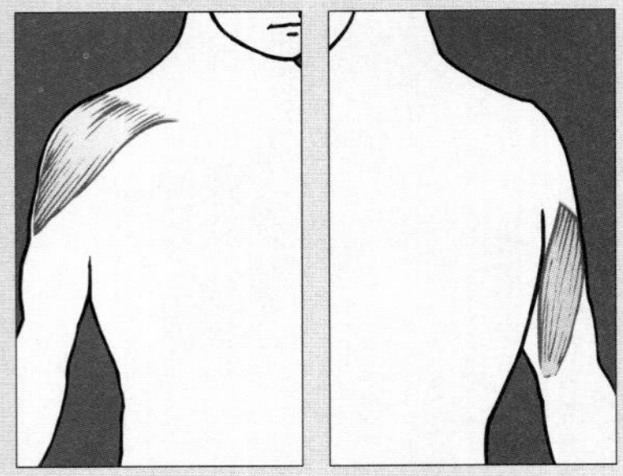

Front   Back

Barbell

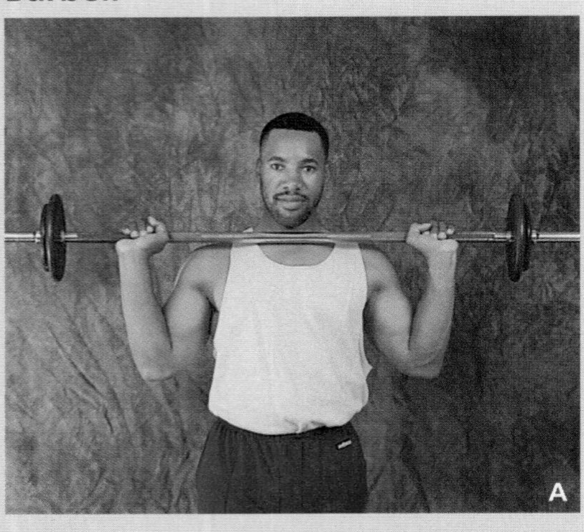

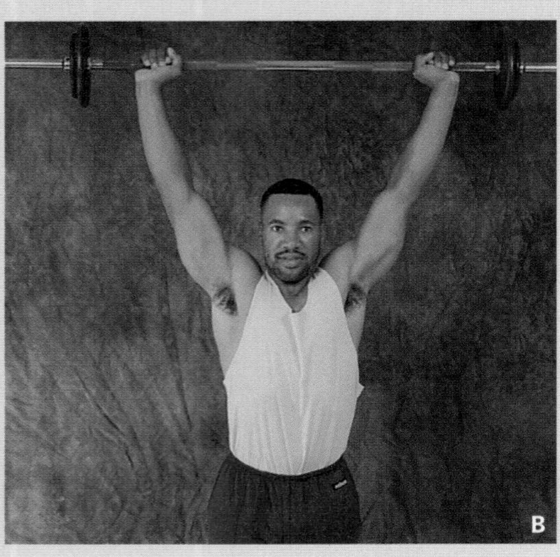

Photos Eric Risberg

Dumbbell

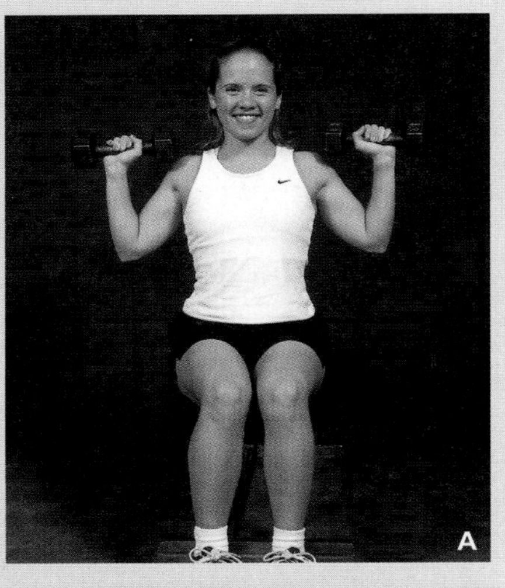

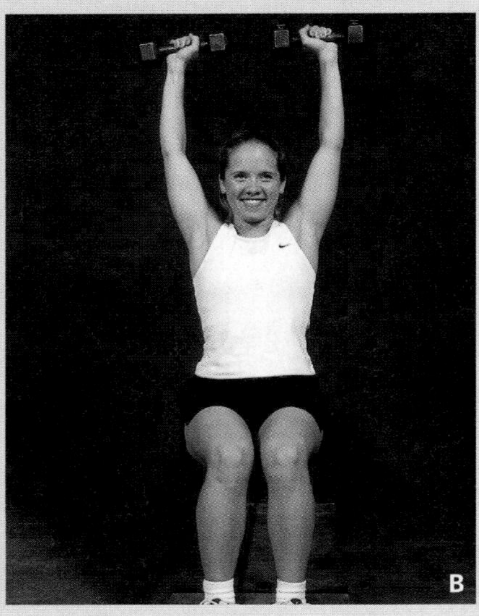

Photos Eric Risberg

Hammer Strength Overhead Press Machine

Muscles developed: Deltoid, triceps.

Starting position: Start in a seated position. Grasp the exercise bars with your hands wider than shoulder-width (A).

Concentric phase: Inhale as you press the exercise bar upward to a straight arm position (B).

Eccentric phase: Exhale as you slowly lower the weight to the starting position.

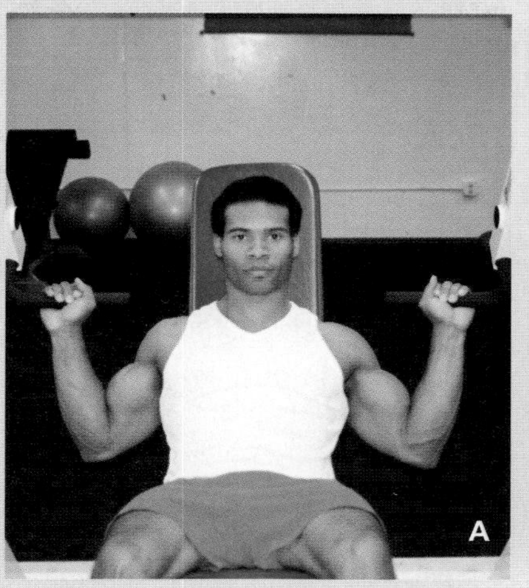

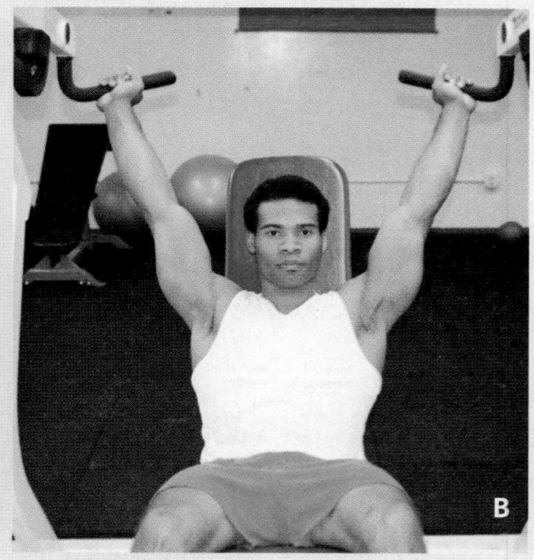

Photos Kristin Dilworth

Boss Overhead Press Machine

Muscles developed: Deltoid, triceps.

Starting position: Start in a seated position with your back against the bench. Adjust the machine so the exercise bar handles are at shoulder-height. Grasp the handles with an overgrip (thumbs in) and with your hands wider than your shoulders (A).

Concentric phase: Inhale and press the bar upward to a straight-arm position (B).

Eccentric phase: Exhale as you lower the weight slowly to the starting position.

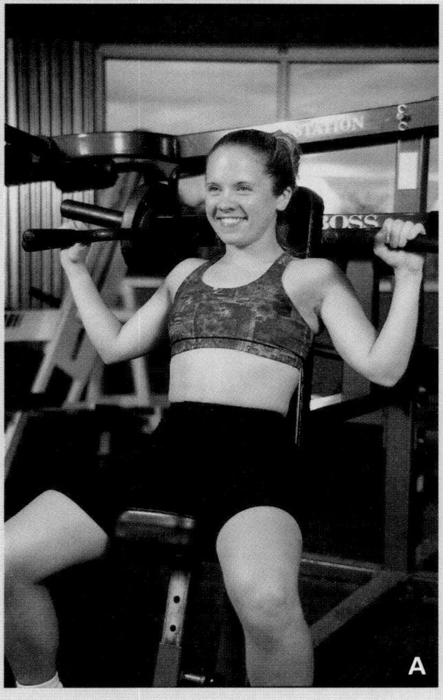

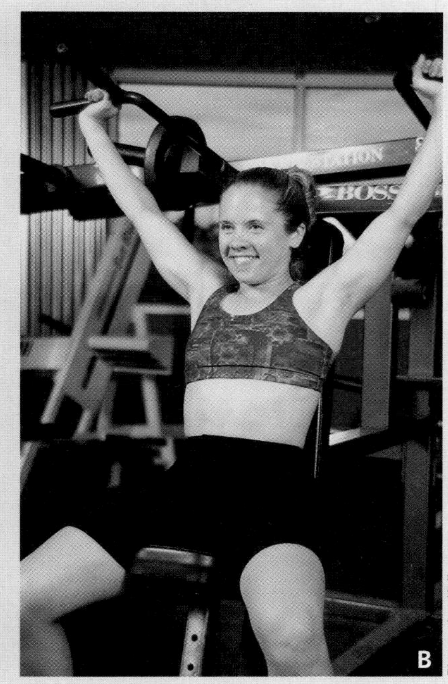

Photos Jon Kelley

Upright Rowing

Muscles developed: Deltoid, trapezius.

Starting position: Start with a barbell hanging at arm's-length in front of your body, hands in a pronated (thumbs in) grip (A).

Concentric phase: Inhale while pulling the elbows as high as possible in a smooth, continuous movement. The bar should reach shoulder level (B).

Eccentric phase: Exhale while lowering the bar slowly to the starting position.

Caution: Concentrate on your deltoid muscles while raising the upper arm and keeping your elbows high. The arm muscles should be as inactive as possible.

Additional information: Upright rowing is like performing lateral raises.

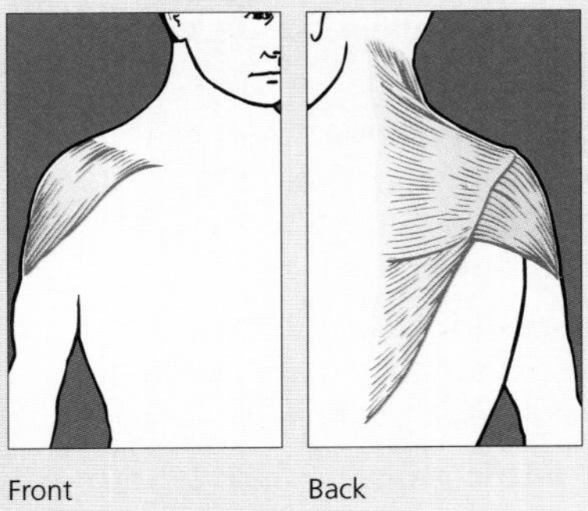

Barbell

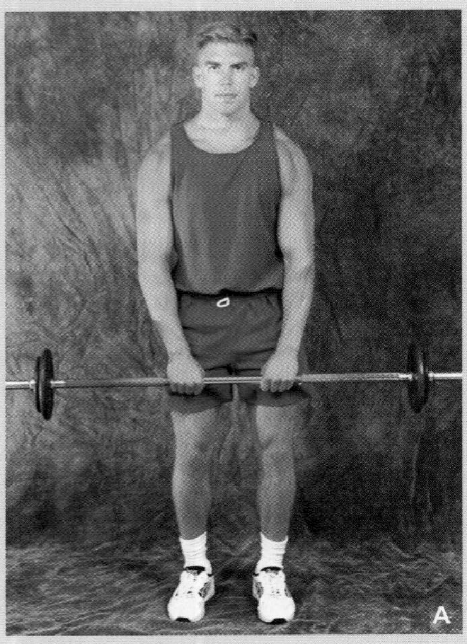

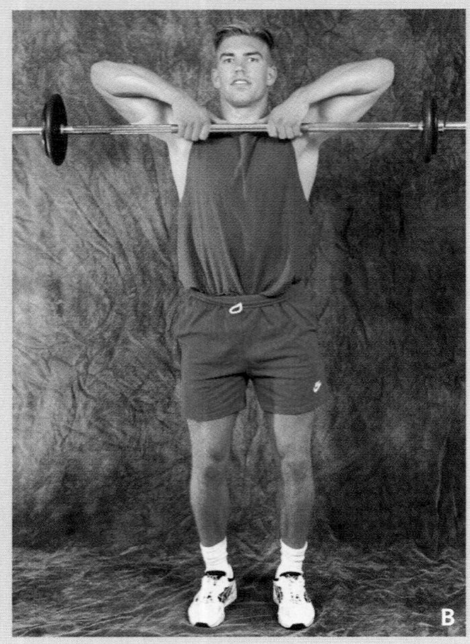

Photos Eric Risberg

Dumbbell

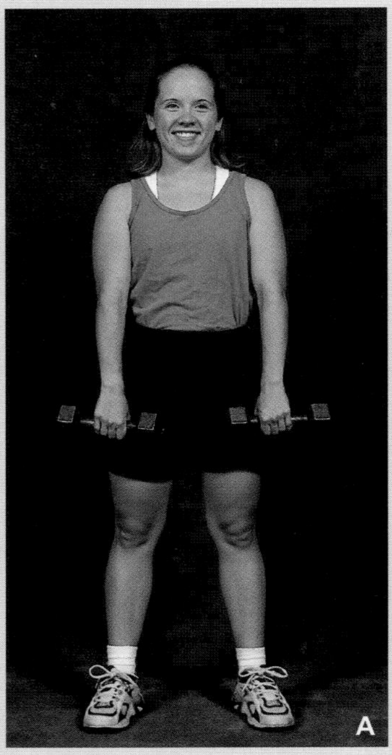

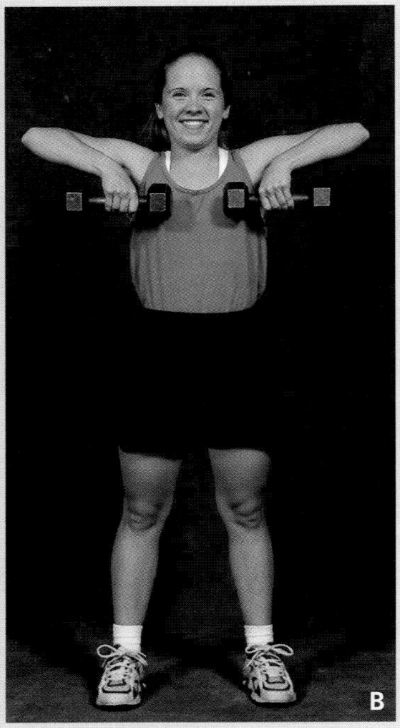

Photos Jon Kelley

Low Pulley Upright Rowing (Curved Bar)

Muscles developed: Deltoid, trapezius.

Starting position: Start in a standing position facing the low pulley station. Hold the exercise handle or handles on the end of the cable (A).

Concentric phase: Inhale as you pull your elbows upward as high as possible in a smooth, continuous movement. Pull your elbows upward until your hands reach shoulder or chin height (B).

Eccentric phase: Exhale as you lower the weight slowly to the starting position.

Caution: Always keep your elbows higher than your hands during this exercise.

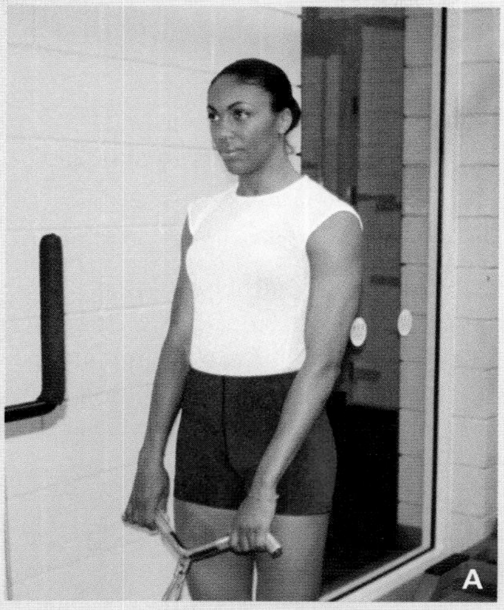
A

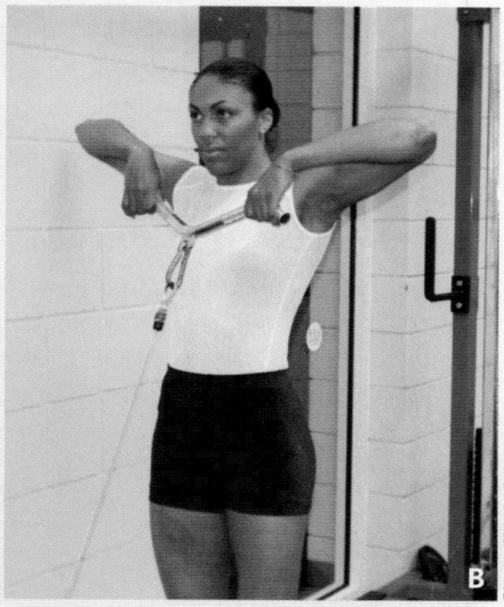
B

Photos Kristin Dilworth

Low Pulley Upright Rowing (Straight Bar)

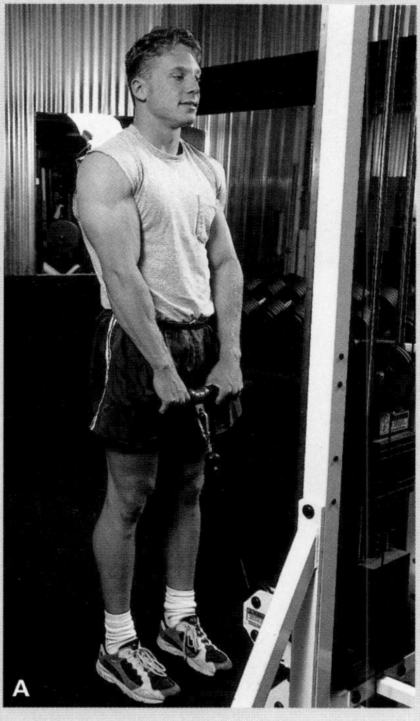
A

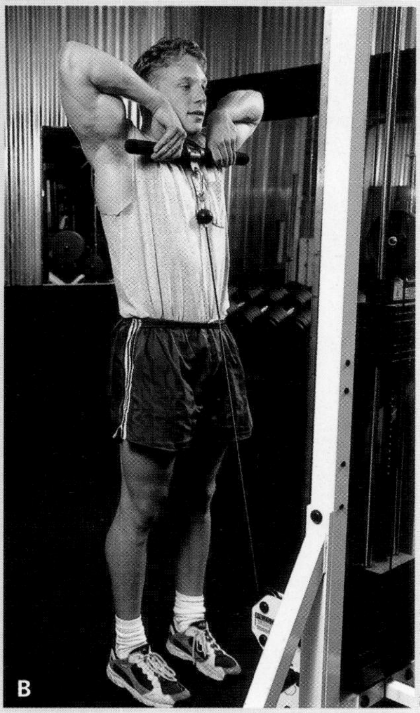
B

Photos Jon Kelley

Dumbbell Lateral Raise

Muscles developed: Deltoid, trapezius.

Starting position: Start with one dumbbell in each hand (A).

Concentric phase: Inhale while lifting the weights away from your body and upward. Keep your arms fairly straight, and raise the weights to shoulder level (B).

Eccentric phase: Exhale while lowering the weights to the starting position.

Variations: Perform the same exercise movement from a sitting position. The deltoid is a muscle with three fairly distinct parts: anterior (front), lateral (middle), and posterior (rear). The lateral raise tends to best develop the lateral part; the front raise develops the front part; and the bent-over lateral raise develops the rear part.

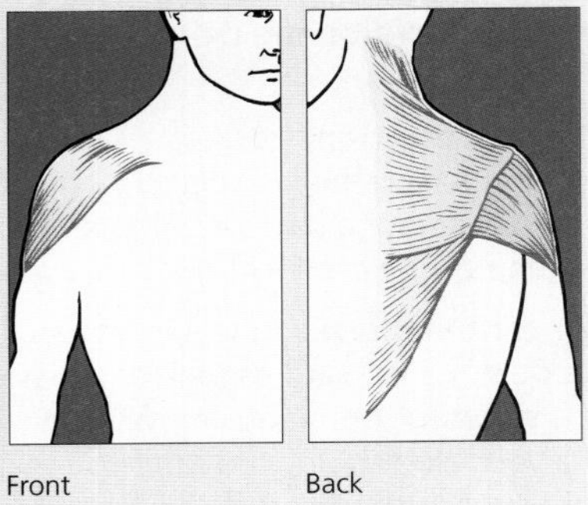

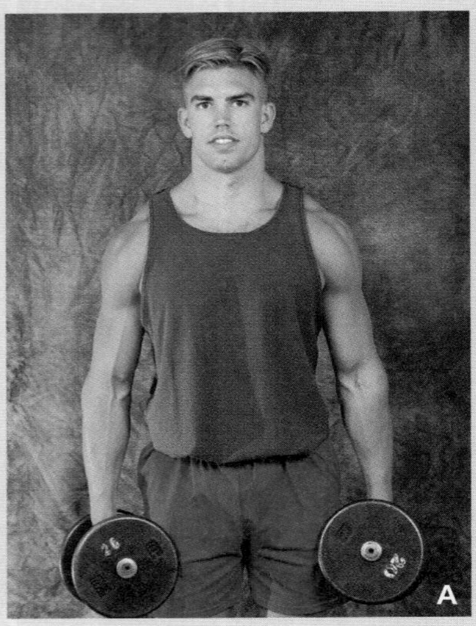

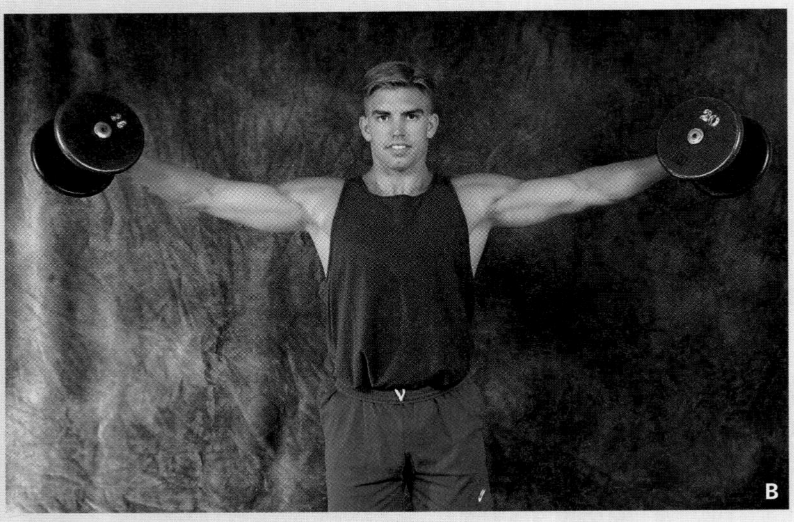

Photos Eric Risberg

Cybex Seated Lateral Raise Machine

Muscles developed: Deltoid, trapezius.

Starting position: Start in a seated position. Adjust the machine so your shoulders are lined up with the pivot points of the machine. Place your arms against the padded portion of the exercise bars (A).

Concentric phase: Inhale as you press your upper arms outward and upward to a position in which your elbows are shoulder height or slightly above (B). Pause briefly at the top.

Eccentric phase: Exhale as you slowly allow your arms to return to the starting position.

Additional information: To focus more on the lateral part of the deltoid, keep your forearms pointing forward. To focus more on the frontal part of the deltoid, have your forearms pointing outward and upward.

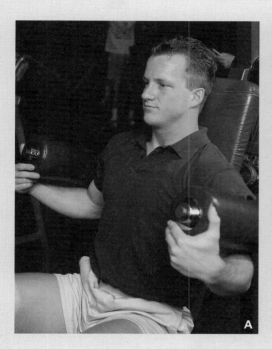

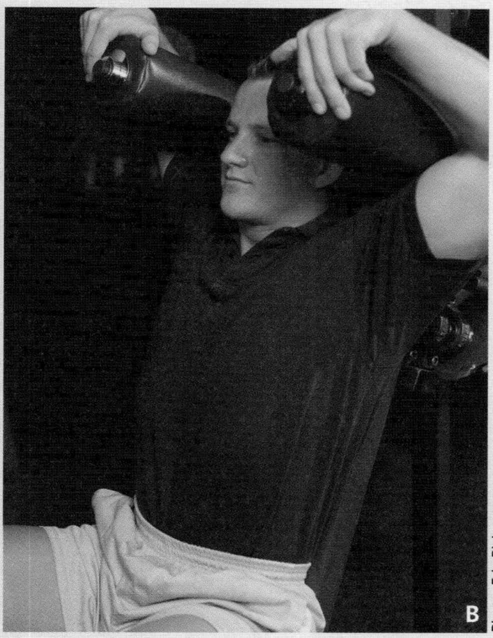

Photos Eric Risberg

Dumbbell Front Raise

Muscles developed: Frontal deltoid, clavicular portion of pectoralis major, coracobrachialis.

Starting position: Stand and hold a barbell or two dumbbells at arms length (A).

Concentric phase: Inhale while raising the weight to shoulder level, keeping your arms straight (B). Pause briefly.

Eccentric phase: Exhale while lowering the weight to the starting position.

Variations: Raise the weight to an overhead position, as long as you do not allow your back to arch or bend.

Caution: On straight-arm exercises a slight bend at the elbow may relieve unnecessary tension or strain in the elbow joint. This is not a problem as long as it makes the exercise more productive for you, but do not bend your elbows to make the exercise easier for the working muscles.

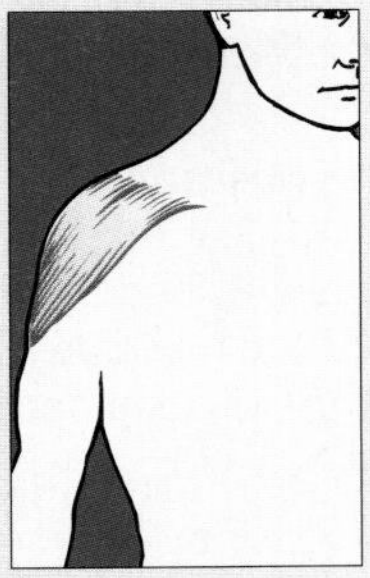

Front

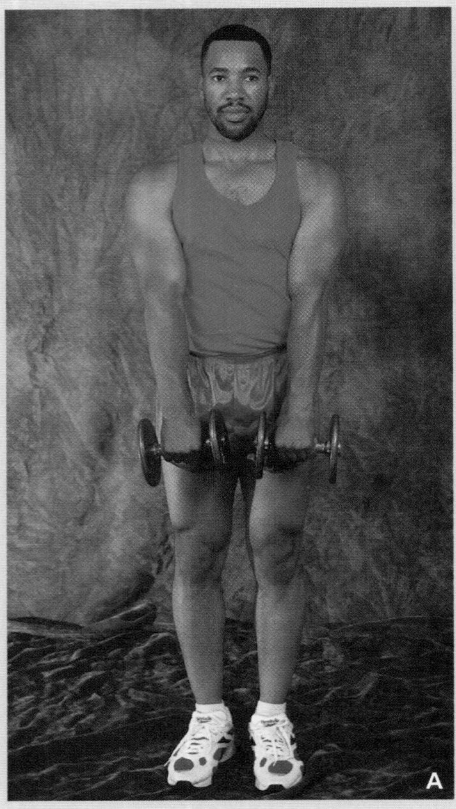

A

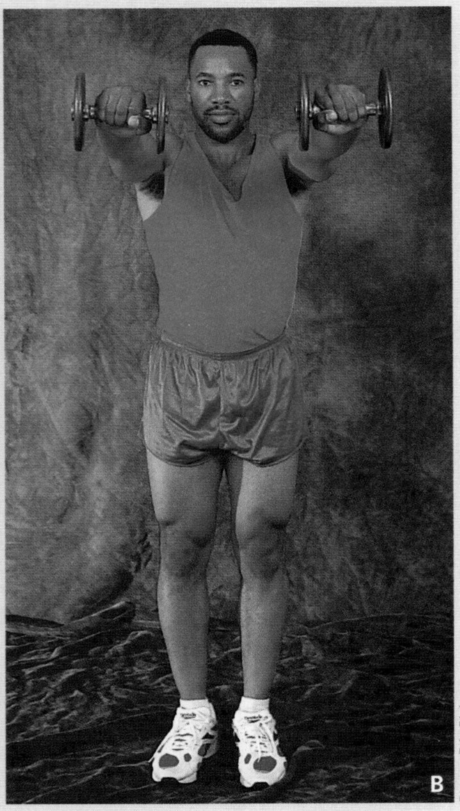

B

Photos Eric Risberg

Dumbbell Bent-Over Lateral Raise

Muscles developed: Posterior (rear) deltoid, rhomboids, trapezius.

Starting position: Bend over with your back flat and knees slightly bent; hold one dumbbell in each hand, arms straight, and dumbbells hanging directly below your shoulder joints (A).

Concentric phase: Inhale while you raise the dumbbells to the side up to shoulder level (B). Pause briefly.

Eccentric phase: Exhale while lowering the weights slowly to the starting position.

Variations: Sit on the end of a bench or lie face down on a flat or incline bench that is high enough to allow your arms to hang fully extended.

Caution: Lift your arms straight to the side or move them slightly forward toward your head as you lift the weight. These muscles also are developed when performing any of the rowing exercises for the back (lats).

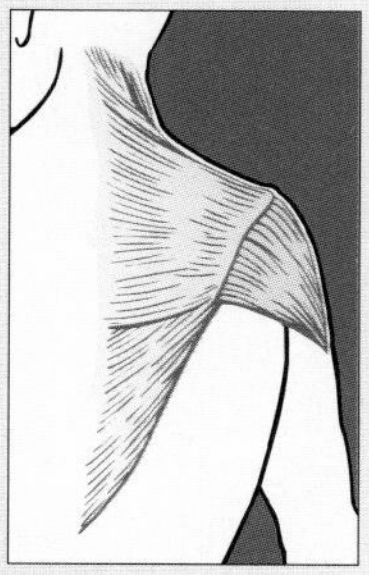

Back

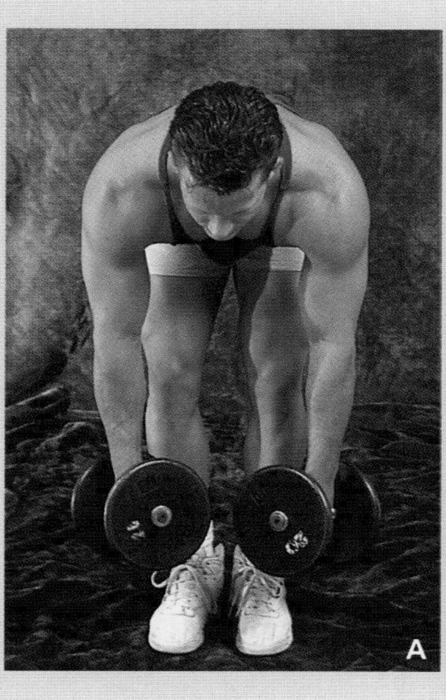

A

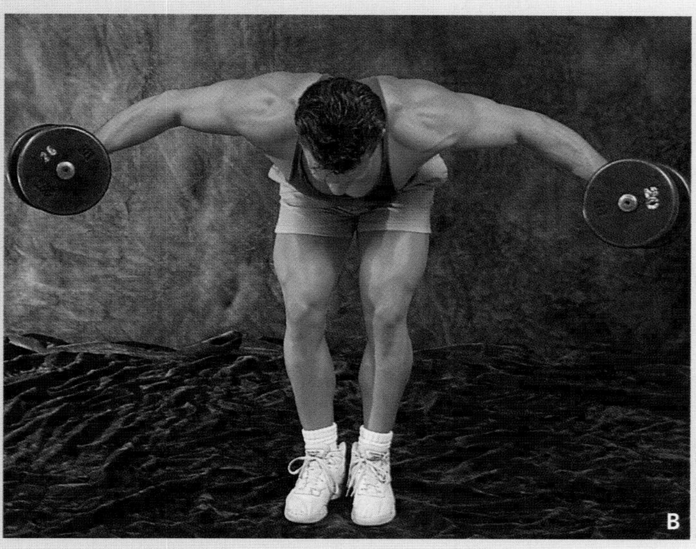

B

Photos Eric Risberg

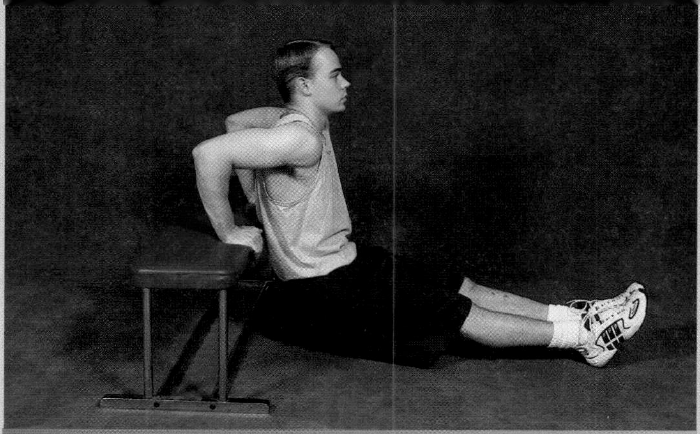

Eric Risberg

11

Arm Exercises

Upper Arm (Elbow flexion, Biceps)

Barbell Curl
Seated Dumbbell Curl
Hammer Strength Arm Curl Machine
Nautilus Arm Curl Machine

Barbell Reverse Curl
Incline Dumbbell Curl
Preacher Curl
Low Pulley Curl

Upper Arm (Elbow extension, Triceps)

Barbell Triceps Extension
One-Dumbbell Triceps Extension
Nautilus Triceps Extension Machine
Triceps Pushdown

Parallel Bar Dips
Bench Dips
Boss Dip Machine
Cybex Weight-Assisted Parallel Bar Dips

Lying Barbell Triceps Extension
Close-Grip Bench Press
Body Master Triceps Extension
Cybex Tricep Extension Machine

Forearm (Wrist flexors and Wrist extensors)

Barbell Wrist Curl
Dumbbell Wrist Curl
Reverse Barbell Wrist Curl
Reverse Dumbbell Wrist Curl

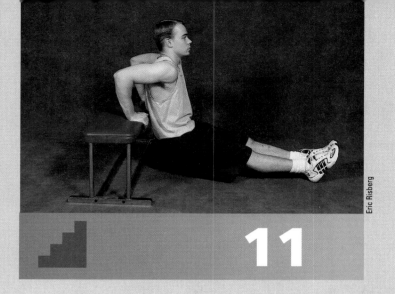

UPPER ARM (ELBOW FLEXION, BICEPS)

Barbell Curl

Muscles developed: Biceps brachii, brachialis, brachioradialis.

Starting position: Stand, holding a barbell in front of your body, hands gripping the bar at shoulder-width with a supinated (thumbs out) grip (A).

Concentric phase: Exhale while raising the weight to your shoulders by moving only at the elbow joint (B).

Eccentric phase: Inhale while lowering the weight to the starting position.

Variations: Any elbow flexion or curling exercise will develop the elbow flexor muscles. Curling exercises have many variations. Vary this standing curl by changing the space between your hands when gripping the bar.

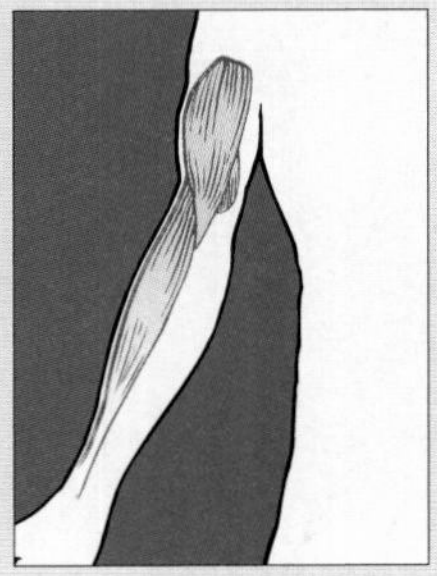

Front

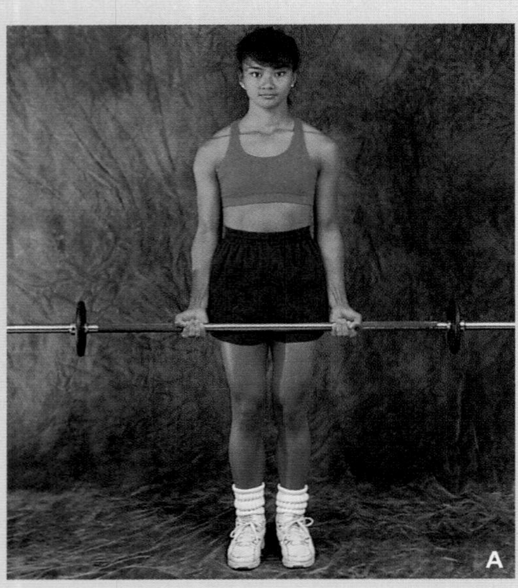

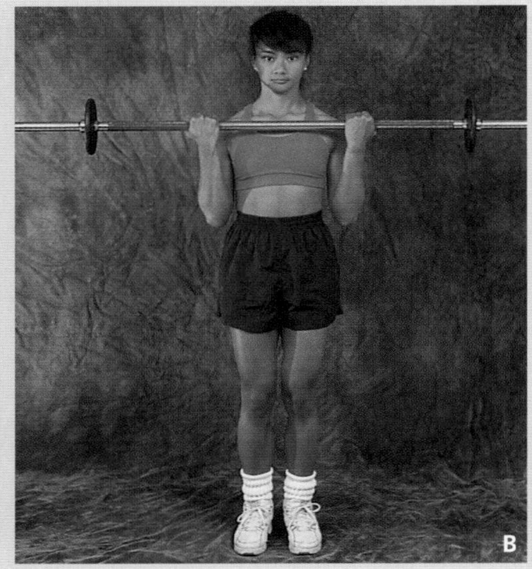

Photos Eric Risberg

Seated Dumbbell Curl

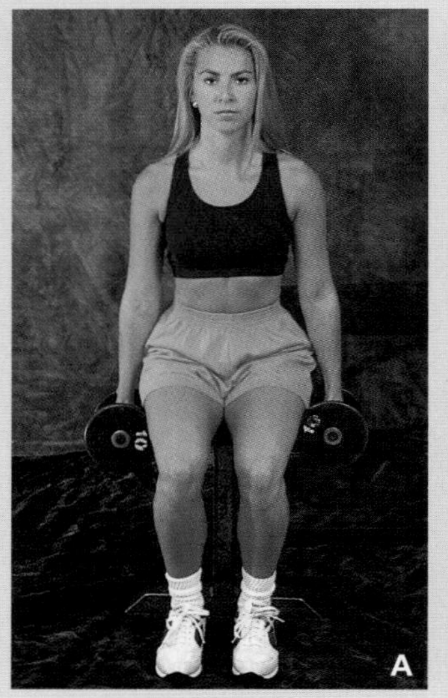

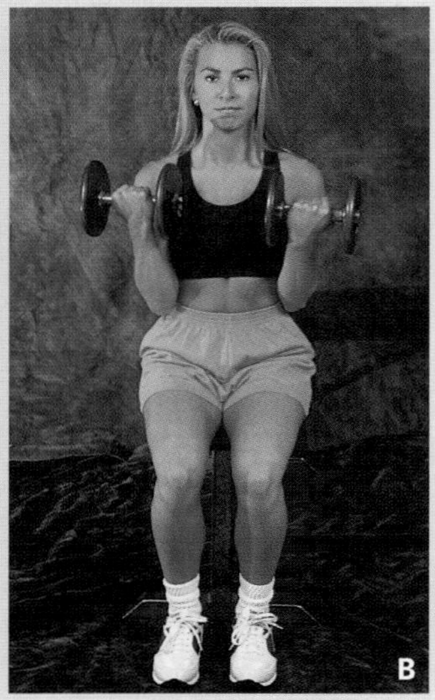

Photos Eric Risberg

Hammer Strength Arm Curl Machine

Muscles developed: Biceps, brachialis, brachioradialis.

Starting position: Grasp the exercise handles of the machine with a palms-up grip; place your elbows on the pad and line them up with the pivot point of the machine (A).

Concentric phase: Exhale as you pull your hands toward your shoulders (B). When you reach the end of your elbow joint range of motion, pause briefly and hold.

Eccentric phase: Inhale as you lower the weight slowly and allow your arms to return to the starting position.

Caution: Do not jerk the weight up or allow it to drop and hyperextend your elbow joints at the bottom. Lift and lower the weight in a smooth, controlled manner.

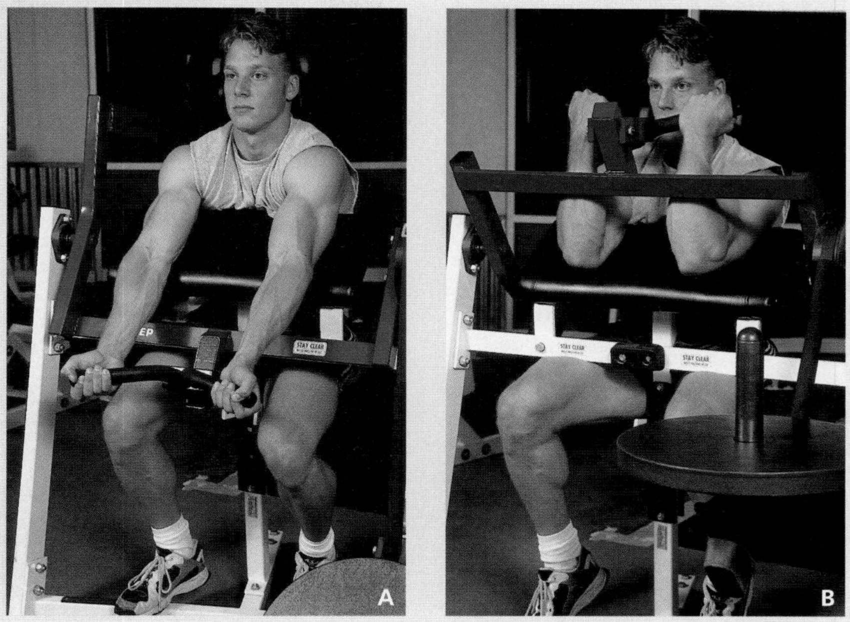

Photos Jon Kelley

Nautilus Arm Curl Machine

Muscles developed: Biceps, brachialis, brachioradialis.

Starting position: Grasp the exercise handles of the machine with a palms-up grip; place your elbows on the pad, and line them up with the pivot point of the machine (A).

Concentric phase: Exhale as you pull your hands toward your shoulders (B). When you reach the end of your elbow joint range of motion, pause briefly and hold.

Eccentric phase: Inhale as you lower the weight slowly and allow your arms to return to the starting position.

Caution: Do not jerk the weight up or allow it to drop and hyperextend your elbow joints at the bottom. Lift and lower the weight in a smooth, controlled manner.

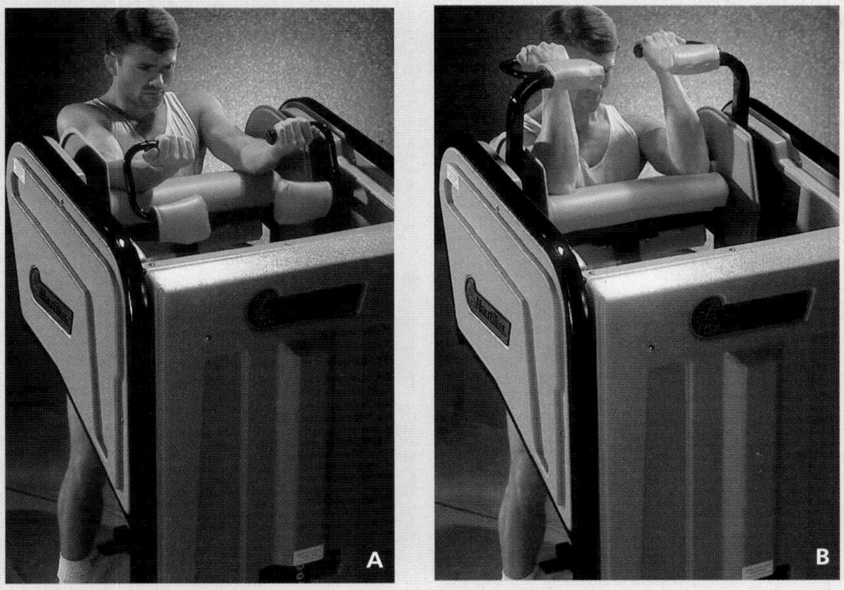

Photos © Nautilus Sports/Medical Industries, Inc.

Barbell Reverse Curl

Muscles developed: Biceps, brachialis, brachioradialis, wrist and hand flexors.

Starting position: Stand and hold a barbell in front of your body with both hands in a pronated (thumbs in) grip (A).

Concentric phase: Exhale while raising the bar to the shoulders by bending only at the elbows (B).

Eccentric phase: Inhale while lowering the bar to the starting position.

Variations: Change the distance between your hands.

Additional information: This exercise provides a strong stimulus to the forearm muscles and often is used as a forearm exercise as well as a variation of the curl.

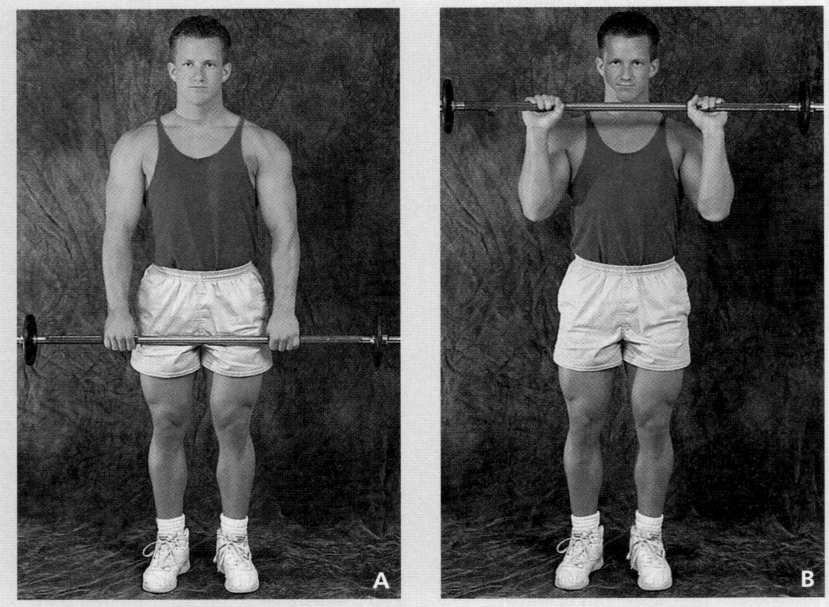

Photos Eric Risberg

Incline Dumbbell Curl

Muscles developed: Biceps brachii, brachialis, brachioradialis.

Starting position: With your back against an incline bench, hold one dumbbell in each hand with your arms extended and hanging directly below your shoulder joints (A).

Concentric phase: Exhale while bending your arms only at the elbow. Pull the weights to your shoulders (B).

Eccentric phase: Inhale while lowering weights to the starting position.

Variations:

1. Alternate your arms so that one is coming up as the other is going down.

2. Turn your arms out so the dumbbells are raised and lowered to the sides of your body instead of in front of your body.

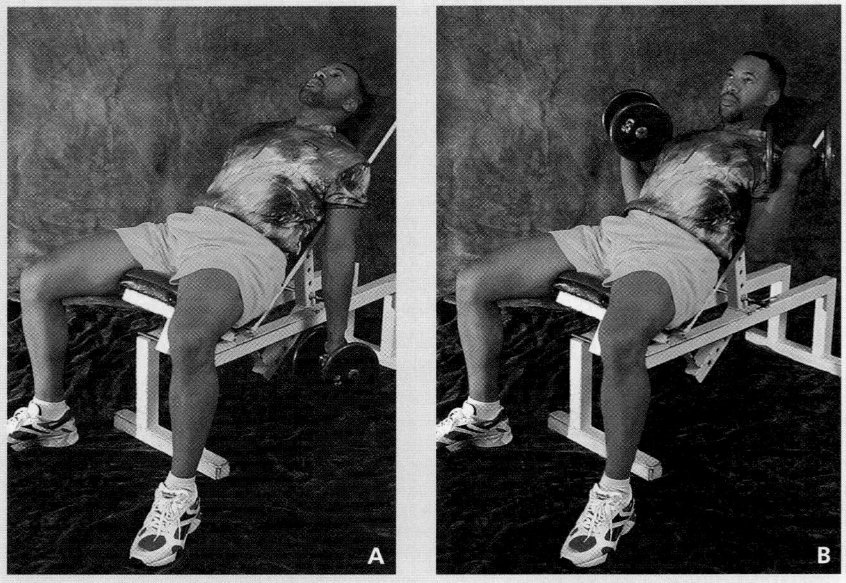

Photos Eric Risberg

Preacher Curl

Muscles developed: Biceps, brachialis, brachioradialis.

Starting position: Grasp the barbell or dumbbells; place your elbows on the pad, and straighten your arms (A).

Concentric phase: Exhale as you pull your hands toward your shoulders (B). When you reach the end of your elbow joint range of motion, pause briefly.

Eccentric phase: Inhale as you lower the weight slowly and allow your arms to return to the starting position.

Caution: Do not jerk the weight up. Do not allow the weight to drop and hyperextend your elbow joints at the bottom. Lift and lower the weight in a smooth, controlled manner.

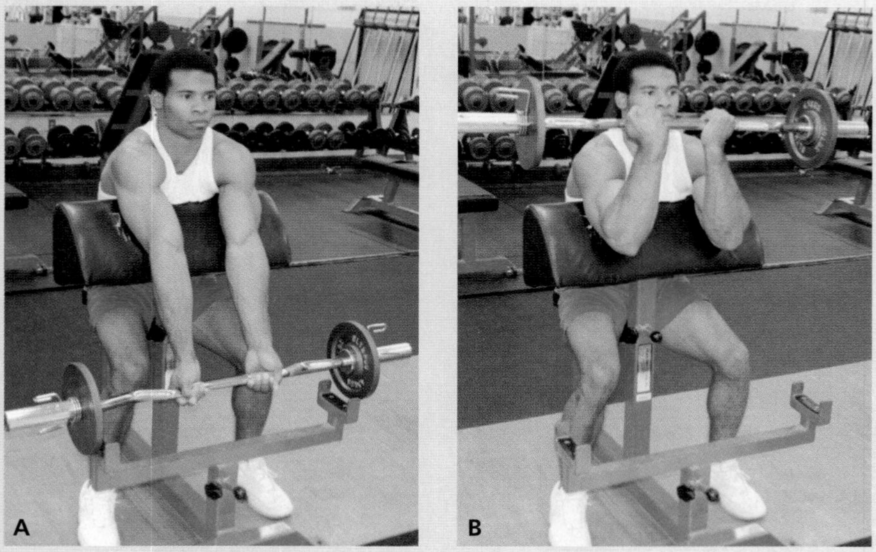

Photos Kristin Dilworth

Low Pulley Curl

Muscles developed: Biceps brachii, brachialis, brachioradialis.

Starting position: Stand in front of the low pulley, facing the weight stack. Hold the exercise bar in a supinated (thumbs out) grip, with both arms straight (A).

Concentric phase: Exhale as you bend only at the elbow joint to bring the exercise bar up toward your shoulders. Move only your forearms; do not allow your upper arms to change position (B).

Eccentric phase: Inhale as you slowly lower the bar to the starting position.

Variations:

1. Change your grip spacing on the bar.

2. Use a pronated (thumbs in) grip and perform reverse curls.

Caution: Bending any joint except the elbow joint will reduce the effectiveness of the exercise and increase the risk of injury.

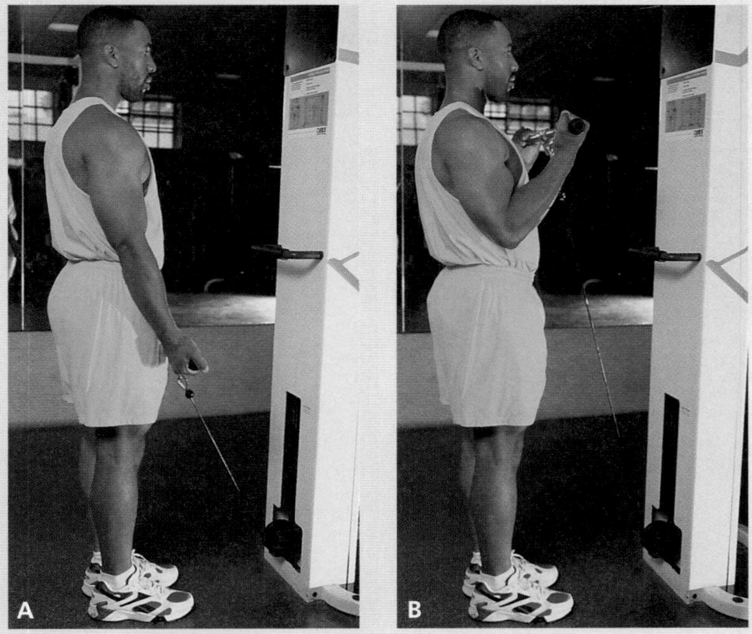

Photos Eric Risberg

UPPER ARM (ELBOW EXTENSION, TRICEPS)

Triceps Extension

Muscles developed: Triceps.

Starting position: Stand and hold a barbell or dumbbell overhead with both hands (A).

Eccentric phase: Inhale as you slowly lower the weight behind your head (B).

Concentric phase: Exhale as you extend both arms and push the weight back to the starting position.

Variations:

1. Perform this exercise with a dumbbell.
2. Perform this exercise from a sitting position.

Additional information: Keep your elbows up throughout the exercise.

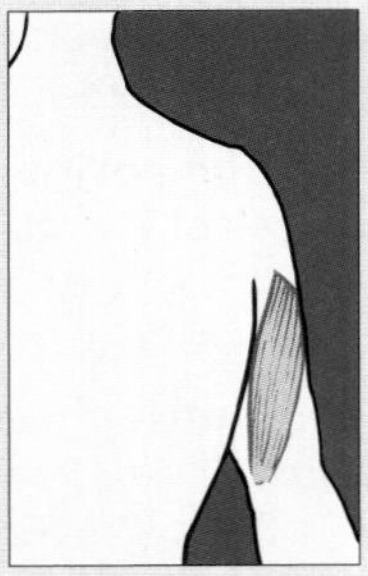

Back

Barbell

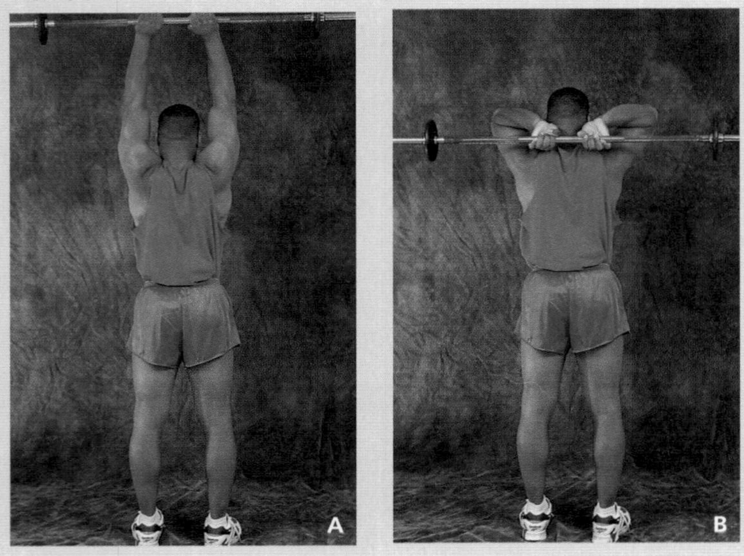

Photos Eric Risberg

One-Dumbbell

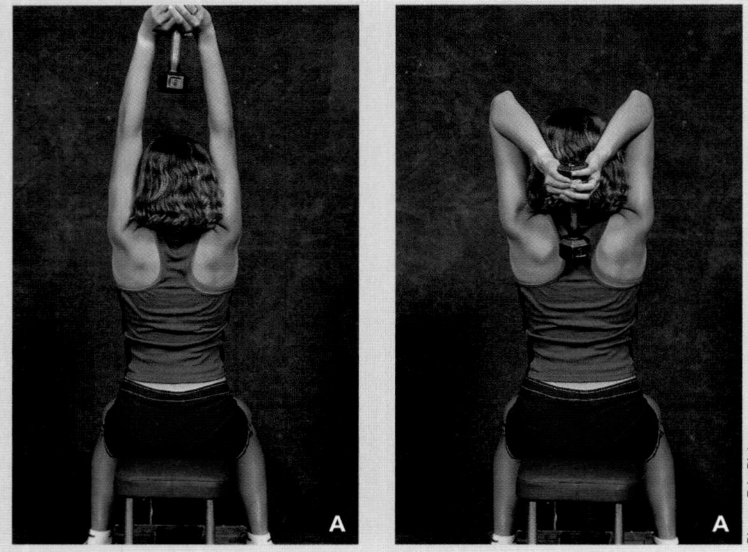

Photos Eric Risberg

Nautilus Triceps Extension Machine

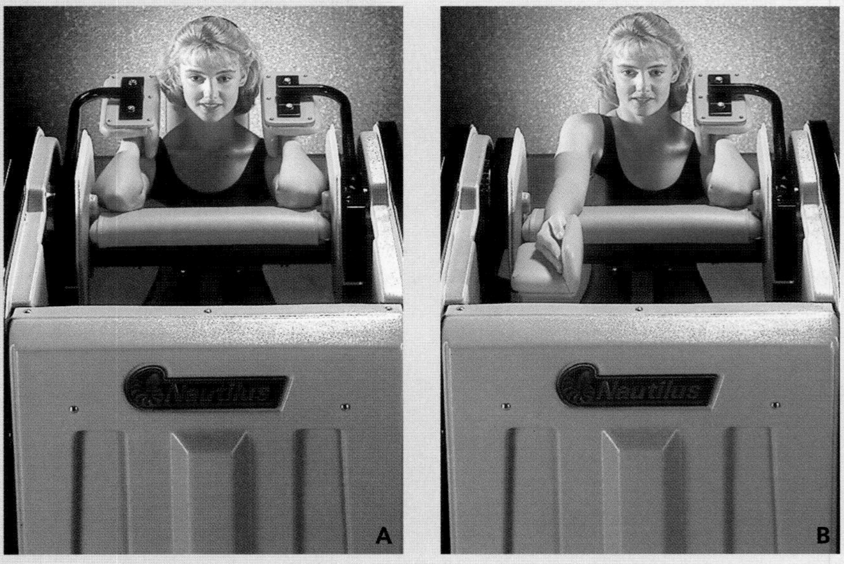

Photos © Nautilus Sports/Medical Industries, Inc.

Muscles developed: Triceps.

Starting position: Place the little finger side of your hands or fists against the padded portion of the exercise bars. With your elbows bent, place the back of your upper arms on the pad provided and line up your elbow joints with the pivot point of the machine (A).

Concentric phase: Exhale as you push both hands forward and downward until your arms are extended. Pause briefly and hold.

Eccentric phase: Inhale as you allow your arms to slowly return to the starting position.

Variations: This exercise also may be performed one arm at a time or alternating arms (B).

Caution: Do not allow the weight to drop during the eccentric phase of the lift. Control the speed of the movement at all times.

Triceps Pushdown

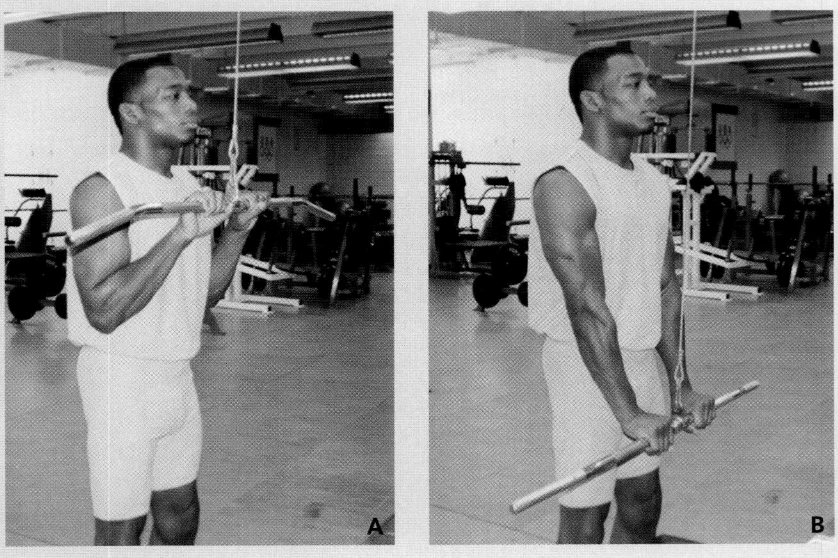

Photos Kristin Dilworth

Muscles developed: Triceps.

Starting position: Place both hands on the high pulley bar (lat machine) with your palms down and your thumbs in (A).

Concentric phase: Exhale as you push the bar down until your arms are straight (B). Throughout the exercise movement keep your upper arms by your sides and move only your hands and forearms.

Eccentric phase: Inhale as you allow your hands and forearms to slowly return to the starting position.

Caution: Keep your head, neck, and chest away from the moving cable.

Parallel Bar Dips

Muscles developed: Triceps, pectoralis major, anterior deltoid.

Starting position: Take a straight-arm support position on two bars parallel to each other and about shoulder-width apart (A).

Eccentric phase: Inhale as you bend your elbows and slowly lower yourself as far as possible (B).

Concentric phase: Exhale as you straighten your arms and return to the starting position.

Additional information: To add weight to this exercise, hang a weight or a dumbbell from a wide strap around your waist and place it between your thighs to stabilize it during the exercise.

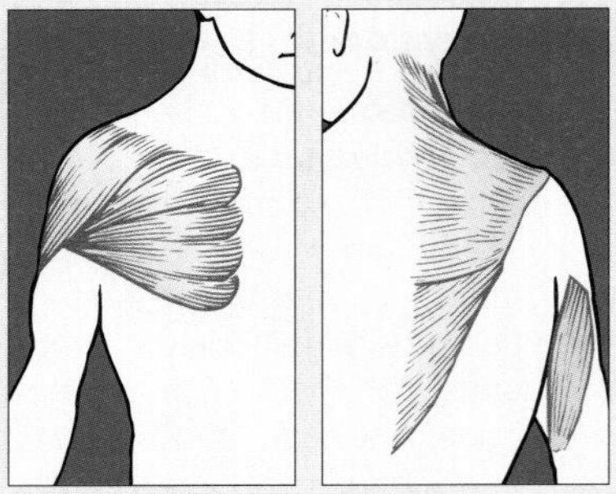

Front Back

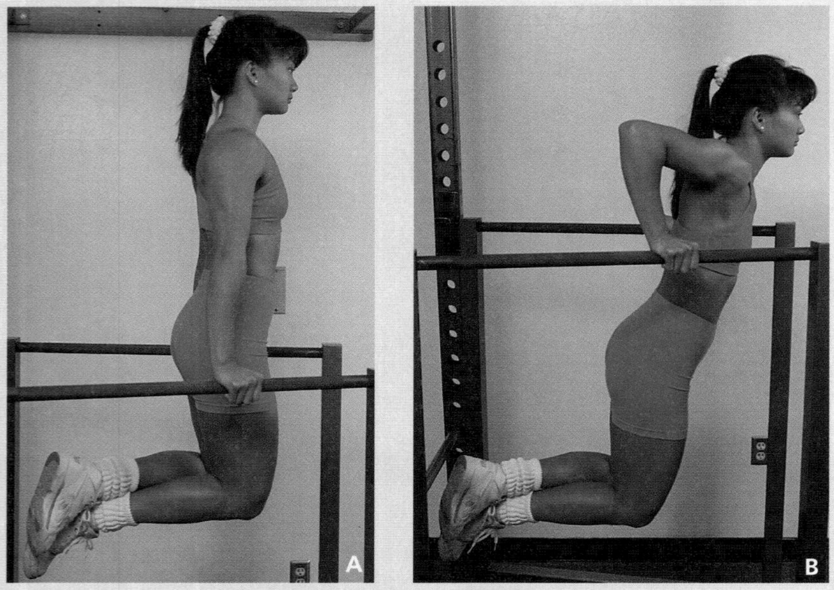

Photos Eric Risberg

Bench Dips

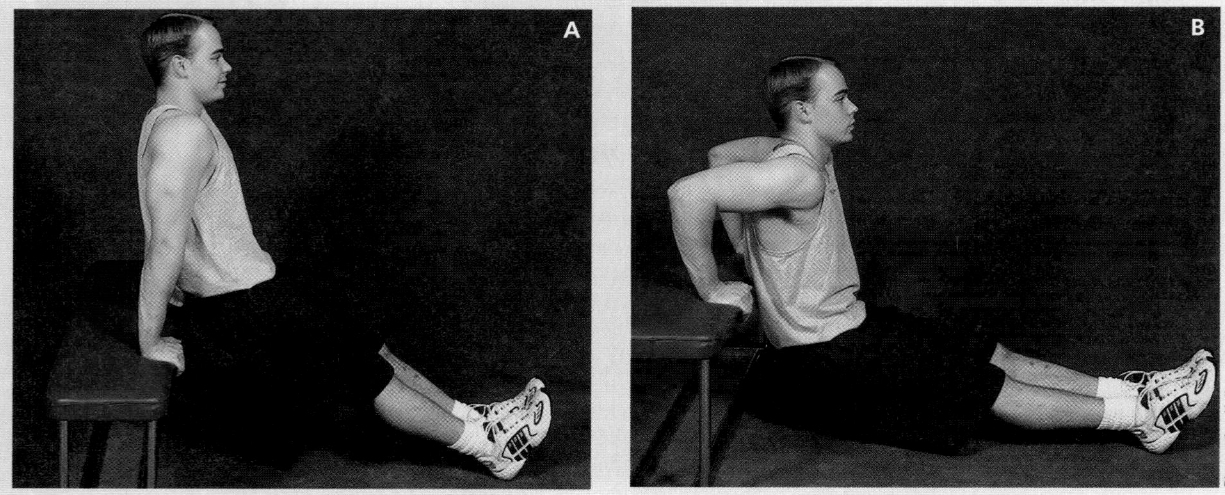

Photos Jon Kelley

Boss Dip Machine

Muscles developed: Triceps, pectoralis major, anterior deltoid.

Starting position: Start with your hands on the exercise bars (A).

Concentric phase: Exhale as you press the exercise bar down until your arms are straight (B).

Eccentric phase: Inhale as you slowly bend your arms and allow the weight to return to the starting position.

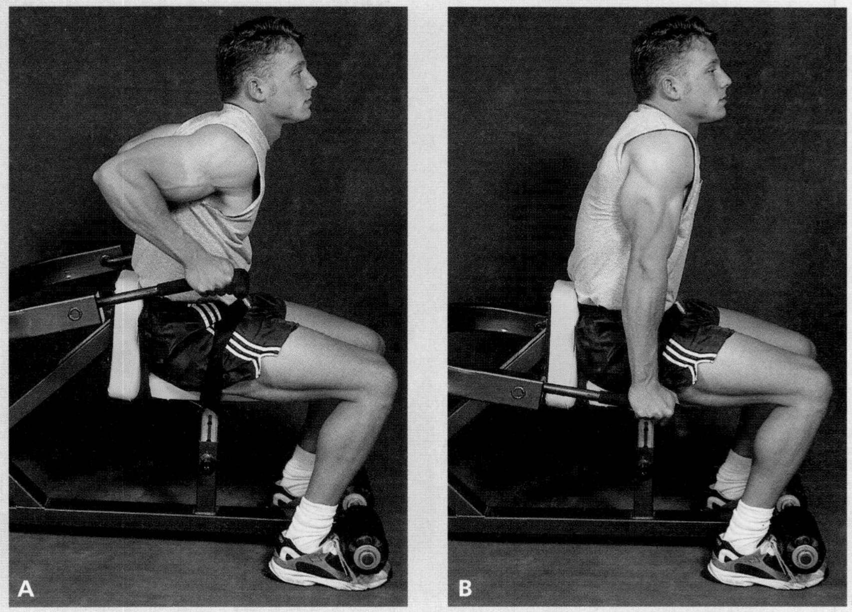

Photos Jon Kelley

Cybex Weight-Assisted Parallel Bar Dips

Muscles developed: Triceps, pectoralis major, anterior deltoid.

Starting position: Select the amount of weight assistance you want from the machine. Place your hands on the parallel bars, step from the platform onto the weight assist bar, and straighten your arms (A).

Eccentric phase: Inhale as you bend your elbows and slowly lower yourself as far as possible (B).

Concentric phase: Exhale as you straighten your arms and return to the starting position.

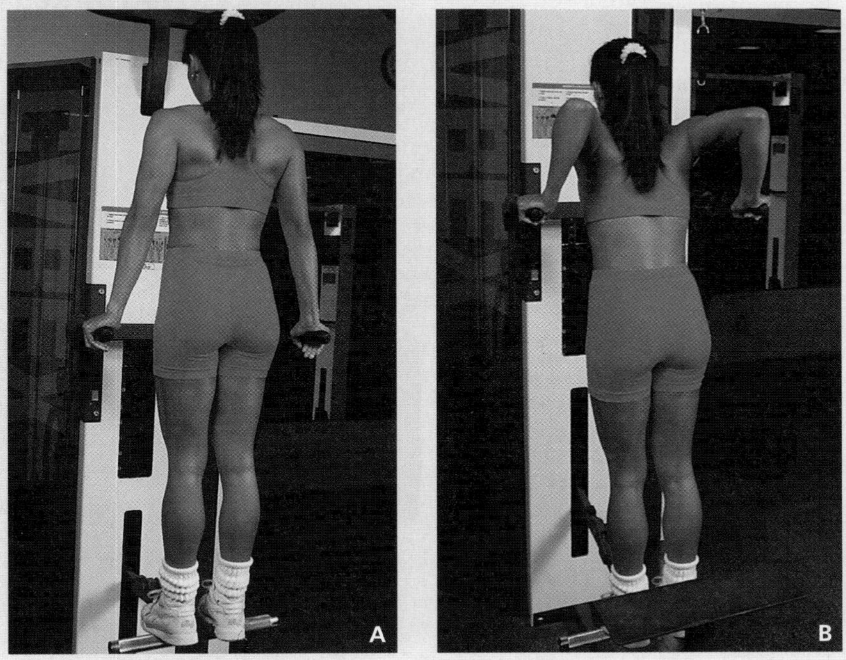

Photos Eric Risberg

Lying Barbell Triceps Extension

Muscles developed: Triceps.

Starting positions: Start on your back on a flat exercise bench and hold a barbell above your shoulders, with both arms straight and your hands 6″ to 8″ apart (A).

Eccentric phase: Inhale while lowering the bar to the top of your head by bending only at your elbows (B).

Concentric phase: Exhale as you push the bar back to the starting position.

Variations: Perform this exercise on an incline bench or a decline bench. Use one or two dumbbells in several variations.

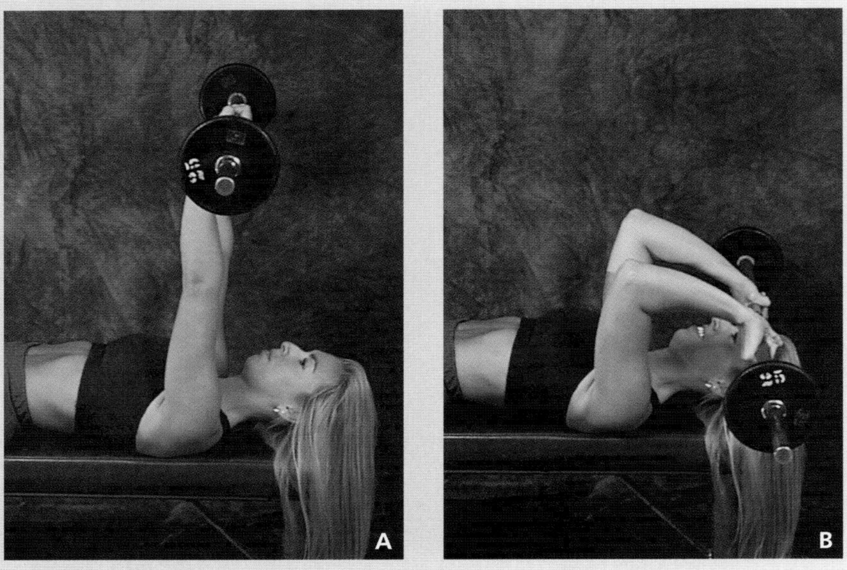

Photos Eric Risberg

Close-Grip Bench Press

Muscles developed: Triceps, anterior deltoid, pectoralis major.

Starting position: Start on your back on a flat bench and hold a barbell directly above your shoulders, with your arms straight and a close grip (hands 6″ to 8″ apart) (A).

Eccentric phase: Inhale as you lower the bar until it touches your chest (B).

Concentric phase: Exhale as you press the weight back to the starting position.

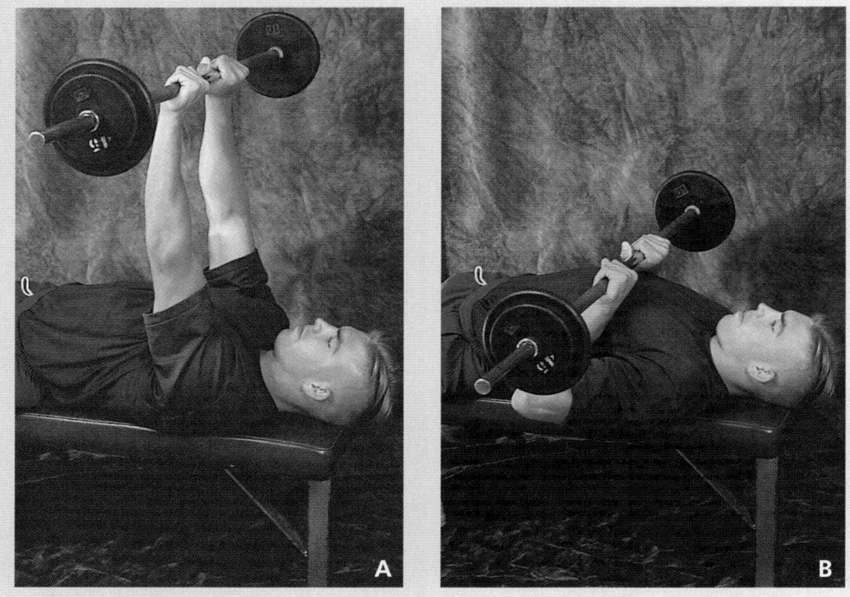

Photos Eric Risberg

Body Master Triceps Extension

Muscles developed: Triceps.

Starting position: Sit on the triceps extension machine and grasp the bar with both elbows pointing up.

Eccentric phase: Inhale as you slowly lower the bar behind your head to the starting position.

Concentric phase: Exhale as you extend both arms and push the bar upward to a straight arm position.

Caution: Keep your elbows pointing up throughout the exercise.

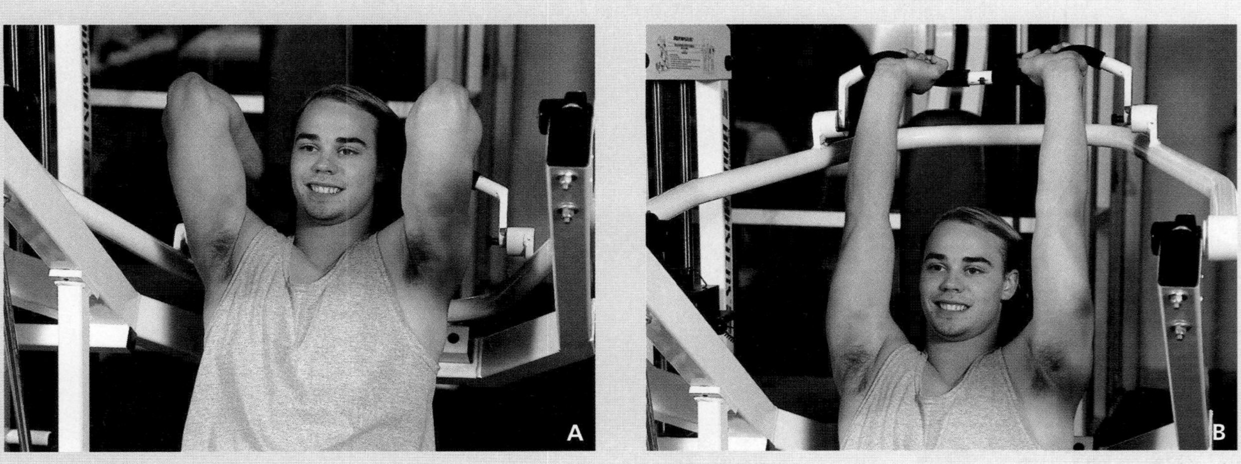

Photos Jon Kelley

Cybex Triceps Extension Machine

Muscles developed: Triceps.

Starting position: Grasp the handles of the exercise machine with your palms facing each other. With your elbows bent, place the back of your upper arms on the pad provided and line up your elbow joints with the pivot point of the machine (A).

Concentric phase: Exhale as you push both hands forward and downward until your arms are extended. Pause briefly and hold (B).

Eccentric phase: Inhale as you allow your arms to slowly return to the starting position.

Caution: Do not allow the weight to drop back to the starting position. Control the speed of movement at all times.

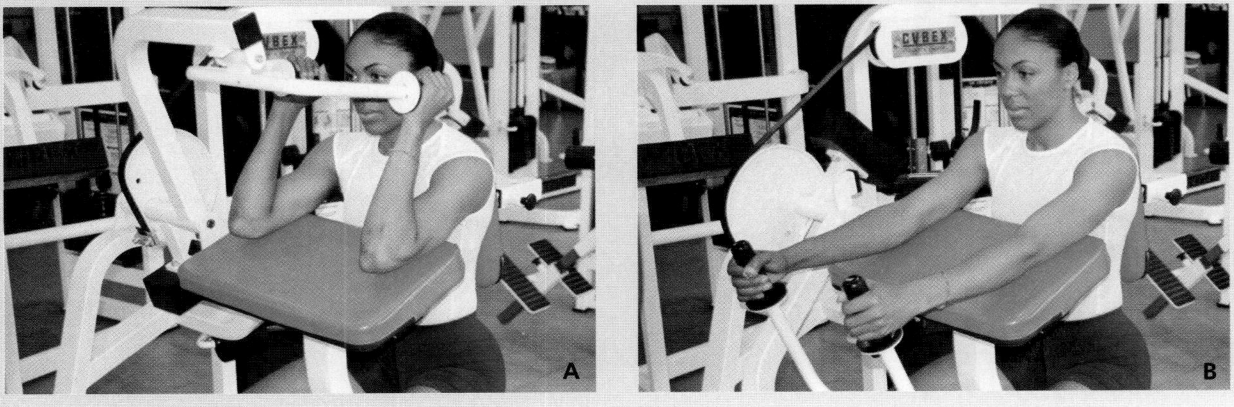

Photos Kristin Dilworth

FOREARM (WRIST FLEXORS AND WRIST EXTENSORS)

Wrist Curl

Muscles developed: Wrist and hand flexors.

Starting positions: Sit on an exercise bench and place your forearms on the bench with your wrists just beyond the end of the bench; hold a barbell with a supinated (thumbs out) grip and allow the bar to hang toward the floor (A).

Concentric phase: Lift the weight, moving only your hands and wrists (B).

Eccentric phase: Lower the bar slowly to the starting position.

Variations:

1. Use one dumbbell in each hand.
2. Use one dumbbell and exercise one arm at a time.

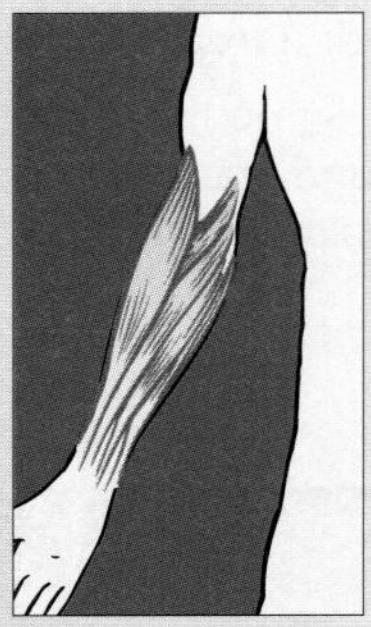

Front

Barbell

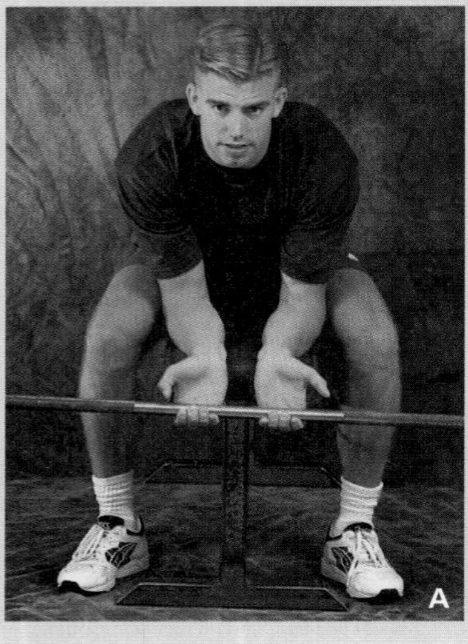

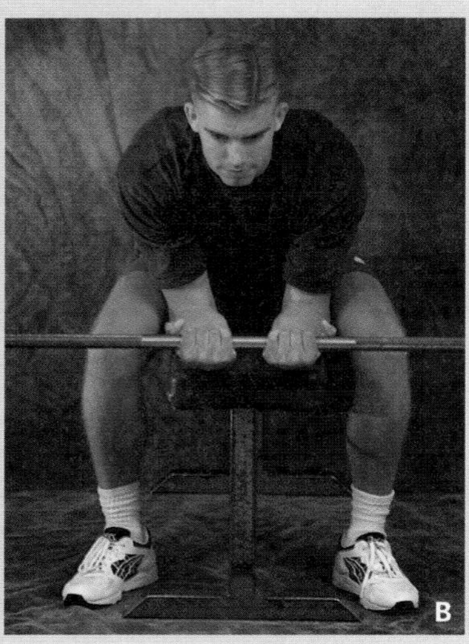

Photos Eric Risberg

Dumbbell

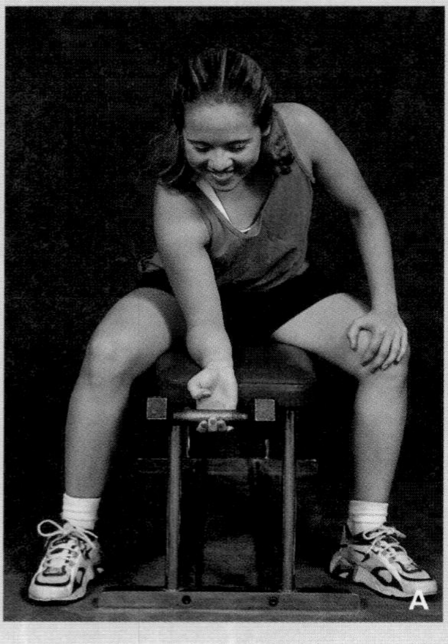

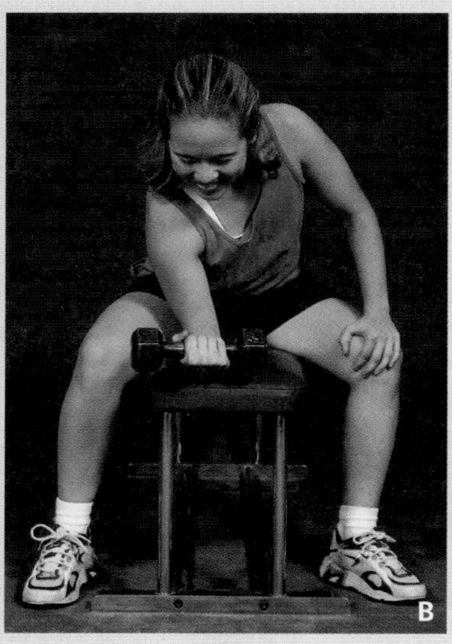

Photos Jon Kelley

Reverse Wrist Curl

Muscles developed: Wrist extensors.

Starting position: Sit on an exercise bench, forearms resting on top of your thighs, wrists just beyond your knees; hold a barbell, using a pronated (thumbs in) grip (A).

Concentric phase: Lift the bar as high as possible, moving only at the wrist joint (B).

Eccentric phase: Slowly lower the bar to the starting position.

Variations:

1. Place forearms across an exercise bench.
2. Use dumbbells.

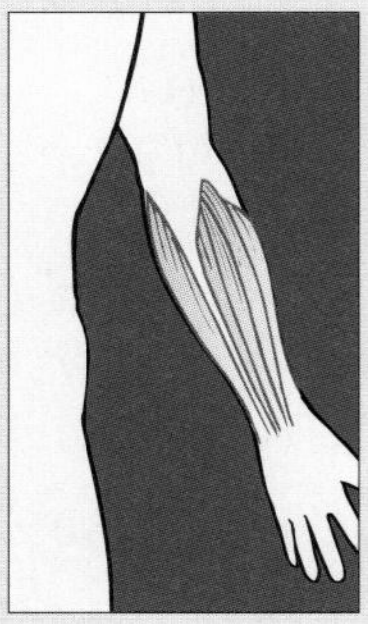

Back

Barbell

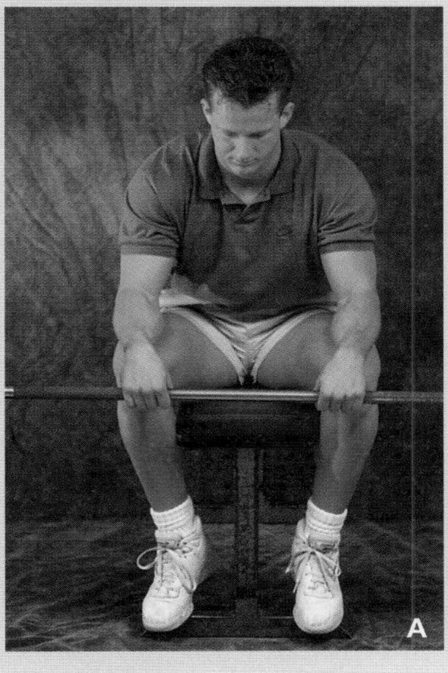

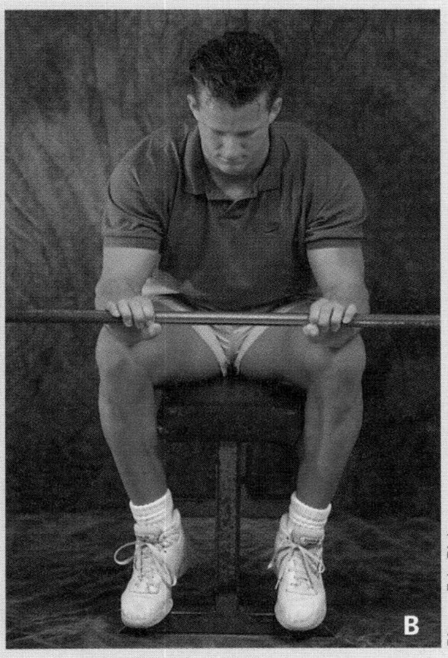

Photos Eric Risberg

Dumbbell

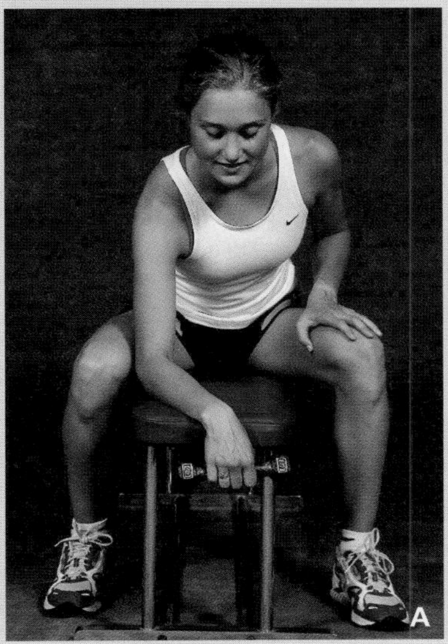

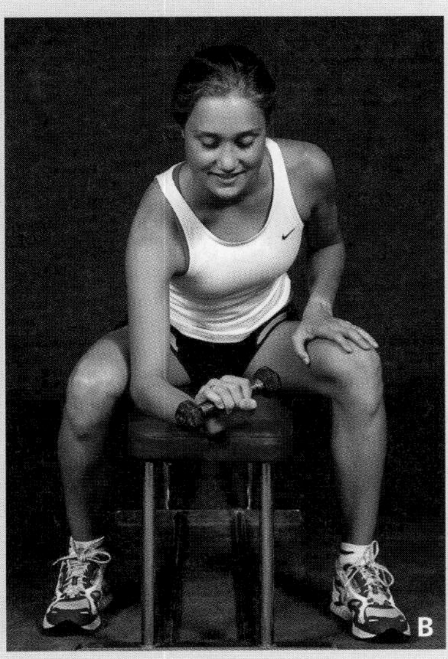

Photos Jon Kelley

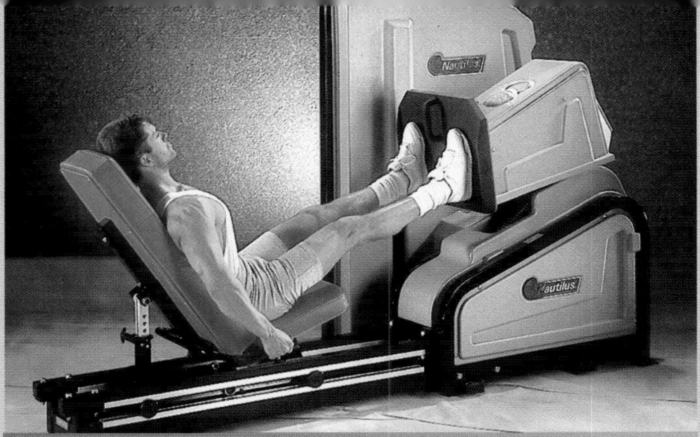

Photos © Nautilus Sports/Medical Industries, Inc.

12

Leg Exercises

Hip and Knee Extension (Gluteus maximus, Quadriceps, Hamstrings)

Barbell Squat
Dumbbell Squat or Dead Lift
Barbell Squat in Power Rack
Dead Lift

Squat Machine
Cybex Leg Press (Weight Stack Machine)
Nautilus Leg Press Machine
Cybex Leg Press (Plate Loaded Machine)

Lunge
Step Up
Leg Press Machine
Hack Squat Machine

Hip Extension (Gluteus maximus)

Cybex Hip Extension Machine

Hip Flexion (Iliopsoas)

Hip Flexion Machine

Knee Extension (Quadriceps)

Cybex Leg Extension Machine
Body Master Leg Extension Machine

Knee Flexion (Hamstrings)

Nautilus Seated Leg Curl Machine
Body Master Leg Curl Machine

Ankle Plantar Flexion

Standing Barbell Calf Raise
Standing Dumbbell Calf Raise
Universal Heel Raise
Cybex Standing Calf Raise Machine

One-Dumbbell Calf Raise
Calf Press on Body Master Leg Press Machine
Calf Press on Cybex Leg Press Machine
Seated Calf Raise

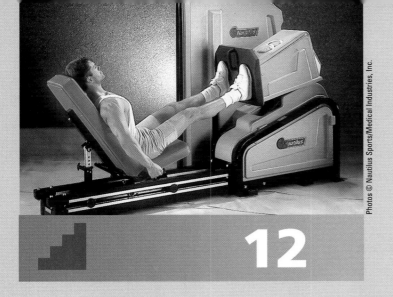

HIP AND KNEE EXTENSION

Squat

Muscles developed: Quadriceps, gluteus maximus, hamstrings, erector spinae.

Starting position: Stand, holding a barbell across your shoulders and upper back (A).

Eccentric phase: Inhale as you bend your knees and hips while keeping your head up and your back flat. Continue bending your knees and hips until your thighs are parallel to the floor (B).

Concentric phase: Exhale as you straighten your legs and hips to return to a standing position.

Spotting: Have one spotter stand directly behind you, or have one spotter stand at each end of the bar and one spotter stand directly behind you.

Caution: Perform this exercise in a squat rack or power rack to guarantee that you will not get stuck under a heavy weight.

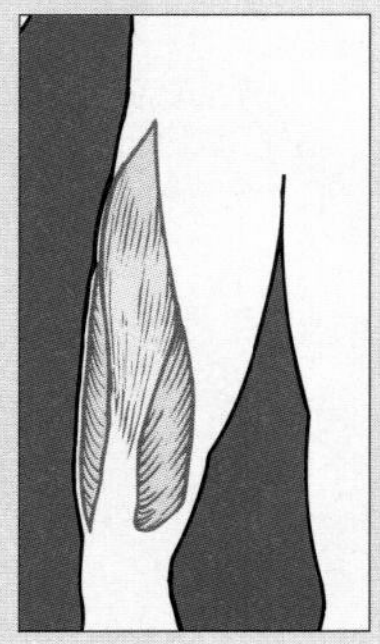
Front

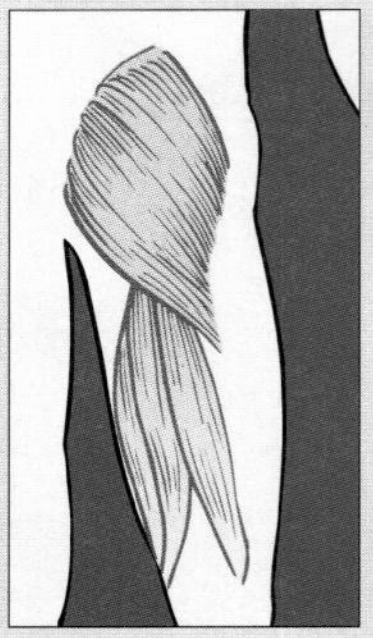
Back

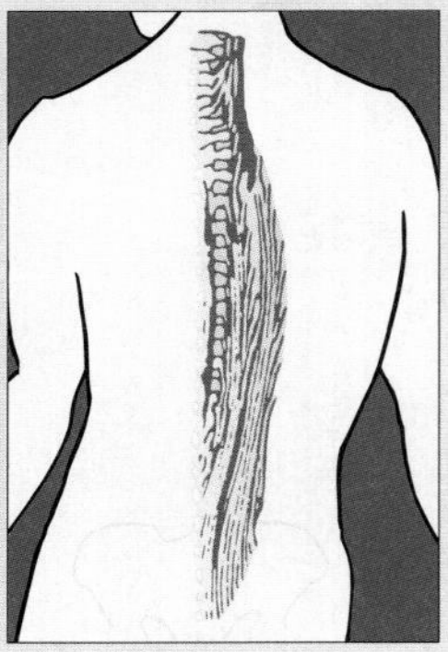
Back

Barbell

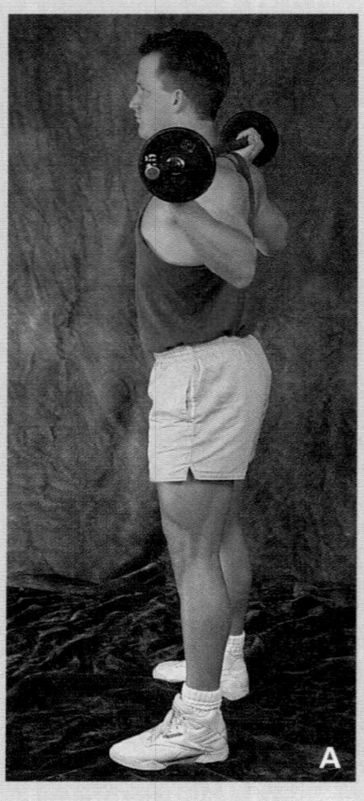

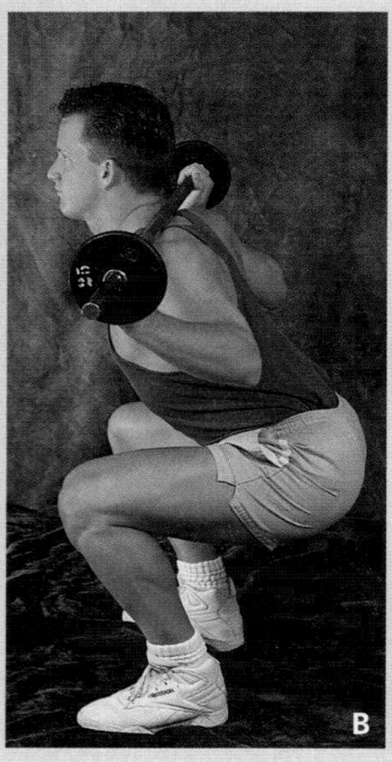

Photos Eric Risberg

Dumbbell Squat or Dead Lift

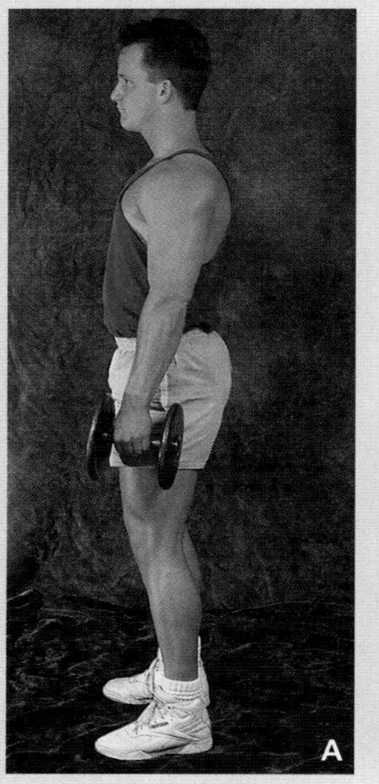

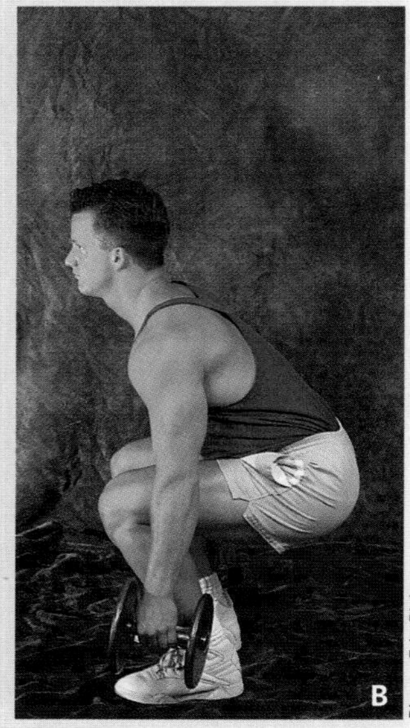

Photos Eric Risberg

Barbell Squat in Power Rack

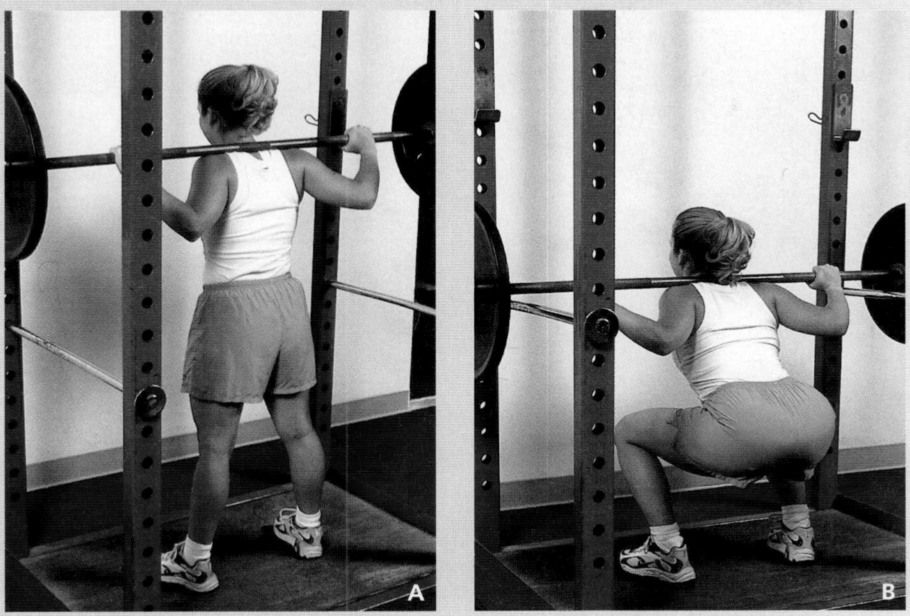

Photos Jon Kelley

Dead Lift

Muscles developed: Erector spinae, gluteus maximus, quadriceps, hamstrings, trapezius, rhomboids, finger flexors.

Starting position: Bend over and assume a mixed grip on a barbell that is lying on the floor. Bend your knees and hips so your hips are approximately knee-level or parallel to the floor. Hold your head up and your back straight (A).

Concentric phase: Keep your neck and back straight while you pull up on the bar (B). Lift the weight by extending your hips and knees.

Eccentric phase: Keep your neck and back straight as you slowly lower the weight back to the floor by bending your knees and hips.

Caution: The dead lift is basically a hand-held squat. It is vital to maintain correct body position and progress slowly to avoid injury. When performed correctly, this is an excellent exercise to strengthen your back extensor muscles as well as your hip and knee extensors.

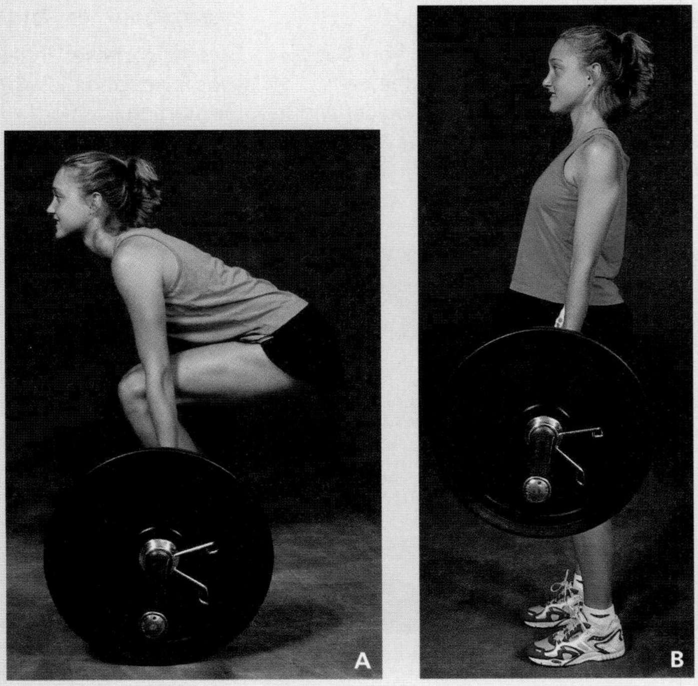

Photos Jon Kelley

Squat Machine

Muscles developed: Quadriceps, gluteus maximus, hamstrings, erector spinae.

Starting position: Place your shoulders under the pads and your hands on the handles. Keep your head up and your back straight. Start with your hips and knees bent (A).

Concentric phase: Exhale as you extend your knees and hips while keeping your back straight (B).

Eccentric phase: Inhale as you lower the weight slowly to the starting position by bending your knees and hips.

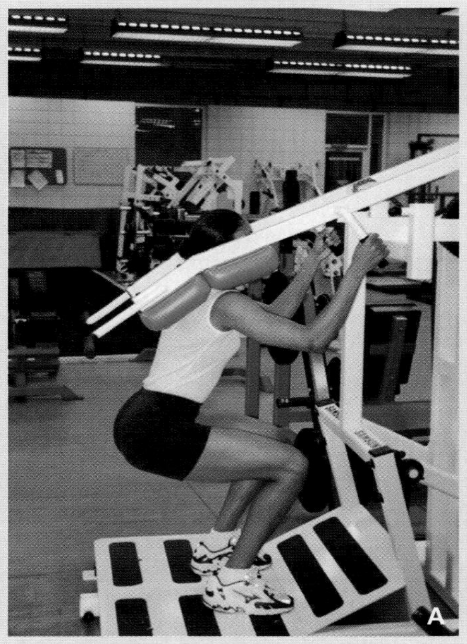
A

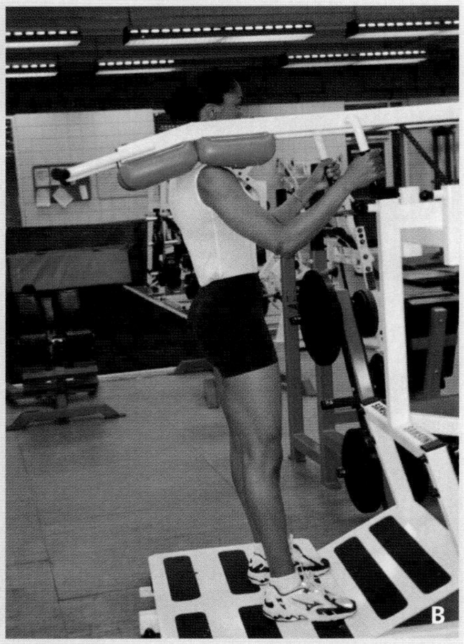
B

Photos Kristin Dilworth

Cybex Leg Press (Weight Stack Machine)

Muscles developed: Quadriceps, gluteus maximus.

Starting position: Start on your back with your shoulders against the pads, your feet on the platform shoulder-width apart, and your knees bent at a 90° angle (A).

Concentric phase: Exhale as you extend your knees and hips (B).

Eccentric phase: Inhale as you bend your knees and hips and slowly return to the starting position.

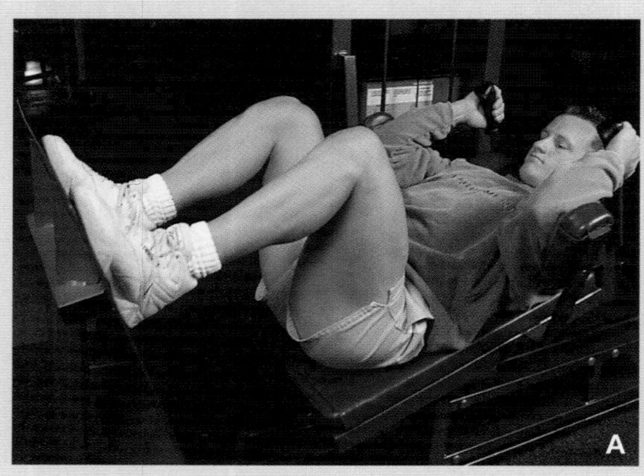
A

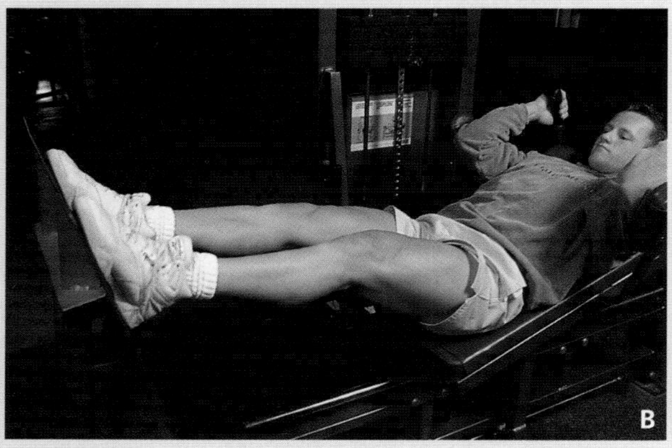
B

Photos Eric Risberg

Nautilus Leg Press Machine

Muscles developed: Quadriceps, gluteus maximus.

Starting position: Start in a sitting position with your knees bent at a 90° angle (A).

Concentric phase: Exhale as you extend your legs (B).

Eccentric phase: Inhale as you bend your legs slowly and allow the weight to return to the starting position.

Additional information: This exercise provides back support and therefore takes the strain off the spinal column, but it will not strengthen the back extensor muscles as the barbell squat and dead lift do.

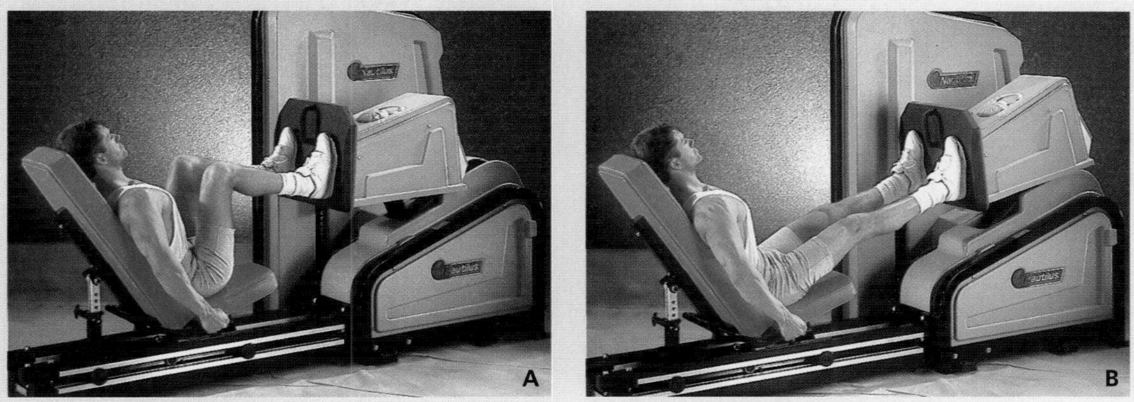

Photos © Nautilus Sports/Medical Industries, Inc.

Cybex Leg Press (Plate-Loaded Machine)

Muscles developed: Quadriceps, gluteus maximus.

Starting position: Start in a position with your knees bent at a 90° angle (A).

Concentric phase: Exhale as you extend your legs (B).

Eccentric phase: Inhale as you slowly bend your legs and allow the weight to return to the starting position.

Additional information: This exercise provides back support and therefore takes the strain off of the spinal column, but it will not strengthen the back extensor muscles as the barbell squat and dead lift do.

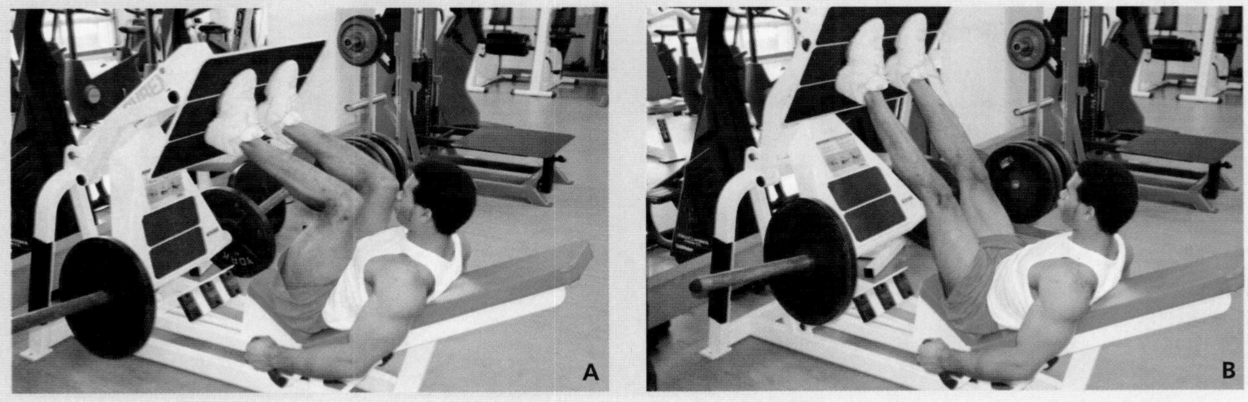

Photos Kristin Dilworth

Lunge

Muscles developed: Quadriceps, gluteus maximus.

Starting position: Assume a standing position with a dumbbell in each hand (A), or a barbell across your shoulders and upper back.

Eccentric phase: Inhale as you take a large step forward with one leg. Bend the knee of your forward leg and lower your body until the thigh of the front leg is parallel to the floor (B). (This is essentially a one-leg parallel squat.)

Concentric phase: Exhale as you extend your forward leg, pushing yourself back to your original standing position.

Spotting: Spotting is not necessary if you are doing lunges with dumbbells. If you are doing lunges with a barbell across your back and shoulders, have one spotter stand at each end of the bar. Or perform the lunges into a squat rack that could support the weight in case you cannot return to the standing position.

Caution: Keep your head up and upper body erect throughout the exercise.

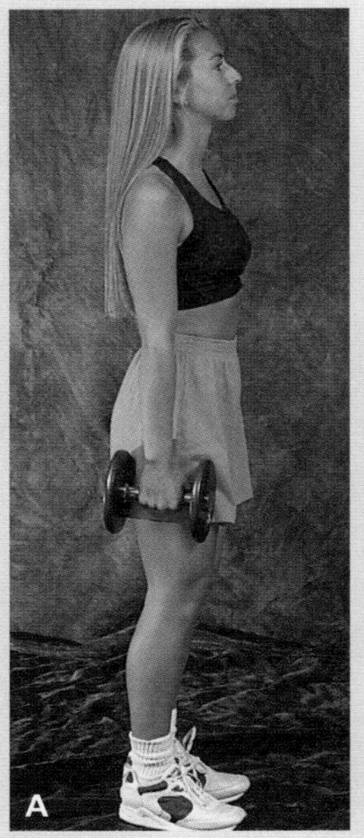

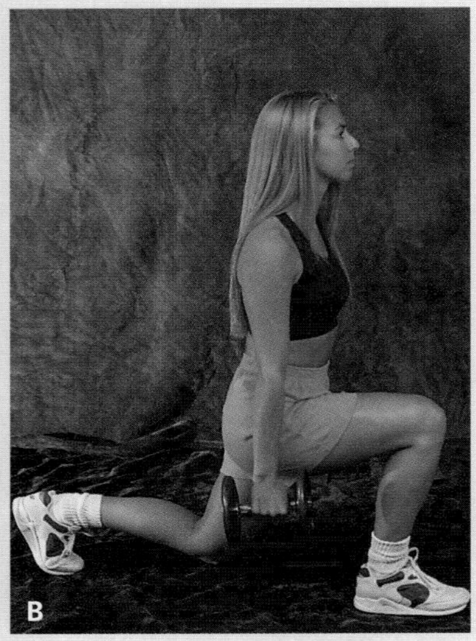

Photos Eric Risberg

Step Up

Muscles developed: Quadriceps, gluteus maximus.

Starting position: Start in a standing position with a dumbbell in each hand (A), or a barbell across your upper back and shoulders.

Concentric phase: Place one foot on the step in front of you. Using your hip and leg muscles, lift yourself up until your leg is straight (B).

Eccentric phase: Lower yourself slowly to the starting position using the same leg.

Spotting: If using dumbbells, you should be all right without a spotter. When using a barbell, have one spotter stand behind you, or a spotter at each end of the bar.

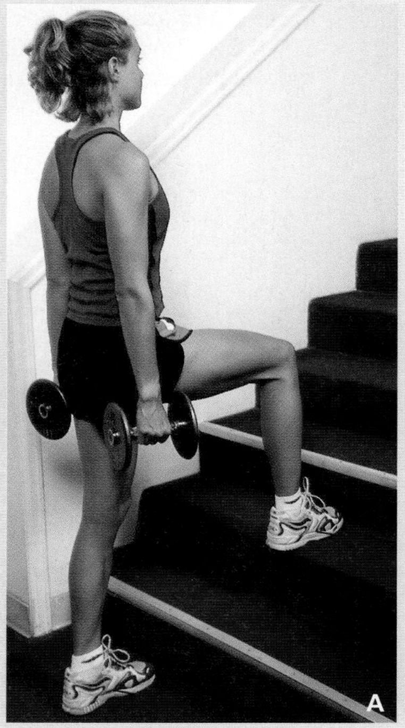

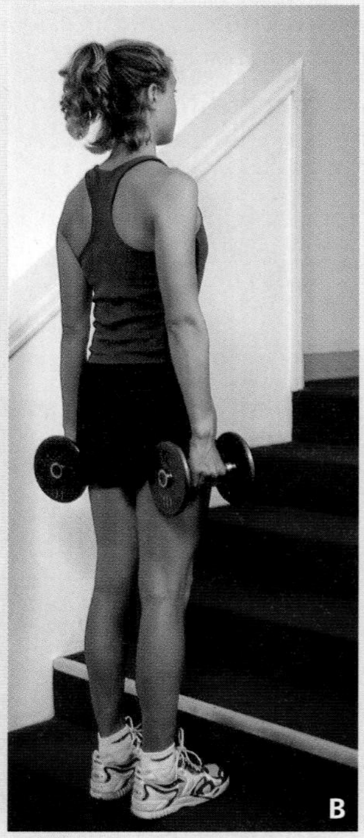

Photos Jon Kelley

Leg Press Machine

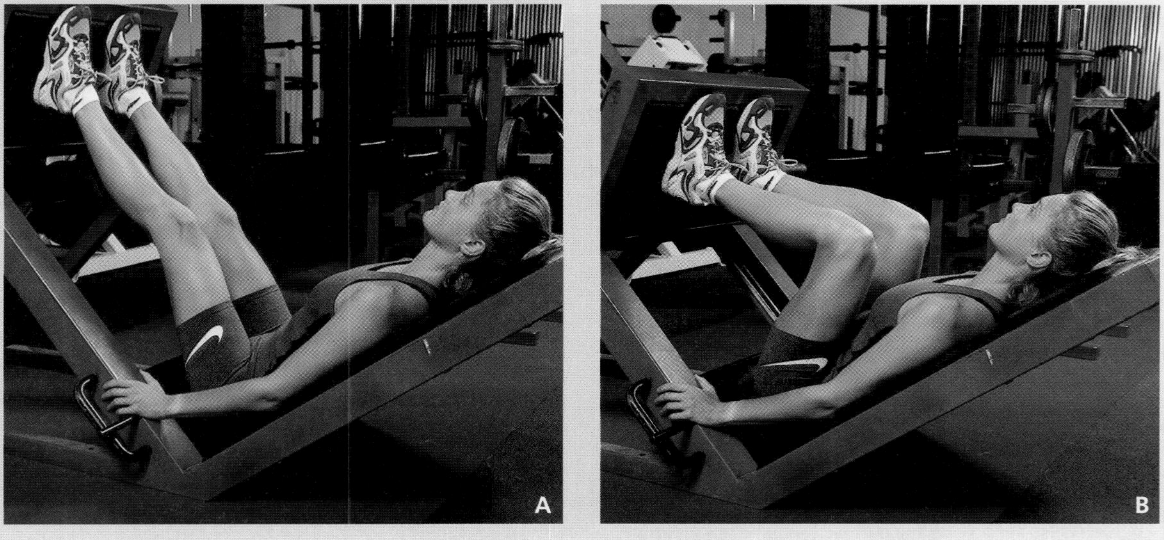

Photos Jon Kelley

Hack Squat Machine

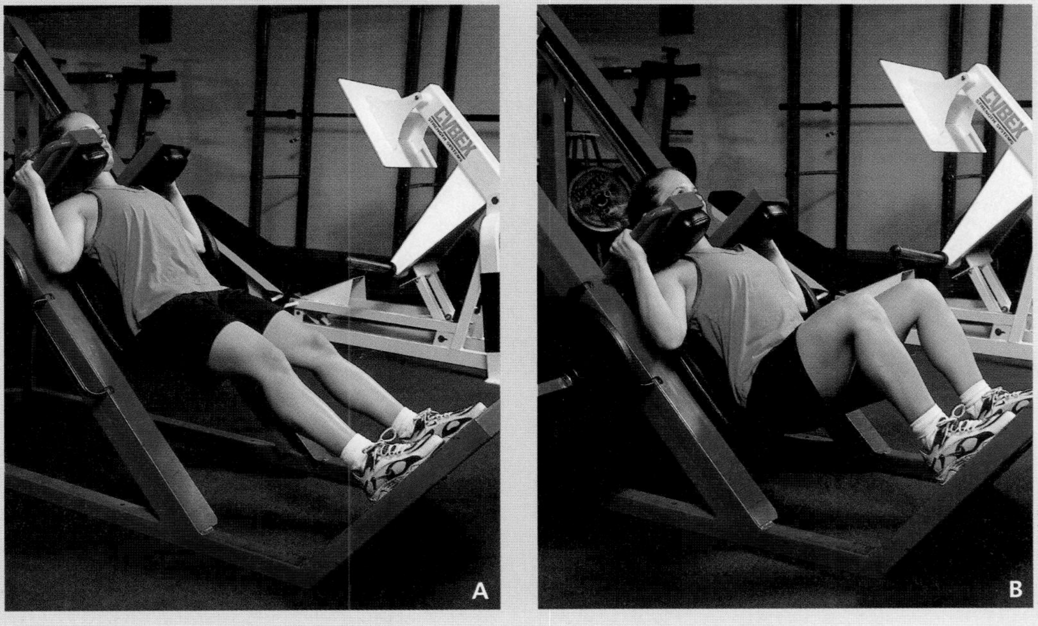

Photos Jon Kelley

HIP EXTENSION

Cybex Hip Extension Machine

Muscles developed: Gluteus maximus, hamstrings.

Starting position: Start in a standing position with one leg over the padded exercise bar, your hands holding the stability bar, and your hip joint lined up with the point of rotation of the exercise machine (A).

Concentric phase: Exhale as you pull your thigh down and back (hip extension) against the resistance (B).

Eccentric phase: Inhale as you slowly allow your leg to return to the starting position.

Additional information: If you keep your knee bent throughout the exercise, your gluteus maximus muscle will do most of the lifting. If you straighten your knee as you extend your hip, the hamstrings will be in a better position to help with hip extension.

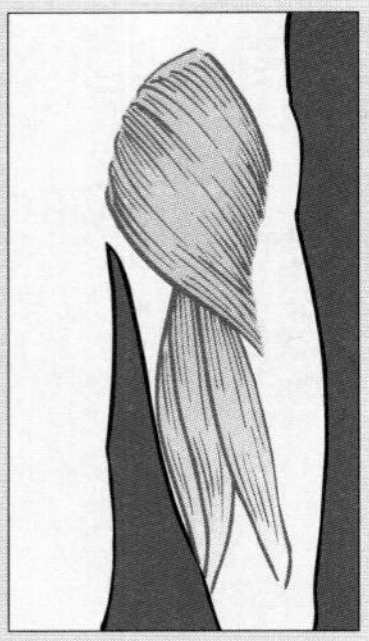

Back

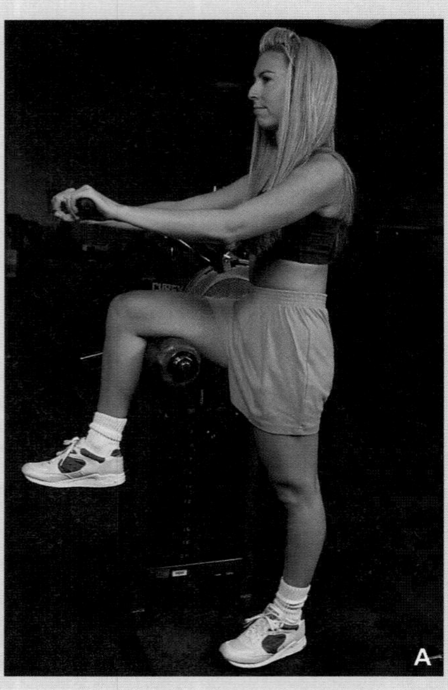

A

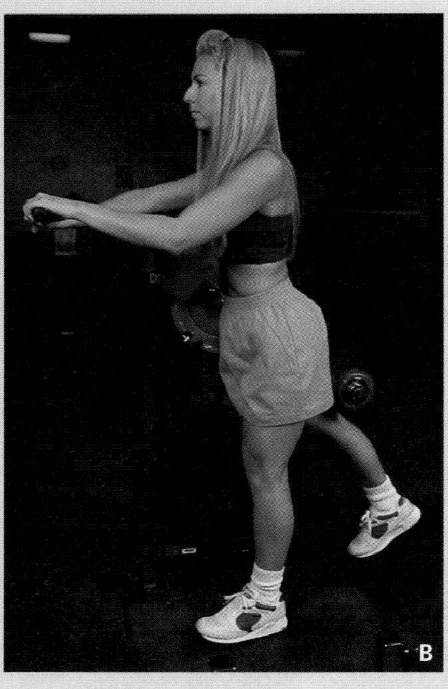

B

Photos Eric Risberg

HIP FLEXION (ILIOPSOAS)

Hip Flexion Machine

Muscles developed: Iliopsoas, rectus femoris.

Starting position: Start in a standing position with one leg against the padded exercise bar and both hands holding the stability bar. The padded exercise bar should be just above your knee joint. Your hip joint should be lined up with the point of rotation of the exercise machine (A).

Concentric phase: Exhale as you pull your bent leg upward against the resistance (B). Tighten your abdominal muscles and keep your lower back flat.

Eccentric phase: Inhale as you lower your leg slowly to the starting position.

Caution: The hip flexors exert a strong pull forward on the lower portion of the spinal column. Therefore, it is important to stabilize the lower spinal column by flexing the abdominal muscles. This exercise is not recommended for individuals with weak abdominal muscles.

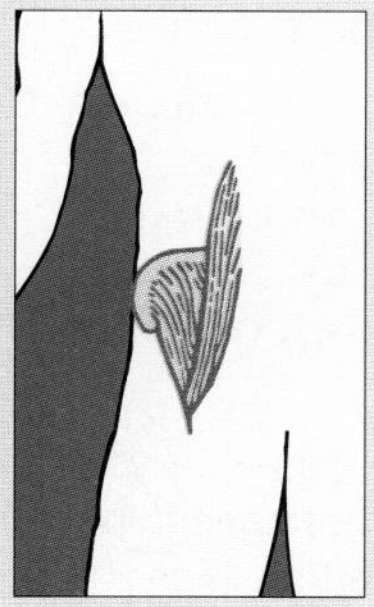

Back

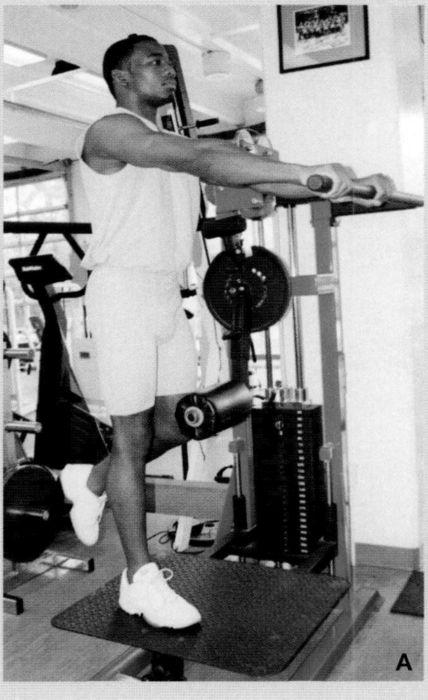

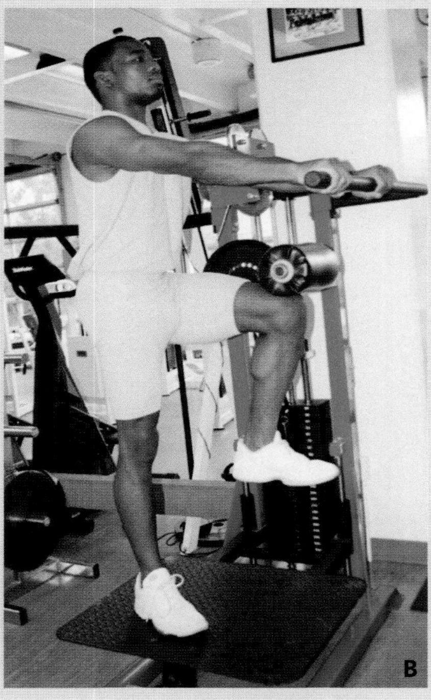

Photos Kristin Dilworth

KNEE EXTENSION (QUADRICEPS)

Muscles developed: Quadriceps.

Starting position: Start in a seated position with your knees bent and the padded exercise bar in front of your ankle or lower leg. Grasp the handles located on each side of the machine (A).

Concentric phase: Exhale as you extend your legs at the knee joints (B). Pause at the extended position, but do not go beyond extension.

Eccentric phase: Inhale as you slowly allow your legs to bend and return to the starting position.

Caution: Control the exercise movement. Do not hyperextend your knee joint. Do not allow the weight to drop.

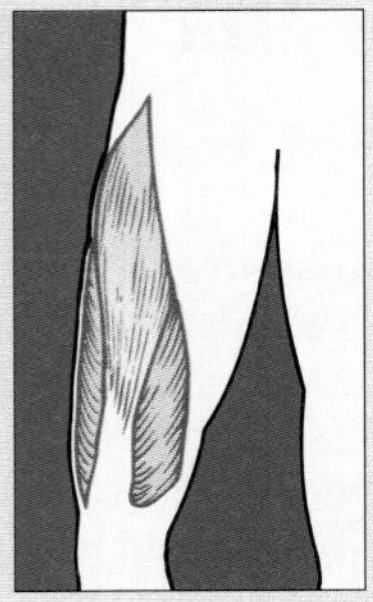

Front

Cybex Leg Extension Machine

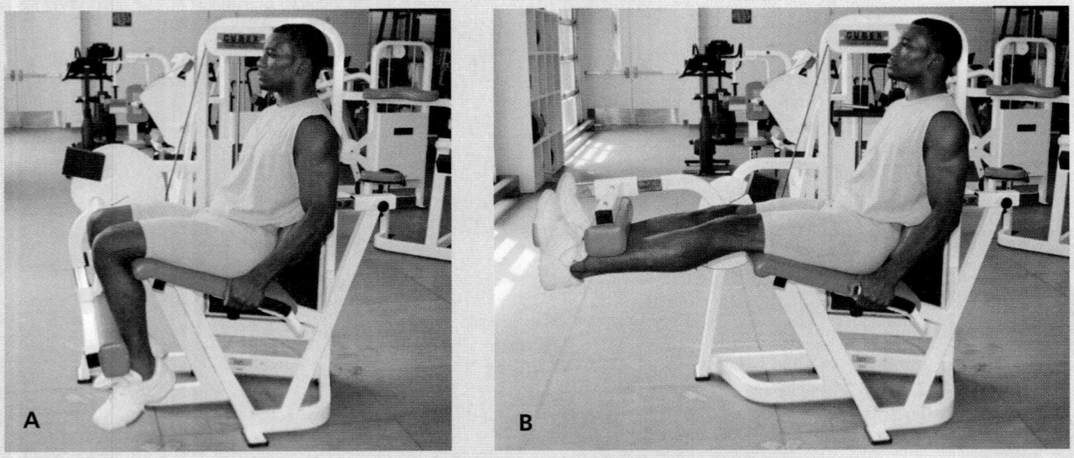

Photos Kristin Dilworth

Body Master Leg Extension Machine

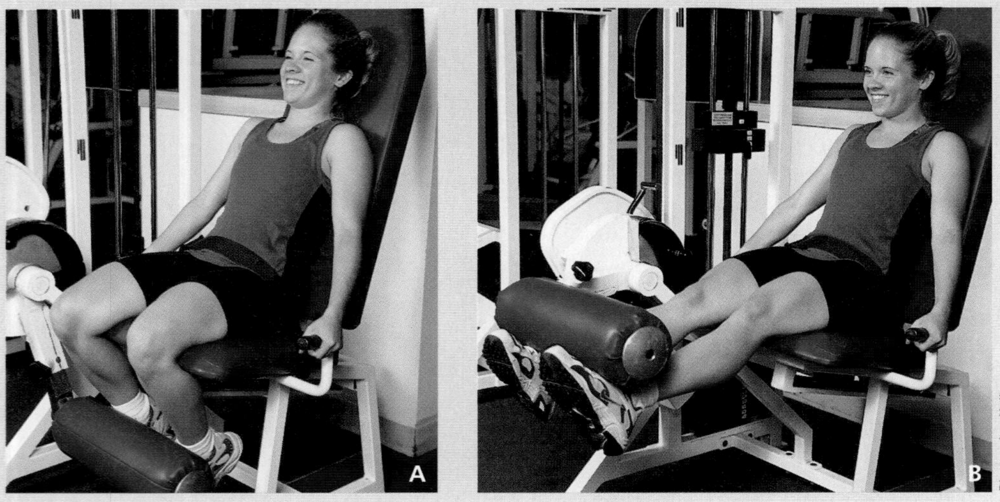

Photos Jon Kelley

KNEE FLEXION (HAMSTRINGS)

Muscles developed: Hamstrings.

Starting position: Start in a sitting or lying position with your legs straight and the back of your lower leg against the padded exercise bar. Line up your knees with the pivot point of the exercise machine. Grasp the handles. On the seated leg curl, fasten the seat belt to hold your hips in the correct exercise position (A).

Concentric phase: Exhale as you bend your knees and pull your lower legs toward the back of your thighs (B).

Eccentric phase: Inhale as you allow your legs to slowly return to the starting position.

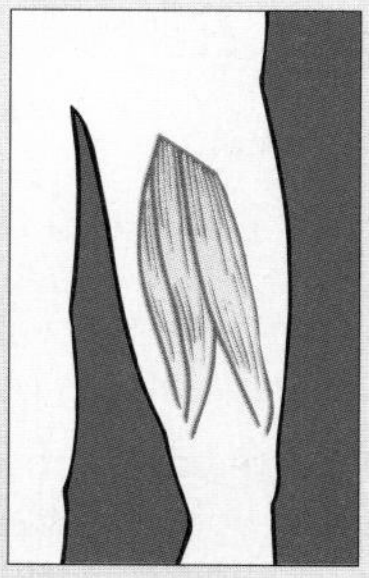
Back

Nautilus Seated Leg Curl Machine

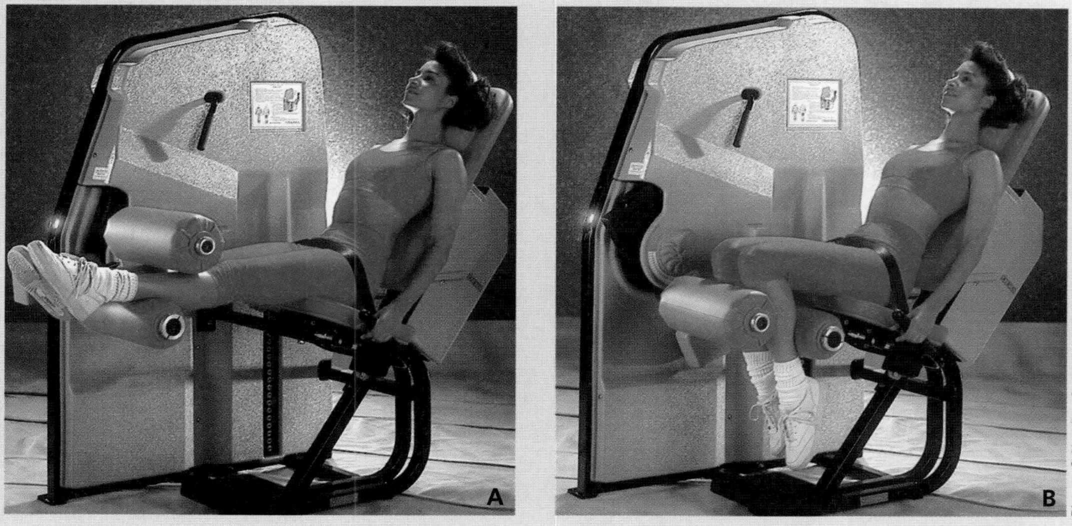

Photos © Nautilus Sports/Medical Industries, Inc.

Body Master Leg Curl Machine

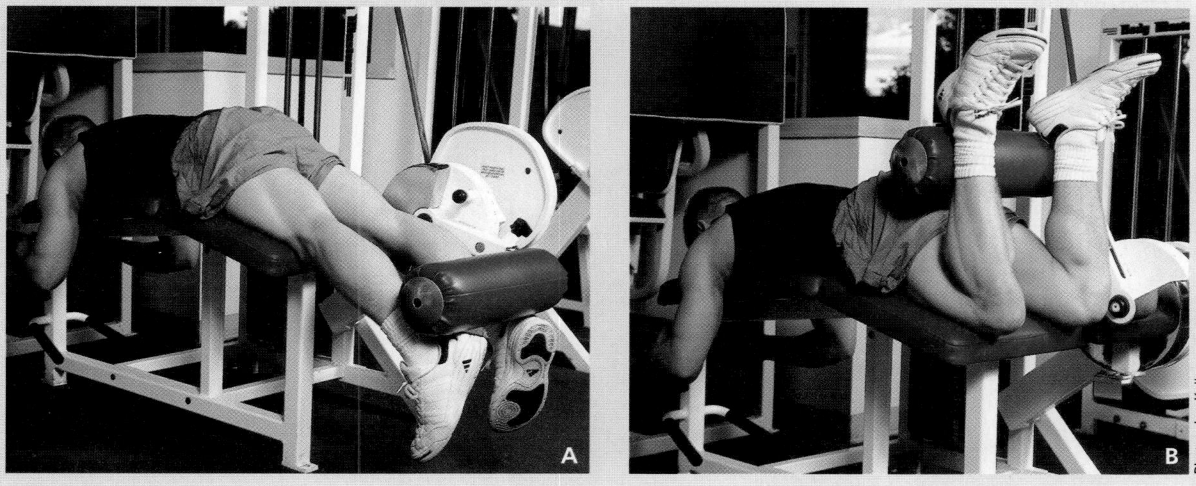

Photos Jon Kelley

ANKLE PLANTAR FLEXION

Standing Calf Raise

Muscles developed: Gastrocnemius, soleus.

Starting position: Take a standing position with a barbell across your shoulders and upper back, the front half of both feet elevated so your heels are lower than your toes (A).

Concentric phase: Exhale while moving only at the ankle joint to raise your heels as high as possible (B). Pause briefly and completely contract the muscles on the back of your legs when you are at the highest position you can reach.

Eccentric phase: Inhale as you slowly lower both heels as far as they can go. The best stretch and maximum range of motion are achieved if your heels cannot touch the floor at the bottom position of this exercise.

Caution: Maintaining balance is difficult during this exercise. Performing the exercise in a power rack or on a standing calf-raise machine usually increases the effectiveness of the exercise because it eliminates the balance problem.

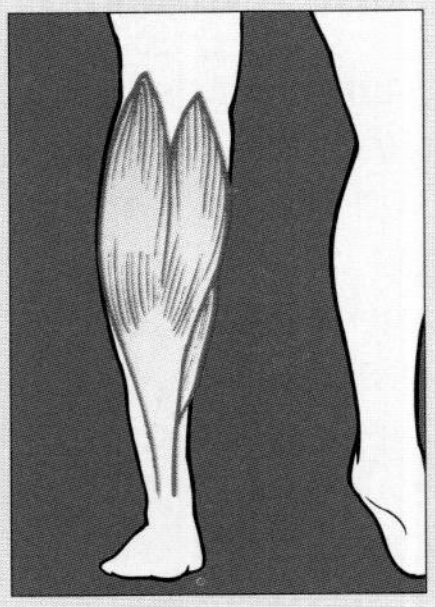

Back

Barbell

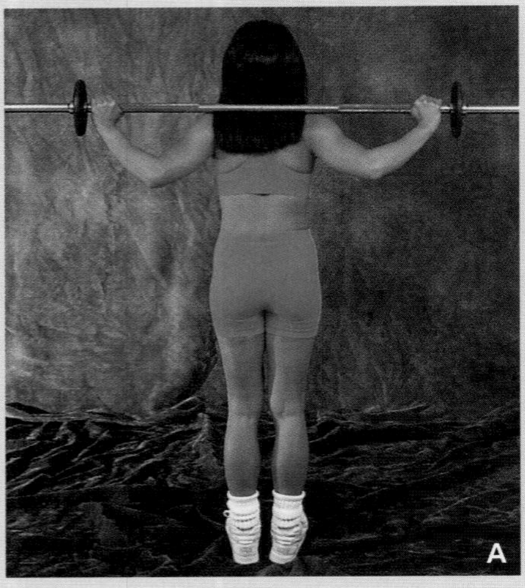

A

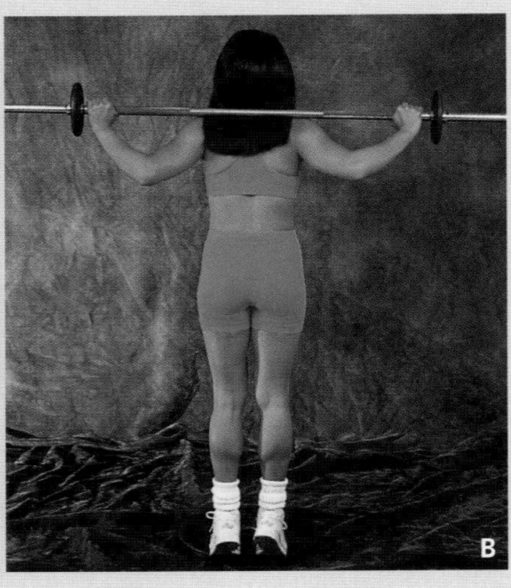

B

Photos Eric Risberg

Dumbbell

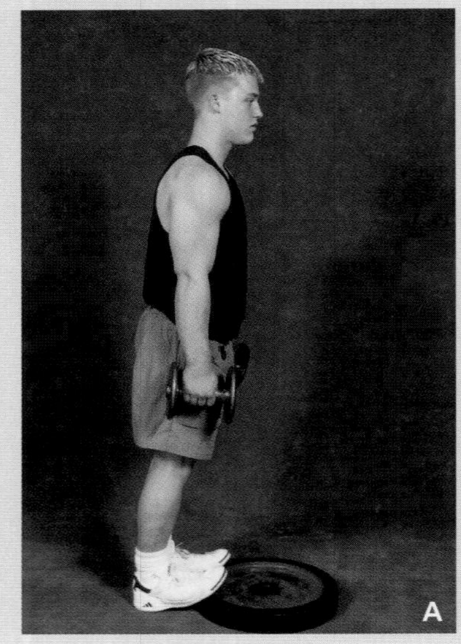

A

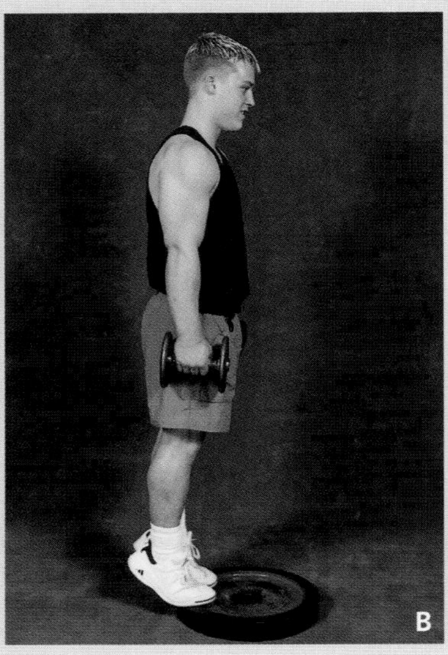

B

Photos Jon Kelley

Universal Heel Raise Machine

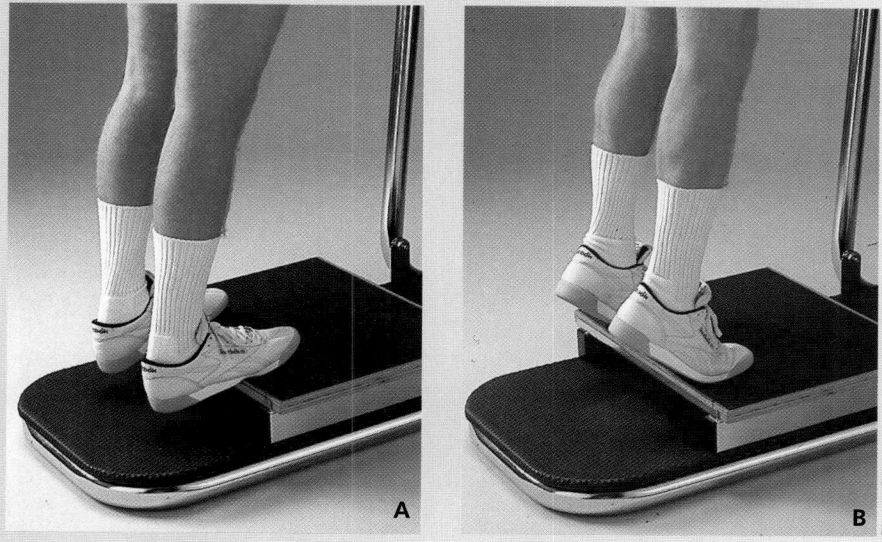

Photos © Universal Gym Equipment, Inc.

Cybex Standing Calf Raise Machine

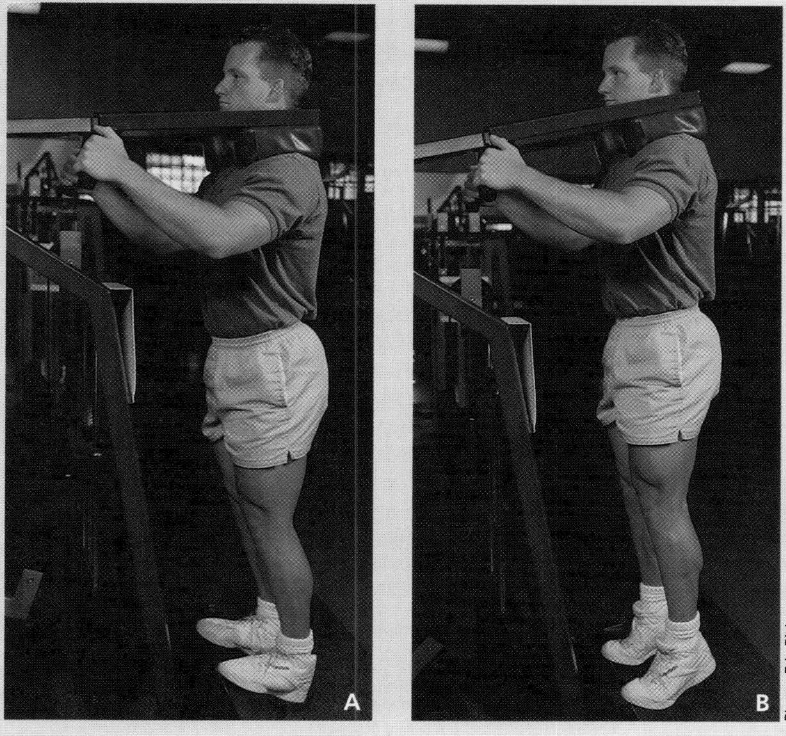

Photos Eric Risberg

One-Dumbbell Calf Raise

Muscles developed: Gastrocnemius, soleus.

Starting position: Stand with a dumbbell in one hand hanging at arm's-length and resting against the side of your thigh. Place all of your body weight on the leg nearest the dumbbell and lift your other foot off the floor (A).

Concentric phase: Exhale as you raise the heel of your support foot as high as possible. Pause at the top.

Eccentric phase: Inhale as you slowly lower the heel of your support foot to a fully stretched position.

Additional information: Place the hand that is not holding the dumbbell on some solid support for balance (B). Use the support hand for balance only; do not pull with that arm to help lift the weight.

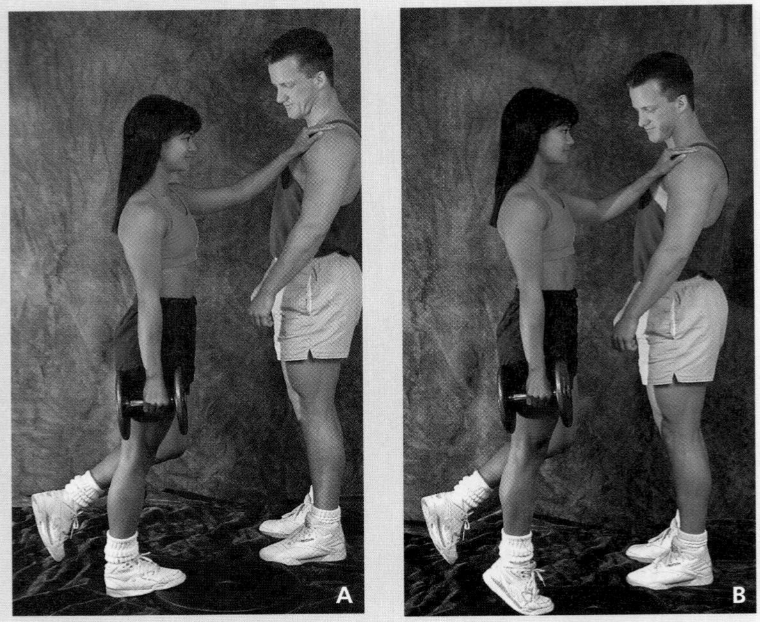

Photos Eric Risberg

Calf Press on Body Master Leg Press Machine

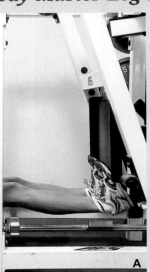

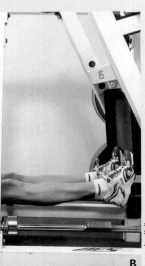

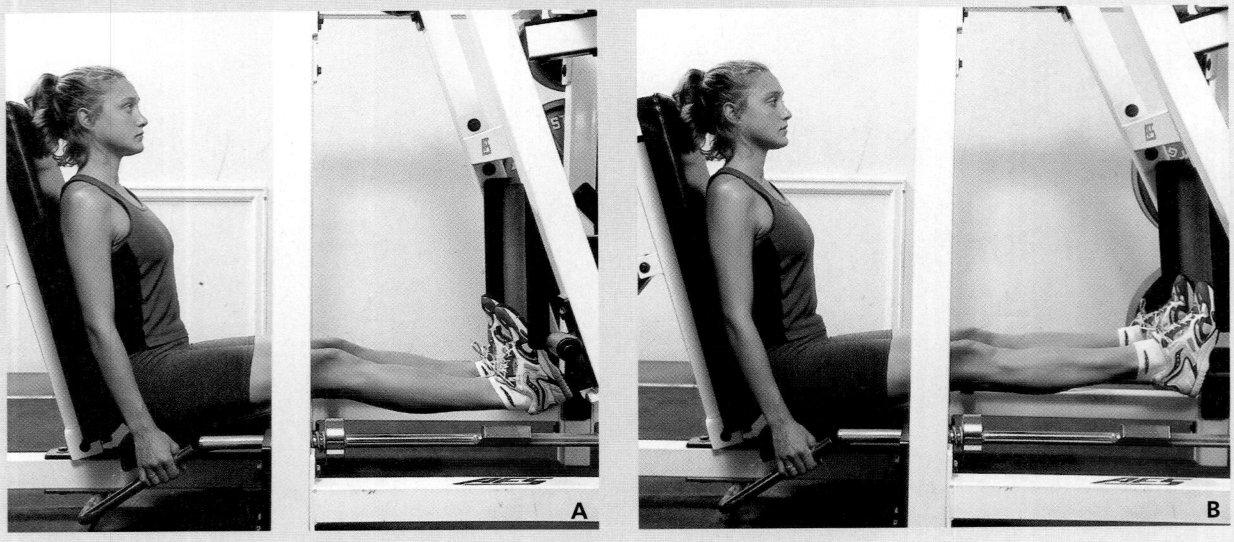

Photos Jon Kelley

Calf Press on Cybex Leg Press Machine

Muscles developed: Gastrocnemius, soleus.

Starting position: Position yourself on a leg press machine. Start with your legs straight, the front half of each foot on the pedals or platform, and your heels lower than the front part of your foot (A).

Concentric phase: Exhale as you press down with the front part of your foot moving only at the ankle joint (B). At the top of your range of motion, hold the muscle contraction and squeeze with your calf muscles.

Eccentric phase: Inhale as you slowly return to the starting position. Stretch the calf muscles in the starting position by allowing the heels to sink as low as possible.

Caution: Do not allow your feet to slip off the pedals or platform.

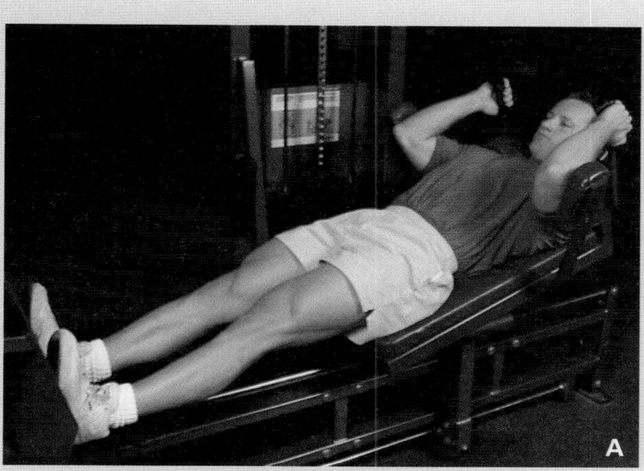

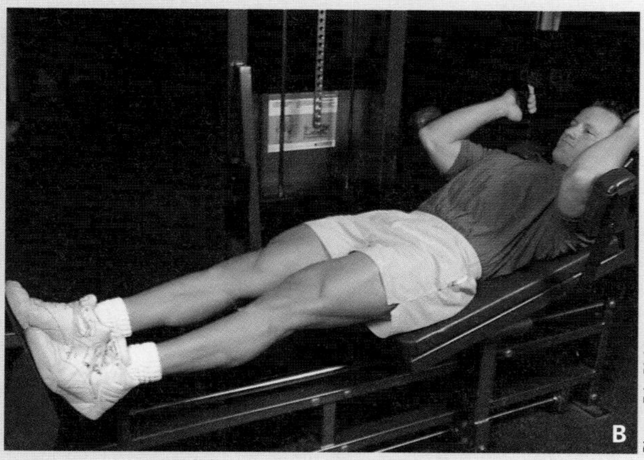

Photos Eric Risberg

Seated Calf Raise

Muscles developed: Soleus (the gastrocnemius becomes much less effective at pulling up on your heel when your knee is bent).

Starting position: Sit with the front half of your foot on the foot plate, your knees under the padded exercise bar and your hands on top of the exercise bar. Your heels should be lower than the front part of your foot (A).

Concentric phase: Lift your heels as high as possible while keeping the front part of your foot on the foot plate (B).

Eccentric phase: Slowly lower your heels to the starting position, and stretch.

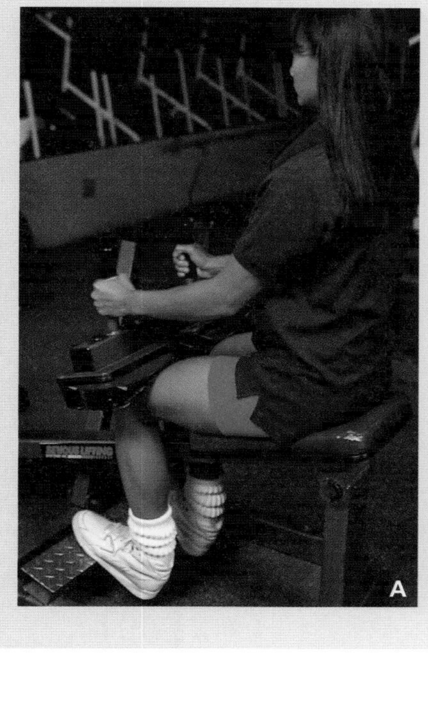

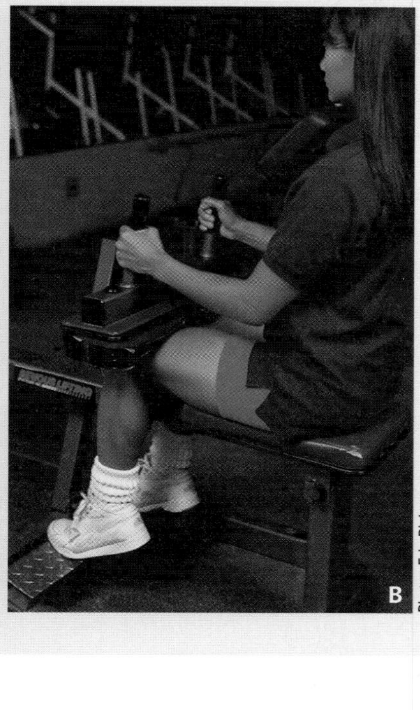

Photos Eric Risberg

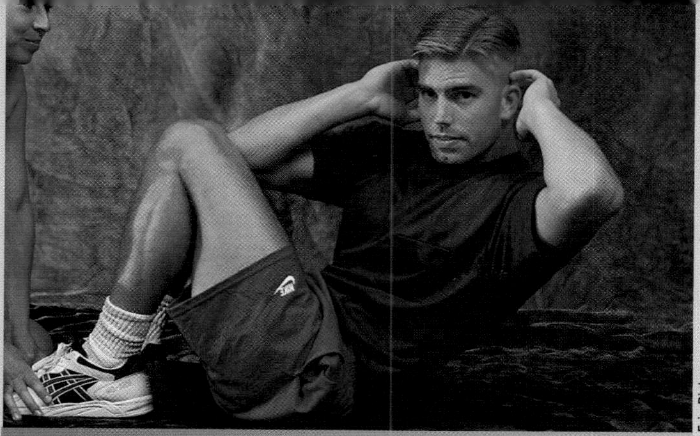
Eric Risberg

13

Trunk Flexion and Extension Exercises

Trunk Flexion (Abdominals)

Crunches, Curl-Ups
Cybex Abdominal Machine
Nautilus Abdominal Crunch Machine

Trunk and Hip Flexion (Abdominals and Hip flexors)

Sit-Ups
Tuck-Ups
Reverse Crunches
Seated Reverse Crunches
Hanging Reverse Crunches or Hanging Knee Raises

Trunk Extension (Erector spinae)

Back Extension
Cybex Seated Back Extension Machine
Cybex Back Extension Machine

The Ab Solution

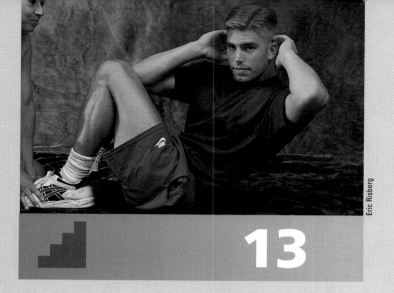

TRUNK FLEXION (ABDOMINALS)

Crunches, Curl-Ups

Muscles developed: Rectus abdominis, abdominal obliques.

Starting position: Start flat on your back. Bend at your knees and hips. Place your feet flat on the floor. Cross your arms over your chest, with each hand touching the opposite shoulder (A).

Concentric phase: Exhale as you "curl up" slowly, pulling your head, neck, shoulders, and upper back off the floor in that order (B). Keep your lower back on the floor throughout the exercise. At the upper limit of this movement, crunch (squeeze) the abdominal muscles by holding this fully contracted position for 3 seconds.

Eccentric phase: Slowly release the curling motion, and inhale as you return to the starting position.

Variations:

1. Keeping your legs straight, place the back of your legs against a wall, with your hips flexed and your back on the floor.

2. Place your lower legs up on a bench with your hips and knees bent.

3. Add a twisting motion to the trunk flexion so that as you curl up, you also move one elbow toward the opposite hip. Alternate the direction of the twist on each repetition.

Additional information: If you want to add weight to this exercise, place it on your upper chest and hold it there by crossing your arms on top of the weight. Or hold a weight in your hands directly above your shoulders with your arms straight. Push the weight straight up toward the ceiling as you curl your trunk.

Caution: Keep your lower back on the floor throughout the exercise.

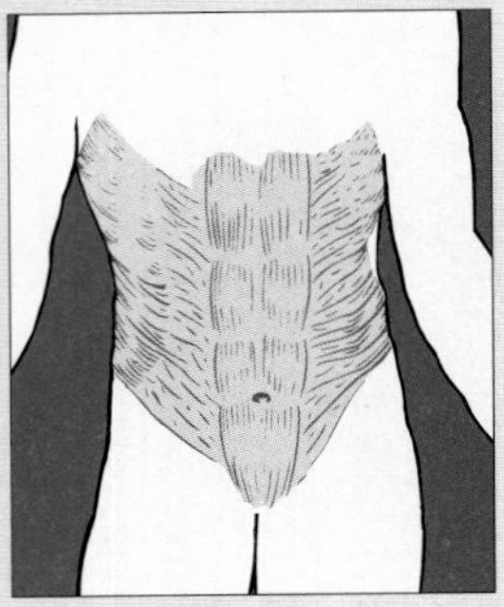

Front

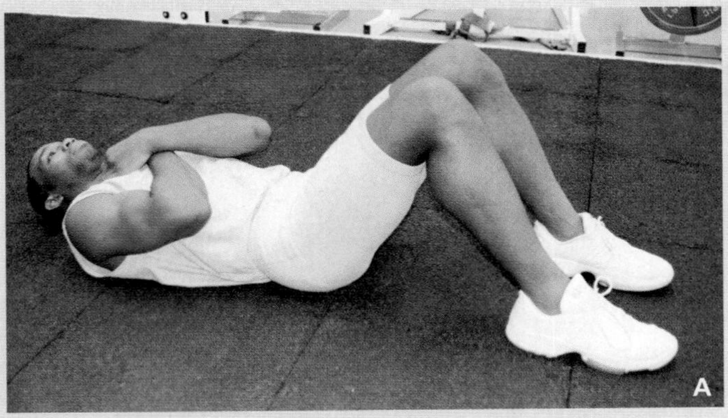

A

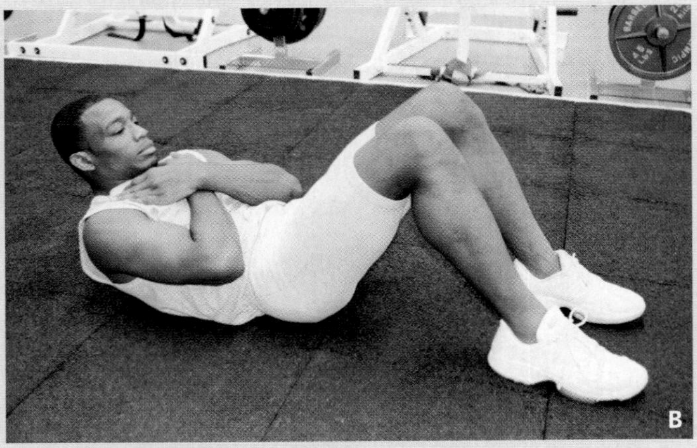

B

Photos Kristin Dilworth

Cybex Abdominal Machine

Muscles developed: Rectus abdominis, abdominal obliques.

Starting position: Start in a seated position with your feet under the anchor straps and your upper chest against the padded exercise bar (A).

Concentric phase: Exhale as you pull with your abdominal muscles to curl your chest toward your hips (B).

Eccentric phase: Inhale as you slowly allow your chest to return to the starting position.

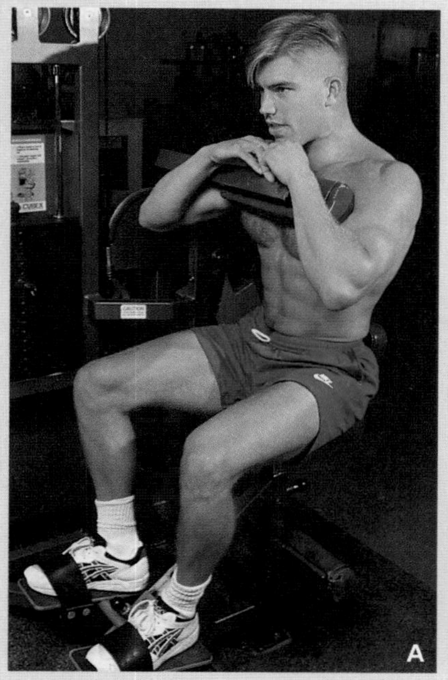
A

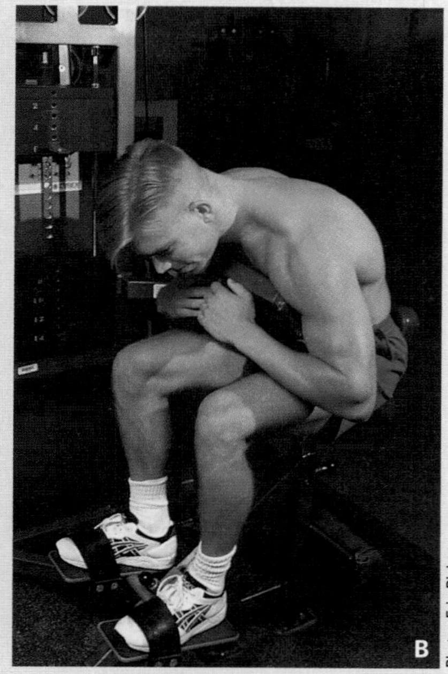
B

Photos Eric Risberg

Nautilus Abdominal Crunch Machine

Muscles developed: Rectus abdominis, abdominal obliques.

Starting position: Start in a seated position with your upper back against the padded exercise bar. Fasten the seat belt and grasp the handles on the exercise bar.

Concentric phase: Exhale as you pull with your abdominal muscles to curl your chest toward your hips.

Eccentric phase: Inhale as you slowly allow your chest to return to the starting position.

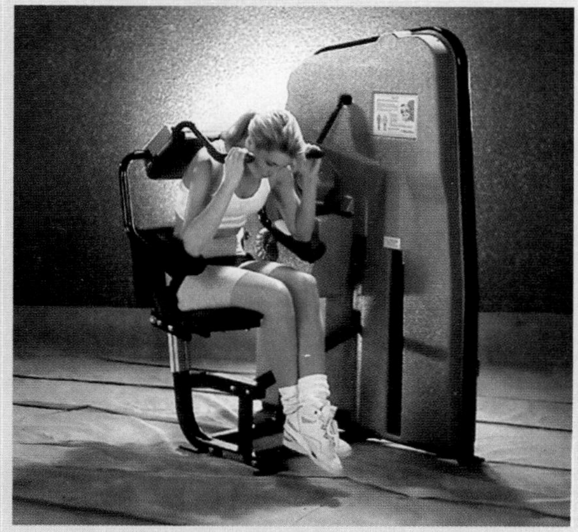

Photos © Nautilus Sports/Medical Industries, Inc.

TRUNK AND HIP FLEXION (ABDOMINALS AND HIP FLEXORS)

Sit-Ups

Muscles developed: Rectus abdominis, iliopsoas, abdominal obliques, rectus femoris.

Starting position: Start flat on your back with your knees bent and both feet flat on the floor; place your fingertips on the opposite shoulder (A).

Concentric phase: Exhale as you slowly pull your head, neck, shoulders, upper back, and lower back off the floor, in that order (B).

Eccentric phase: Slowly return to the starting position by placing your lower back, upper back, shoulders, neck, and head back on the floor, in that order. Inhale as you near the starting position.

Variations:

1. Twisting sit-ups (require trunk flexion and trunk rotation): Curl up and twist, touching one elbow to the opposite knee. Alternate the direction of the twist on each repetition.

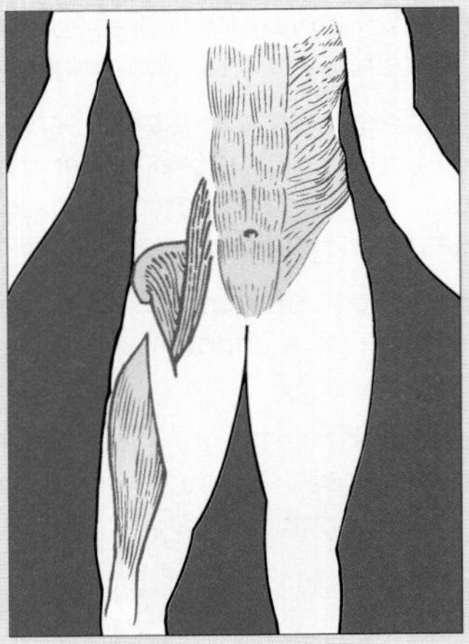

Front

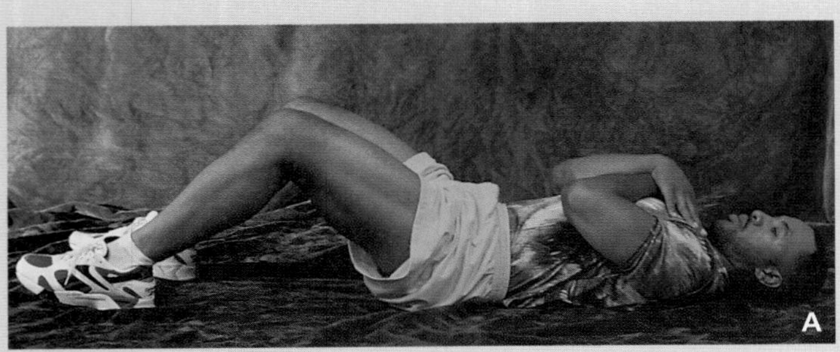

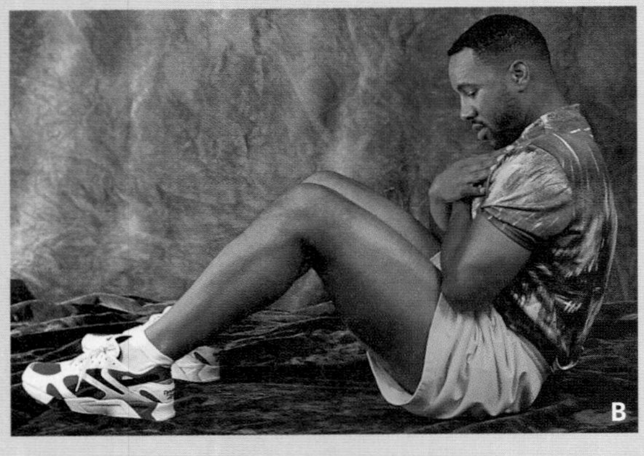

2. Change your arm position, or add weight. If you add weight, place it on your upper chest and hold it in place with your hands.

3. As you add weights, you probably will have to anchor your feet by placing them under something or by having someone hold them.

Additional information: This exercise requires the use of the hip flexors near the end of the concentric phase of the exercise, which does not seem to be a problem if the trunk is fully flexed first.

Caution: Do not pull with the hip flexor muscles until the abdominal muscles are fully contracted. Do not pull on your head with your arms.

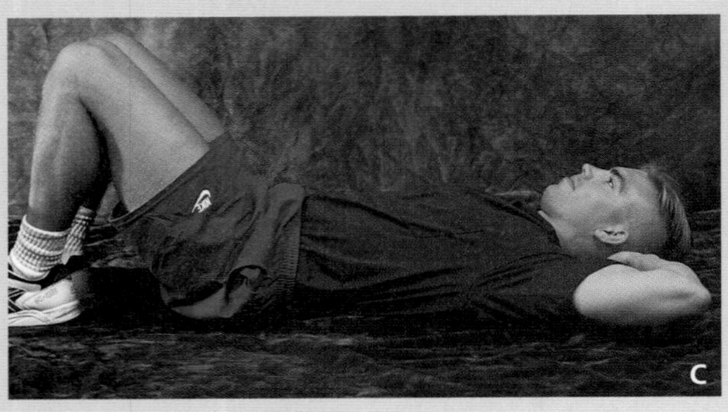

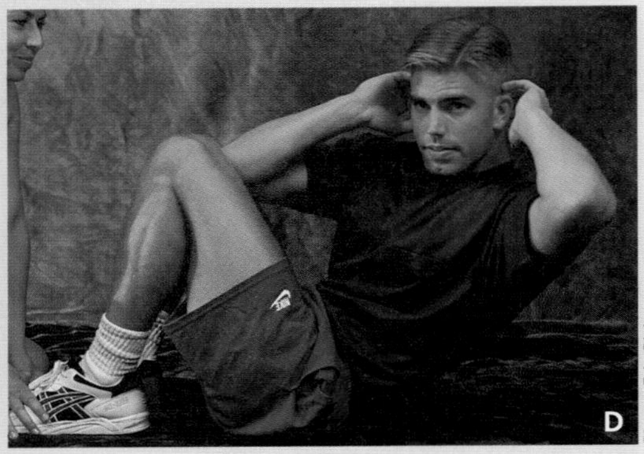

Photos Eric Risberg

Tuck-Ups

Muscles developed: Rectus abdominis, abdominal obliques, iliopsoas.

Starting position: Start on your back with your legs extended and your arms extended overhead (A).

Concentric phase: Exhale as you flex your trunk, hips, and knees while bringing your arms and chest toward your legs. Finish in a tucked sitting position (B).

Eccentric phase: Inhale as you return slowly to the starting position.

Variations: The "V Sit-Up": Keep your arms and legs extended as you raise them, and touch your fingers to your toes as they reach the top of the upward motion.

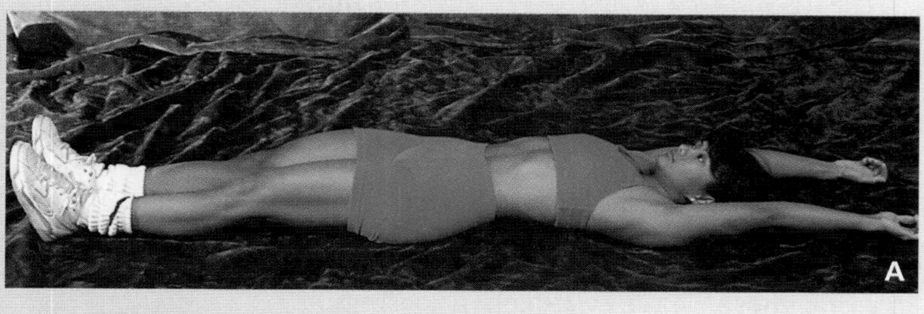

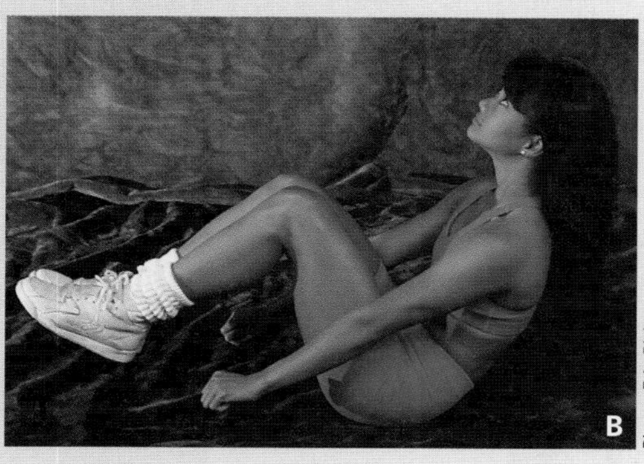

Photos Eric Risberg

Reverse Crunches

Muscles developed: Rectus abdominis, abdominal obliques.

Starting position: Start on your back, and bend your hips and knees so that your feet are flat on the floor; place your arms by your sides (A).

Concentric phase: Exhale as you slowly pull your knees toward your shoulders. Lift your hips and lower back off the floor. Focusing on the abdominal muscles, pull the pelvic girdle toward the rib cage (B).

Caution: Do not roll back on your head and neck; stay on your upper back and shoulders.

Eccentric phase: Inhale as you slowly return to the starting position.

Variations:

1. Start with your legs straight. Pull your heels toward your hips first, then pull your knees toward your shoulders.

2. Twisting reverse crunches. Try to pull one knee toward the opposite shoulder. Alternate the direction of the twist on each repetition.

Caution: Perform this exercise in a controlled manner. Vigorous twisting of the trunk can result in injury to the spinal column.

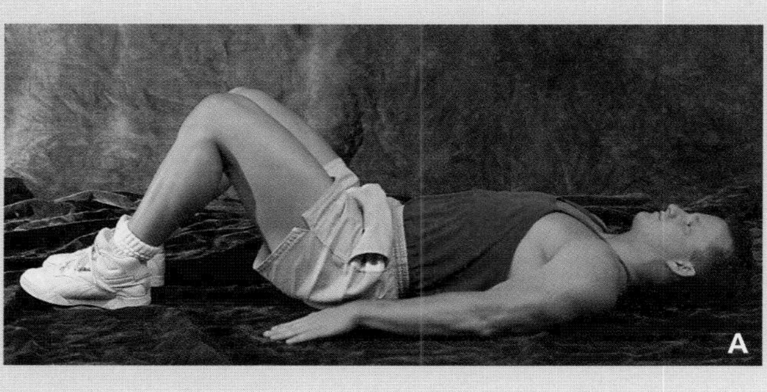

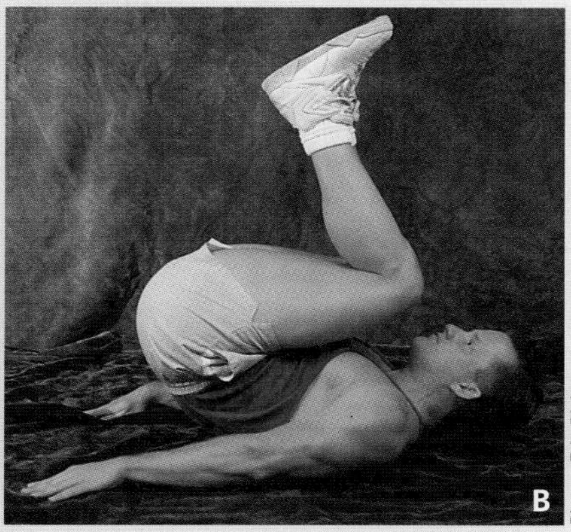

Photos Eric Risberg

Seated Reverse Crunches

Muscles developed: Rectus abdominis, abdominal obliques, iliopsoas.

Starting position: Sit on the edge of a bench or chair. Lean back with your shoulders, straighten your legs, and lift both feet off of the floor (A).

Concentric phase: Exhale as you bring your knees up toward your shoulders (B).

Eccentric phase: Inhale as you return your legs slowly to the starting position.

Variations:

1. Keep your hips and knees bent throughout the exercise. From this position with your legs tucked up, curl or crunch the pelvic girdle toward the rib cage, then return to the starting position but do not extend at the knee or hip joints.

2. Follow variation 1, except twist the torso so that you pull one shoulder toward the opposite knee. Alternate the twisting motion on each repetition.

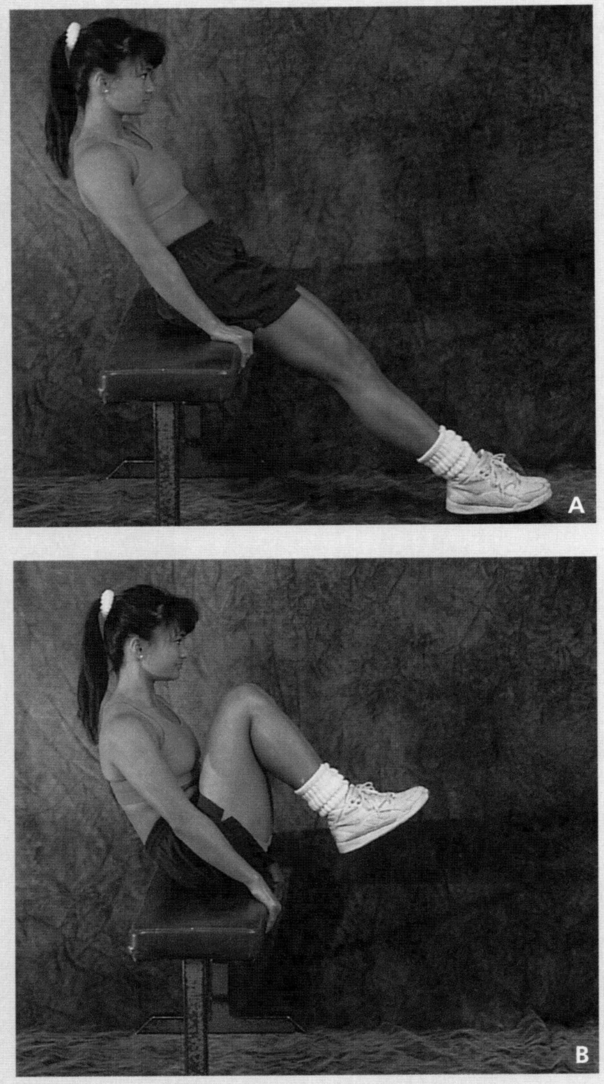

Photos Eric Risberg

Hanging Reverse Crunches or Hanging Knee Raises

Muscles developed: Rectus abdominis, abdominal obliques, iliopsoas.

Starting position: Hang from your hands (A).

Concentric phase: Exhale as you bring your knees up toward your shoulders (B).

Eccentric phase: Inhale as you return your legs slowly to the starting position.

Variations:

1. Lift your knees up and keep them up while you do abdominal crunches.

2. Add a twisting motion as you near the completion of the knee raise so that one knee is pulled toward the opposite shoulder. Alternate the twisting motion on each repetition.

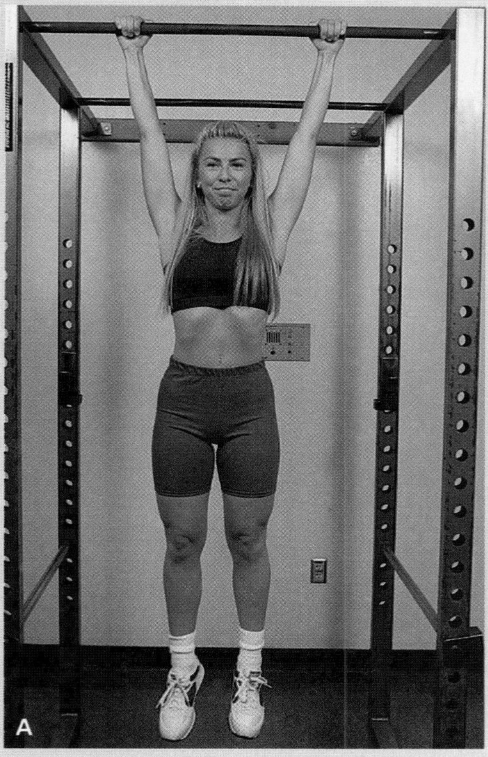

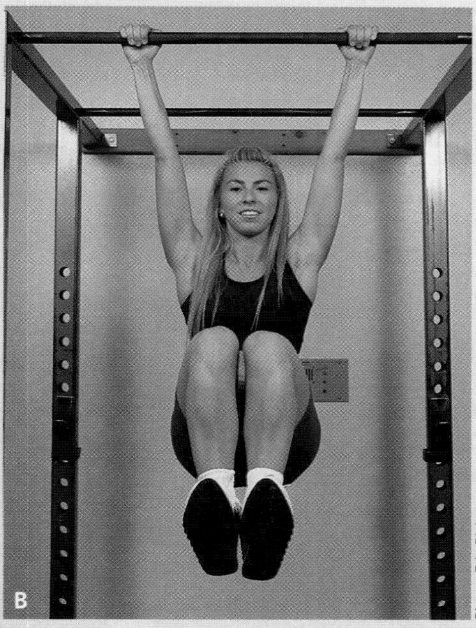

Photos Eric Risberg

TRUNK EXTENSION (ERECTOR SPINAE)

Back Extension

Muscles developed: Erector spinae.

Starting position: Start on a flat exercise bench with the front of your legs and hips on the bench and with your upper body beyond the end of the bench (A). Have someone hold your feet.

Concentric phase: Inhale as you raise your upper body to a position in which your back is parallel to the floor (B).

Eccentric phase: Exhale as you return slowly to the starting position.

Additional information: You may use a specially designed back extension bench if you have one available.

Variations:

1. Place your hands on your lower back with your palms up.

2. Cross your arms on your chest

3. Place your hands behind your head. As your arms move away from your waist and toward your head, the resistance increases.

4. If you wish to add additional resistance, hold a barbell plate behind your head or on your chest.

Caution: Perform this exercise in a smooth and controlled manner. Do not raise your head and shoulders above parallel or arch your back.

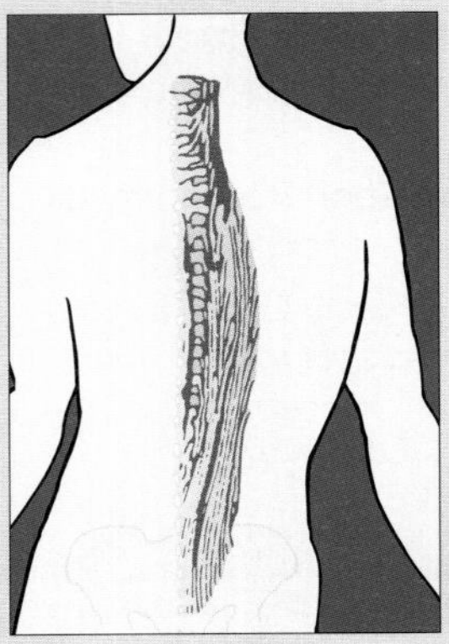

Back

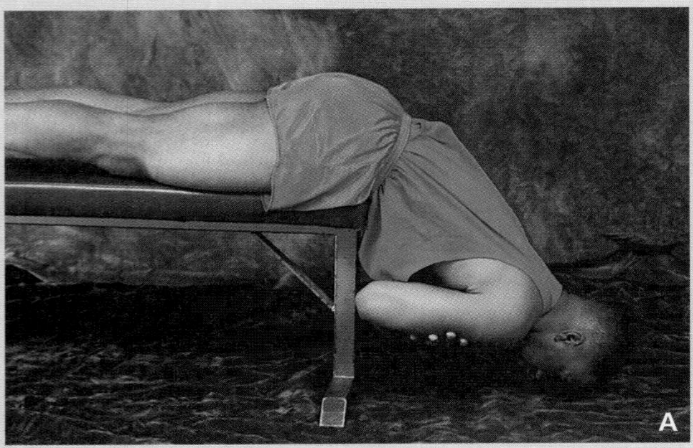

A

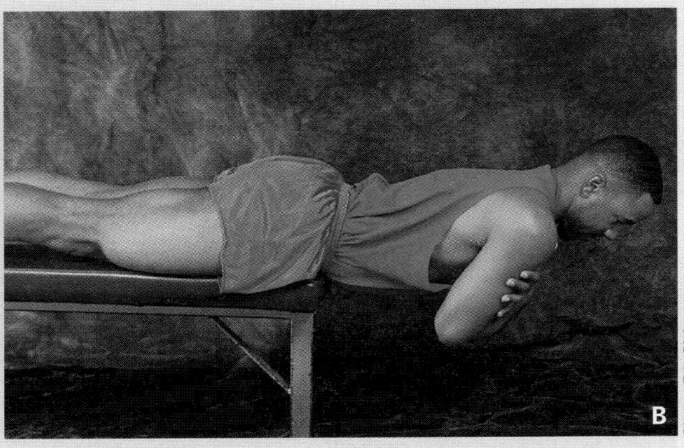

B

Photos Eric Risberg

Cybex Seated Back Extension Machine

Muscles developed: Erector spinae.

Starting position: Start in a seated position leaning forward with your feet on the foot plate. Cross your arms on your chest or place your hands on the front of your thighs (A). Your upper back should be against the padded exercise bar.

Concentric phase: Inhale as you press backward and extend your back (B).

Eccentric phase: Exhale as you return slowly to the starting position.

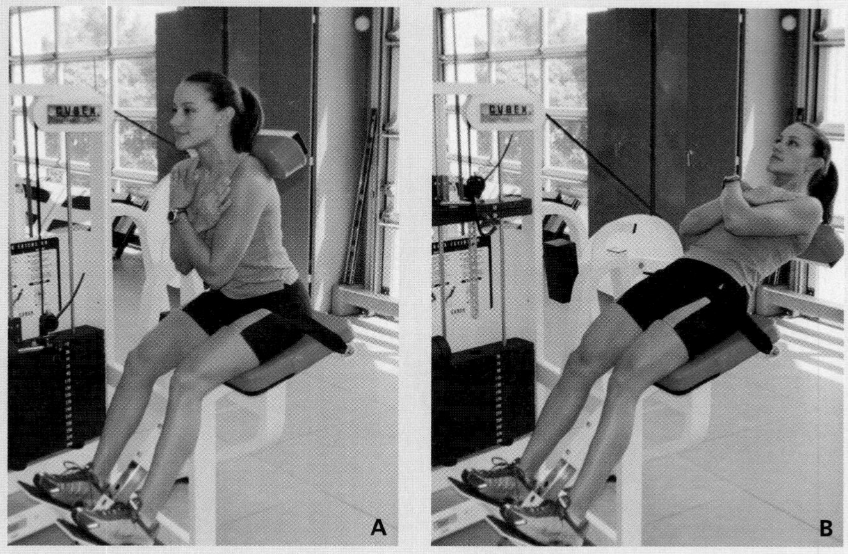

Photos Kristin Dilworth

Cybex Back Extension Machine

Muscles developed: Erector spinae.

Starting position: Start in a seated position, leaning forward with your feet on the foot plate. Cross your arms on your chest or place your hands on the front of your thighs (A). Your upper back should be against the padded exercise bar.

Concentric phase: Inhale as you press backward and extend your back (B).

Eccentric phase: Exhale as you return slowly to the starting position.

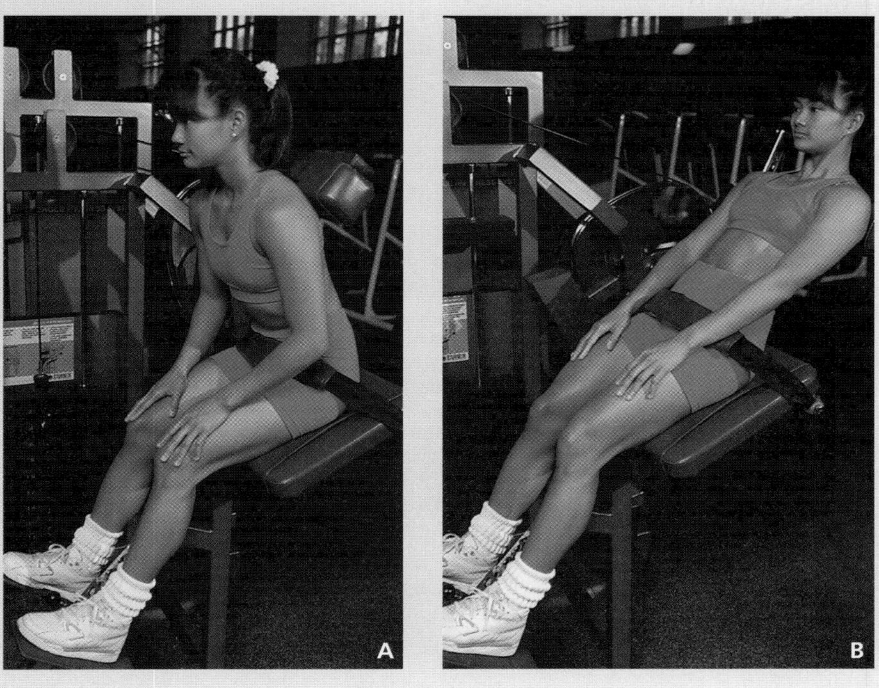

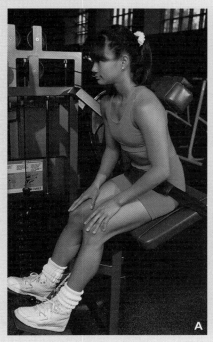

Photos Eric Risberg

The Ab Solution

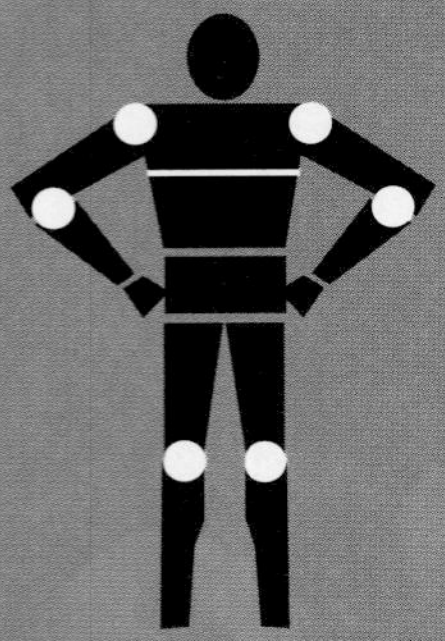

A question people frequently ask, while pointing to their protruding abdomen, is: "How can I get rid of this?" If you want to reduce your waist circumference, you will need to work on the following three things. You probably are aware of the first two already, but the last one might surprise you.

1. Reduce your stored body fat.
2. Increase your abdominal muscle strength and muscle tone.
3. Improve your posture.

Reduce

If you have excess body fat on your abdomen, you should:

- Burn more calories than you consume.
- Eat healthy, but eat less than you do now.
- Increase your aerobic activity to burn more calories per day.
- Engage in a progressive resistance exercise program (weight training) to build more muscle, and to increase your metabolic rate.

Strengthen

Your abdomen also might be bulging because of weak abdominal muscles. The earlier part of this chapter contains exercises to strengthen your abdominal muscles.

Posture

Change, as you probably know, takes a long time, but if you would like to reduce your waist by 1 or 2 inches immediately, try this: stand up straight, lift your chest, pull your shoulders back, and pull your abdomen in. Poor posture is a major contributing factor for a protruding abdomen. To reinforce good posture, add the following exercises to your regular weight-training program.

1. Perform deep-breathing straight-arm pull-overs with a light to moderate weight to lift and stretch your rib cage. Refer to Chapter 8, Chest Exercises, to learn the steps in performing this exercise.
2. Perform a rowing exercise with a moderate weight and concentrate on squeezing your elbows together and pulling your shoulders back in the fully contracted position. Hold this position for 3 seconds and squeeze your shoulder blades together to develop the muscles that pull your shoulders back. Refer to Chapter 9, Back Exercises, to learn how to perform rowing exercises.
3. Perform a back extension exercise to develop the erector spinae muscles, which—as the name implies—cause the spine to be erect and pull the spine into good posture. Refer to the back extension exercises in this chapter.
4. For a few minutes each day, probably in a private place, put a hardbound book on the top of your head and practice standing, sitting, and walking with good posture.

The Ab solution, in sum, is a combination of

- reducing your stored body fat,
- increasing your abdominal muscle strength,
- improving your posture.

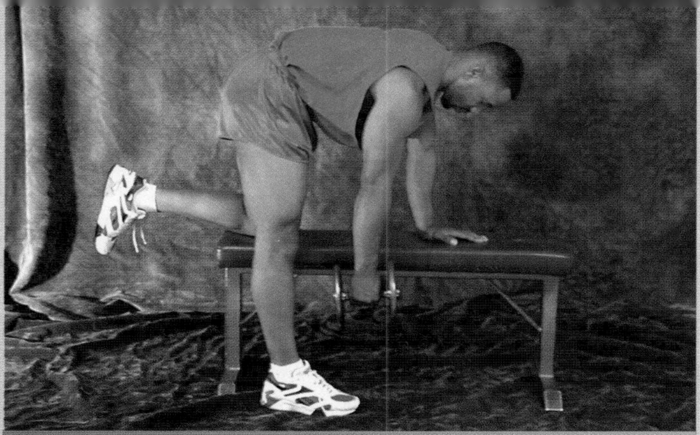
Eric Risberg

14

Record Keeping and Measuring Progress

Accurate record keeping is necessary to measure your progress and evaluate the success of your training program.

Record Keeping

It is important to record each training session. Write down what you do during each workout immediately after you do it.

Weight training is not an exact science. Although weight training adheres to some general guidelines, many variables affect your progress. Each individual is different and responds differently to a weight training stimulus. The information you record during your training sessions can be a valuable source of information about your personal response to a variety of weight training exercises. From this, you will be able to look back through your records and compare your progress using various training methods and exercises. This will help you find which exercises and training methods work best for you. The important things to record are:

- Name of each exercise.
- Order in which exercises are performed.
- Resistance used in each set.
- Repetitions completed in each set.
- Day of the week.
- Date.
- A general comment about how you felt or anything that might have influenced your training that day, positive or negative (for example, "felt tired, 2 hours sleep").

Keeping track of your weight training sessions helps to provide motivation and to ensure the correct exercise stimulus. From the written record of what you were able to do during the previous training session comes a challenge to

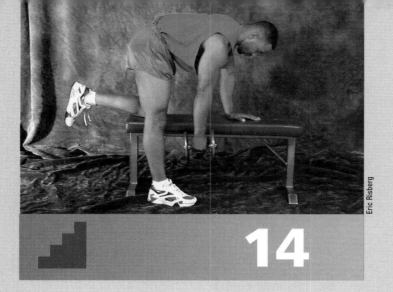

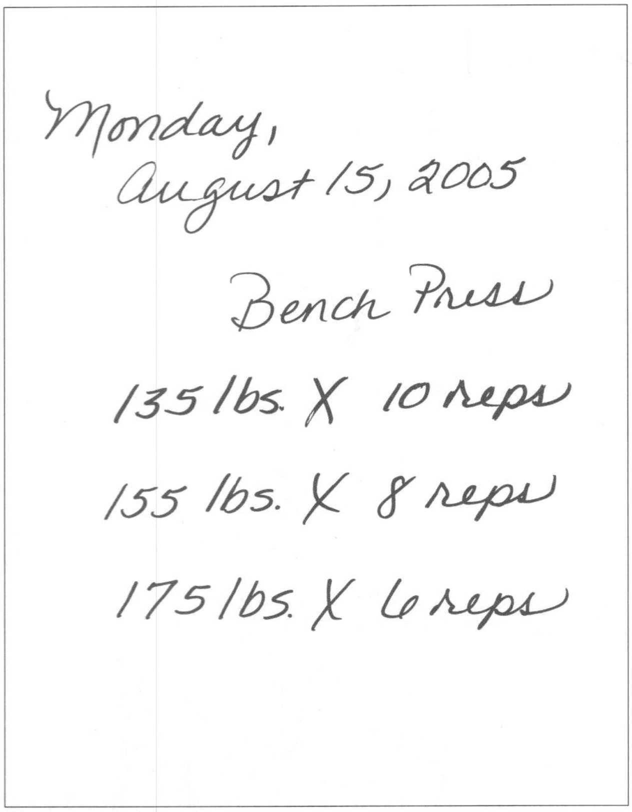
Monday,
August 15, 2005
Bench Press
135 lbs. X 10 reps
155 lbs. X 8 reps
175 lbs. X 6 reps

Figure 14.1 Open-page log.

do a little bit more—one more repetition or 5 more pounds. Figures 14.1 and 14.2 provide examples of written record keeping—the first informal and the second a printed form.

Measuring Progress

The specific measurements recorded are strength, muscular endurance, size, body weight, and body fat.

Measuring Strength

Strength is the ability of a muscle to exert force. If you are training with weights to gain strength, you can measure your progress in at least two common ways:

1. Workout repetition maximums.
2. One-repetition maximums.

Weight training for maximum strength gain requires that you lift relatively heavy weight (85% to 100% of your one-repetition maximum) for relatively low repetition maximums (1-RM to 6-RM). Your repetition maximum (RM) is the maximum amount of weight you can lift for a given number of repetitions. For example, if you can complete 5 repetitions with 155 pounds but cannot do another repetition, your 5-RM is 155 pounds. After a few more workouts, if you can complete 5 repetitions with 160 pounds, you have increased your strength as indicated by the increase in your 5-RM.

Another way to test your progress is by testing your one-repetition maximum (1-RM) periodically using the exercises you perform in your training program. Your 1-RM is the heaviest weight you can lift one time while maintaining correct exercise technique. You will be limited to the heaviest weight you can lift through the weakest point in the range of motion. But you will still find the heaviest weight you can lift one time, and this is a measurement of your ability to exert force (strength).

The first time you test your 1-RM, start with a light weight and perform 10 repetitions to warm up. Then add weight to each subsequent set and perform one repetition in each set until you find the heaviest weight you can lift correctly one time. Try to find your 1-RM within five or six sets. To find your maximum strength, you need to perform enough sets for the muscles to be warmed up but not so many that the muscles are fatigued.

To perform 1-RM strength tests after the first time, start with a warm-up set of 10 repetitions with 60% of your previous 1-RM. Then perform one repetition each at 80%, 85%, 90%, and 95% of your previous 1-RM. After these progressively heavier sets, try for a new personal record based upon how the 95% load felt. If the 95% felt easy, you may want to try 10 pounds more than your previous 1-RM. If the 95% set was very hard, you may want to try just 2½ pounds or 5 pounds more than your previous 1-RM. Rest about 2 minutes between each set, and 3 to 5 minutes before attempting your new personal record.

If you fail to maintain correct exercise form on a strength test so you can lift a heavier weight, you are lying to yourself about your true strength. You also have a greater risk of injury when you attempt to lift a weight heavier than you can really handle. Always use spotters for the exercises in which you could get trapped under a heavy weight.

As a beginning weight trainer, you might want to test 1-RMs once a month for the first 6 to 12 months. After that, increases come more slowly, so testing once every 2 or 3 months might be adequate. You also may choose not to test your 1-RM strength at all. If 1-RM strength is not important, interesting, or motivating to you, you probably have no reason to test it. You need not risk injury or failure attempting 1-RM lifts if it is not important to you.

STRENGTH AND MUSCULAR ENDURANCE PROGRESS LOG

Name: ______________________ Section: ______________________

Date	23 Sept 2005													
Exercise	Wt	Rep	Wt	Rep	Wt	Rep	Wt	Rep	Wt	Rep	Wt	Rep	Wt	Rep
Bench Press	135	10												
	155	8												
	175	6												

Figure 14.2 Sample form for record keeping.

Measuring Muscular Endurance

Muscular endurance is the ability of a muscle to exert force for a long time or for many repetitions. If you are training with weights to gain muscular endurance, you can measure your progress by performing as many consecutive repetitions as possible with an established weight.

Select a weight that is at least 50% but not more than 70% of your 1-RM. Perform as many continuous repetitions as possible without pausing between repetitions. Maintain strict exercise form. Repeat this test once a month, using the same weight every time. An increase in the number of repetitions you can complete is evidence of an increase in your muscle endurance.

Measuring Size

The most common way to measure changes in muscle size is to measure the circumference of various body parts using a tape measure. Although circumference measurements include many other kinds of tissue (bone, fat, blood vessels, skin, and so on), muscle and fat are the two tissues that change the most. If you are training your muscles hard and eating properly, circumference gains should be a result of increased muscle and losses should be a result of decreased fat.

If you measure yourself, you can take measurements anytime you want and the same person will be taking the measurements in the same way every time. A Gulick tape measure is ideal if one is available, as it has a spring tension device on the end that enables you to take all measurements with the same tension on the tape. If a Gulick tape is not available, you can take measurements with a standard cloth tape measure. Place the tape around the circumference so it is firm but not so tight that the skin is indented. Measure to the nearest eighth of an inch or half centimeter.

Measurements commonly taken by men and women who wish to change their appearance are given here. These represent the circumference measurements that are most likely to change in response to a weight training program. For some body parts two measurements—relaxed and flexed—are described. If you are trying to lose excess body fat, use the relaxed measurements. If you are trying to gain muscle size, use the flexed measurements. Take the measurements while you are in a standing position with your feet about 6 inches apart. The tape measure should be horizontal unless the directions for a body part specify something different.

Neck *relaxed*: Measure the horizontal circumference midway between the shoulders and the head.

Chest *relaxed*: Measure at the largest circumference during relaxed breathing. Do not lift your chest or flex your muscles.

Chest *flexed* (expanded): Measure at the largest circumference of the chest with the lungs filled, rib cage lifted, and muscles flexed.

Waist *relaxed*: Measure the horizontal circumference at the level of the navel. The abdominal muscles should be in their normal state of tonus for a relaxed standing position.

Waist *flexed*: Measure the horizontal circumference with the abdomen pulled in as far as possible.

Hips *relaxed*: Measure at the largest horizontal circumference.

Hips *flexed*: Tighten the muscles in the hip region, and measure at the largest horizontal circumference.

For all of the following arm and leg measurements, hold the tape perpendicular to the limb segment being measured. Measure both arms and both legs.

Thigh *relaxed*: Measure the horizontal circumference midway between the hip joint and the knee joint.

Thigh *flexed*: Slightly bend the knee joint and contract all of the thigh muscles. Measure midway between the hip joint and the knee joint.

Calf or leg *relaxed*: Measure at the largest circumference.

Calf or leg *flexed*: Measure the largest circumference with the muscles of the leg flexed.

Upper arm *relaxed*: With the arms hanging relaxed, measure the horizontal circumference midway between the shoulder joint and the elbow joint.

Upper arm *flexed*: Raise your arm to shoulder height and to the side of your body. Bend your elbow and flex all of the muscles of the upper arm. Measure the largest circumference.

Forearm *relaxed*: With your arm hanging in a normal relaxed position, measure the largest circumference of the forearm, between the wrist and the elbow.

Forearm *flexed*: Bend your elbow and wrist so that as many forearm muscles as possible can be contracted. Measure at the largest circumference between the wrist and the elbow.

All of these measurements should be taken the first time you measure. After that you may choose to measure just the ones in which you are the most interested. Beginning weight trainers might want to measure once a month for the first year. After the first year, changes tend to come more slowly, so you might want to take measurements once every 2 or 3 months. How often you measure is up to you. It is your training program.

The measurements suggested here are ones that are commonly used. Because they are used to measure your progress—muscle gain or fat loss—they should be taken exactly the same way each time and, if possible, with the same tape measure. These measurements are taken to provide information about the effectiveness of your training program.

Measuring Body Weight

If your goal is to change your body weight, this can be measured on an accurate scale. It is best to use the same scale, at the same time of day, wearing as little clothing as possible and the same clothing each time. A scale measures your total body weight but does not differentiate between muscle and fat.

Estimating Body Fat

The percentage of total body weight that is stored as body fat, called *percent body fat*, can be measured in many ways. All of the methods have advantages and disadvantages, and many factors can affect the accuracy of body fat estimates. You should keep in mind that this measurement is an estimate, with an error range.

Rather than estimating percent body fat, you can have *skinfold measurements* taken at the sites where you are most interested in losing excess subcutaneous body fat. If they are taken by someone who is trained and experienced, skinfold measurements can be highly accurate. A reduction in your skinfold measurement at a given site is a fairly certain indication of a loss of stored subcutaneous body fat at that site.

Photographs

Changes in appearance take place gradually and cannot be seen as they occur. Taking photographs of various poses can be an excellent means of periodically checking your progress. A photograph is a good way see yourself as you really are. The photograph should be taken while you are wearing as little clothing as possible, such as a swimsuit. Subsequent photographs should be taken with the same camera, location, position, and distance. Photographs taken before you start training can be highly motivating, and they are fun to have after you have gotten into better shape.

Evaluating Progress

Physical changes take time. Changes usually appear faster in beginners than more experienced exercisers. How often you measure to evaluate your progress is up to you. It is your training program. You are in control.

Genetic Potential

Each individual has some upper limit to the amount of strength or size or muscle endurance he or she can gain. For the beginning weight trainer, gains are relatively easy and fast. As progress continues and gains get close to a person's genetic limit, the gains become more difficult and slower.

One of the most intriguing aspects of weight training is that you have no way of knowing when you have reached your genetic limit, or if *anyone* has ever reached his or her limit. After years of weight training, body builders and strength athletes continue to improve, though the rate of improvement slows.

Problem Solving

When you have not made progress for a long time (2 or 3 months), problem solving is in order. What might be the cause of your lack of progress? Change the one thing that you think is most likely for your lack of progress. Allow 3 or 4 weeks for the change to start making a difference. If you have not progressed after a month, try changing a different variable. Give it time to work.

Changing more than one variable at a time may leave you with more questions than answers. Changing too often (less than 4 to 6 weeks) might not allow enough time to find out what works for you and what does not. Keep in mind that what works for you now may not work when your body adapts to it. Some of the factors to consider in solving a lack of progress in weight training are:

- amount of resistance
- number of repetitions
- number of sets
- rest between sets
- number of exercises per body part
- total number of exercises performed
- order of exercises
- frequency of training
- concentration when exercising
- intensity of training
- regularity of training—hour and day
- motivation level
- nutrition
- rest
- other activities
- mental stress
- drugs
- alcohol
- tobacco

Name ______________________________ Section ______________

Size Measurement

Directions:

Read the discussion on Measuring Size in Chapter 14, Record Keeping and Measuring Progress.

		1st Measurement Date:		2nd Measurement Date:		3rd Measurement Date:		4th Measurement Date:	
Height ⟶									
Weight ⟶									
Neck	(relaxed) ⟶								
Chest	(relaxed) ⟶								
	(flexed) ⟶								
Waist	(relaxed) ⟶								
	(flexed) ⟶								
Hips	(relaxed) ⟶								
	(flexed) ⟶								
Right (R) Left (L)		R	L	R	L	R	L	R	L
Thigh	(relaxed) ⟶								
	(flexed) ⟶								
Calf	(relaxed) ⟶								
	(flexed) ⟶								
Upper Arm	(relaxed) ⟶								
	(flexed) ⟶								
Forearm	(relaxed) ⟶								
	(flexed) ⟶								

Name ______________________________ Section ______________

Strength Measurement

Directions:

1. Read the section Measuring Strength, in Chapter 14, Record Keeping and Measuring Progress.
2. Train with weights for at least 2 weeks before testing your strength.
3. Test your strength every 4 weeks after the first test.
4. Move the weight in a smooth, continuous manner.
5. Maintain strict exercise form.
6. Do **not** hold your breath.
7. Increase the weight for each set.
8. Rest between sets.
9. Rest 3 to 5 minutes before your final record attempt.
10. Start with a light weight that you can lift 10 times. After that first warm-up set, continue increasing the weight and performing one repetition until you reach your one-repetition maximum (1-RM). Try to reach your 1-RM within five or six total sets.
11. Record the date, the exercise, and your 1-RM.
12. Always remember "Safety First." Don't injure yourself attempting 1-RM lifts.

Strength Test	1st Test	2nd Test	3rd Test	4th Test
	Date:	Date:	Date:	Date:
Exercise	Weight	Weight	Weight	Weight

Name ______________________________ Section ______________

Muscle Endurance Measurement

Directions:

1. Read the section on Measuring Muscular Endurance in Chapter 14, Record Keeping and Measuring Progress.
2. Test your strength to find your one-repetition maximum.
3. Select a weight that is approximately 60% of your 1-RM.
4. Perform as many continuous repetitions as possible, with absolutely no pause to rest between repetitions.
5. Move the weight in a smooth, controlled manner.
6. Maintain strict exercise form.
7. Test your muscle endurance every 4 weeks after the first test.
8. Use the same weight for each exercise every time you test yourself for muscle endurance on that exercise. An increase in repetitions using the same weight should indicate an increase in muscle endurance.

Muscle Endurance Test		1st Test Date:	2nd Test Date:	3rd Test Date:	4th Test Date:
Exercise	Weight	Reps	Reps	Reps	Reps

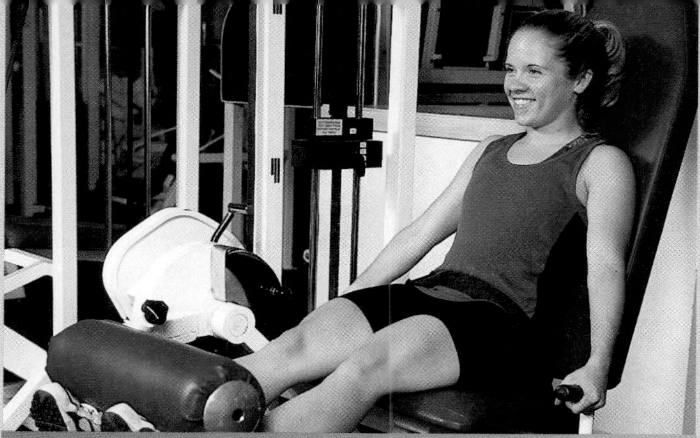

15

Success

"Success" has a different meaning for each person. In this chapter, success is defined as *setting a goal and achieving it*. Successful people achieve goals they have set for themselves. A successful person reaches big success as a result of many smaller successes. Success breeds success. Achieving smaller goals leads to achieving larger goals. This process results in a lifestyle that is as enjoyable as the attainment of each goal. People with personal goals are people with a passion for living. People with goals know what they want out of life and they are going after it.

A Formula For Success

Written Goals

Goals are an extremely important part of any successful weight training program. Putting the necessary effort into weight training is difficult without some desirable goal to be reached. A successful weight training program cannot be planned without a goal. All successful training programs are based on a desired outcome. If you don't have a desired outcome, how can you plan to reach it?

Goals should be as specific as possible. This may be difficult if you are just beginning a new activity such as weight training, but try to be as specific as possible.

Once you decide on a goal, write it down. This is an important step. Make a contract with yourself. Your thoughts and spoken words tend to become modified with the passing of time, but your written goal will remain the same every time you read it. Once you have written your goal, you may begin to steer a course rather than drift aimlessly. Knowing where you want to go, before and during your journey, is important.

After you have a clearly defined written goal, you will find that making decisions is easier. If you know exactly where you want to go, it is a matter of deciding, "Yes, this will take me toward my goal" or "No, this will not take me toward my goal."

To obtain great success or achievement, goals must take into consideration your unique individual qualities. Your goals should be challenging, but attainable, based upon where you are starting and what you believe is possible.

Most people find happiness in striving for and attaining worthwhile goals. Boredom is often the result of not having goals. Some say weight training is boring, or life is boring. People who are bored are probably not working toward goals they are passionate about. If you know what you are trying to accomplish, weight training and life, become exciting adventures—not easy, but certainly not boring. When you stop striving for goals you stop growing.

Positive Thinking

Positive thinking is such an essential ingredient in success that some people have identified it as the *only* ingredient. One reason is that the goal-setting stage is primarily an internal process others do not see. Positive thinking, by contrast, is obvious to everyone who comes in contact with the individual.

Your subconscious mind works on what you feed it. One sure way to short-circuit your success is to set a goal and not believe you can make it. Instead, you should fill your mind with positive thoughts, send out positive thoughts, and resist the negative thoughts of others. Positive people see the good side of bad situations and the bright side of every situation. Is the half glass of water half full or half empty? Your answer to that simple question may reveal a lot about your attitude. Many people dwell upon what they don't have and can't do; others focus upon what they do have and can do.

Your should not strive for success without happiness. It would be an empty success even if your goal is achieved. Successful people enjoy what they are doing. Most people are as happy as they decide to be. Your happiness is based on your internal reaction to external events.

Imagination is stronger than willpower. Form a clear detailed image of what you want. Every creation starts with an idea. If you focus on success, you will succeed. If you focus on failure, you will fail. Positive thoughts create positive results.

Desire is the power behind human action. Successful people have a burning desire to reach their goals. Positive thinking includes belief. Belief is more than wishing, it is knowing.

The Subconscious Mind

We don't know much about the subconscious mind, but we do know it is extremely powerful and it can help solve our problems. The subconscious mind works day and night to bring about what you imagine or visualize. The subconscious mind is the reason positive thinking is so important. If you expect to fail, you will fail. If you expect to succeed, you will succeed.

Your subconscious mind can be programmed through repetition. Repetition can accomplish great tasks. Therefore, you should read your goals aloud at least twice each day, morning and night. Read your weight training goals before each training session so you know why you are there and what you need to do.

You have an opportunity to participate in your own creation. You can become what you want to become. You can be the person you want to be. To put your subconscious mind to work to help you reach the goals you set, use autosuggestion and repeat your desire or goal to yourself regularly. Once an idea is deeply embedded in your subconscious mind it will go to work to help you achieve your goal. Keep a notepad and pencil near for ideas. Solutions will come to you. Write these ideas immediately so you can expand on them later. Often, if they are not written, they are gone. You may remember that you had a great idea but not be able to remember what it was.

A Written Plan

Everyone has the same amount of time each week. Why do some people accomplish more than others? They learn to manage themselves and use their time wisely. Lack of time indicates a lack of organization. Some people say they don't have time to exercise. What they should say is that exercise is less important to them than anything else they do.

Effectiveness means doing the right things. This requires a focus on *results*. Your time should be spent on the things that make a difference. In your weight training program, be sure you are doing the things that lead to the achievement of your goal. Don't waste your time on things that don't matter.

Efficiency means doing things right. This requires a focus on *methods*. Once you are doing the right exercises and you are doing the exercises right, you will be well on your way to reaching your goals.

Time should be planned to continue learning about weight training. The more you learn, the better you can plan to reach your goals.

Take time to plan how you will reach your goals. Evaluate your progress toward your goals. After evaluation, make the necessary adjustments in your plan.

Do It!

All of the previous steps are useless unless you do it. You never get anywhere unless you move. Decide what activities will lead to your goals, then act upon your decision. Learn to act and make things happen instead of reacting to things that happen.

Work and sacrifice are required to reach your goals. There is always a price to pay for anything worthwhile. You almost always have to pay the price in advance. Don't expect to get something for nothing. You must work at success. Once you have decided what must be done, discipline yourself to do it.

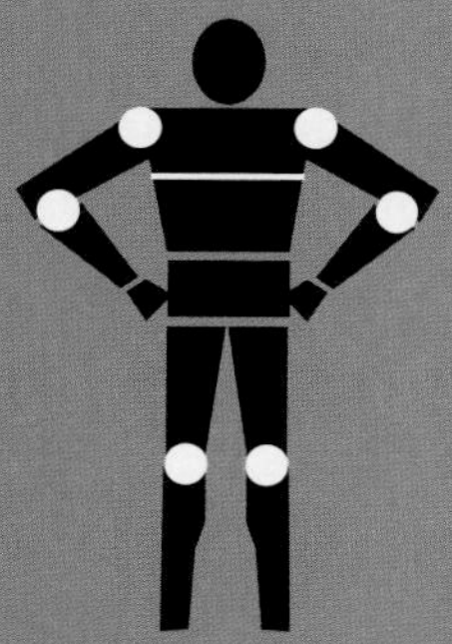

Steps in the Formula for Success

- Develop written goals
  - Set short-term goals that you can achieve that will lead to your long-term goals.
  - Fix in your mind exact, measurable goals.
  - Write your goals.
- Use positive thinking.
  - Believe you can reach your goals.
  - Have faith in your ability to achieve your goals.
- Use your subconscious mind.
  - Read your goals aloud at least twice each day, morning and night.
  - Read your weight training goals before each training session.
- Develop a written plan.
  - Take time to plan so your efforts are directed toward your goals.
  - Evaluate your progress and modify your plan.
- Do it.
  - Start working toward your goal, and don't stop until you reach it.
  - Enjoy the journey as much as the arrival.

Poorly Written Goals	Well Written Goals
Increase my bench press. *(no set amount, no time limit)*	I will bench press 240 pounds one time by ______ (day, month, year)
Firm up my muscles. *(too general; how will you know?)*	I will perform 30 repetitions of the barbell curl using 60 pounds by ______ (day, month, year)
Get in shape. *(too general; how will you measure this?)*	I will have a 28-inch waist by ______ (day, month, year)

Table 15.1 Examples of Poor Goals and Good Goals

One of the most common reasons for failure is failure to take action. Procrastination has caused more failure than any other single factor. Now is the time to take action. The clock is already running and it cannot be stopped or reversed.

Once you get started, you must persist. Persistence is a familiar word but a rare quality. Many who take the first step fail because they do not continue working toward their goal. Stick with it, don't give up, never give up. If your goal is worthwhile, it is worth your best effort.

This formula for success will work for almost anything you want. It is presented in this book to help you reach your weight training goals.

Writing Weight Training Goals

Your goals must be believable, achievable, reasonable, and attainable (Table 15.1). Don't set yourself up for failure by setting unbelievable goals. A goal to bench press 1,000 pounds by the end of this year is not reasonable. A goal to lose 20 pounds of fat by the end of this week is not possible. Set goals that you can sincerely believe in. Once you reach a goal, you can always set a higher goal. Success breeds success.

Goals must be compatible. Running a marathon in 2 hours and performing squats with 800 pounds on the same day are not compatible training goals.

Your weight training goals should be specific and measurable. Set a specific time for their attainment. Complete the "Goal Setting" assignment at the end of this chapter. If you have too many goals at one time you may not be able to reach them all. Rather than setting too many goals at one time, focus on a few goals that are most important to you. However, you can have several short-term goals that all contribute to the same long-term goal.

The goals you set must be your own, not someone else's goals for you. They must be *your* goals, something *you* want.

If you do not want to increase your muscular strength, muscular size, or muscular endurance; if you do not want to perform better, look better, or feel better; if you cannot think of any goal that weight training can help you achieve—you may perceive weight training to be difficult, time-consuming, and boring. However, if you want to increase your muscular strength, muscular size, or muscular endurance; if you want to perform better, look better, or feel better; if you can think of a goal that weight training can help you achieve—you will perceive weight training to be worthwhile and interesting.

Name ______________________________ Section ______________

Goal Setting

Directions:

1. Read Chapter 15, Success.
2. Set weight training goals that are specific, measurable, believable, and compatible.
3. Set a specific date by which you will reach your goals.
4. Set goals that are something you want very much. The greater your desire to reach your goals, the greater your chance of achieving it.
5. Set goals for measurable changes in muscular strength or size or endurance.
6. Write at least one, but no more than three, personal weight training goals. These should be short-term goals that can be reached in the next 3 months.

Goal 1: I will ______________________________

____

____

by ______________________________
(day, month, year)

Goal 2: I will ______________________________

____

____

by ______________________________
(day, month, year)

Goal 3: I will ______________________________

____

____

by ______________________________
(day, month, year)

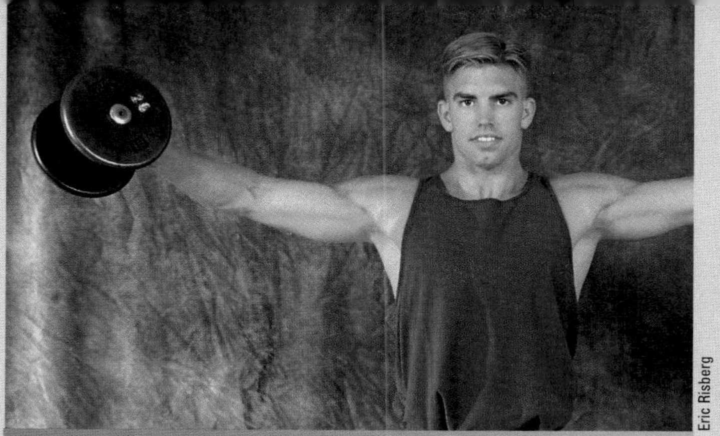

16

Planning Your Personal Weight Training Program

Before planning your personal weight training program, you should review the basic principles that underlie weight training. Then you can proceed to develop a program based on your unique needs.

Basic Weight Training Principles

Three basic principles underlying all weight training progress are specificity, overload, and progression.

Specificity

The *specificity* principle states that you must exercise the specific muscles that you want to develop. You also must follow specific exercise guidelines to produce the specific type of change you want—muscle strength, muscle size, or muscle endurance.

Overload

The *overload* principle is the basis of all training programs. In weight training, overload means that a muscle must be forced to work harder than normal.

Progression

Once your muscles adjust to a given workload, they are no longer overloaded. The workload must be increased gradually as the muscle adapts to each new demand. This is the principle of *progression.*

Considerations in Planning Your Weight Training Program

Your Goals

Planning a weight training program must begin with what you wish to accomplish. You can train for three basic aspects of muscle fitness:

1. Muscle strength.
2. Muscle size.
3. Muscle endurance.

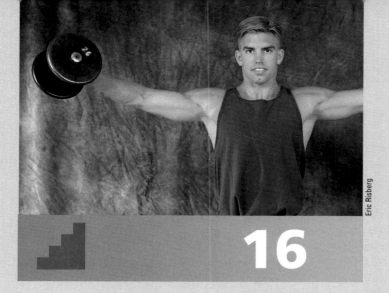

Any weight training program you choose will result in some increase in all three areas. Untrained beginners gain on almost any weight training program as long as it applies the principle of progressive overload. Some general guidelines that have emerged from research and experience will help you focus on developing the aspect of most interest to you.

Which Exercises

Which exercises are the best? The best weight training exercises are *compound exercises.* These exercises require more than one joint and more than one group of muscle to move the weight. With compound exercises, such as the squat and the bench press, large amounts of muscle are exercised at the same time. Exercises that require both arms or both legs to work together allow the use of more weight and maintain a balance of development on both sides of the body.

Almost all weight trainers use the same basic exercises. Some of these common exercises are included in the beginner or basic weight training program in this book.

Overall balanced development should be the goal. This means not ignoring certain body parts or overdeveloping one or two body parts. You should develop both sides of your body equally, and exercise the opposing muscle or muscle group.

In the beginning, if you don't know much about the muscles, the underlying principle is that, for every exercise action or movement you perform, another exercise should produce an opposite action or movement. For example, if you perform an exercise that develops elbow flexion, you also should perform an exercise that develops elbow extension.

Number of Exercises

One exercise per body part is enough for the beginning weight trainer. In fact, one exercise per body part is enough for all but the most advanced, high-level-strength athletes and body builders. One exercise for each major muscle group or body part translates to about 8 to 12 basic exercises in your training program.

Order of Exercises

You should exercise the largest muscles first, then work your way down to increasingly smaller muscles. This is because the largest muscles require the most energy and need the smaller muscles to assist. If the smaller muscles are fatigued first, you will have difficulty handling enough weight to exercise the larger muscles properly. For example, most back exercises require grip strength. If the finger and forearm flexors have been exercised already, they will become fatigued sooner than the larger back muscles. The largest muscles are located on the torso. Proceeding outward on the arms and legs, the muscles get smaller.

The order of exercises also may be based on a *work-rest principle*: If a muscle is worked during an exercise, it is allowed to rest during the next exercise. If you are exercising opposing muscle groups, you may work a muscle, then let it rest as you work on the opposing muscle. This will allow you to complete more work in less time.

Another consideration in the order of exercises is whether to perform a *circuit* or to do the exercises in a traditional (non-circuit) manner. When you perform a circuit, you do each exercise in your training program once in a specified order. Then you perform each exercise again (and possibly again) in that same order. The traditional way of lifting weights is to do all of the sets of one exercise before moving to the next exercise.

Resistance

The amount of weight you use depends upon what you want to develop. The general rule is that for *strength*, you need a heavy weight and few repetitions. For muscle *endurance*, you need a light weight and more repetitions. Muscle *size* development calls for moderate weight and repetitions. Before using heavy weights, you should warm-up with lighter warm-up sets.

Strength
85% to 100% of 1-RM

Muscle size
70% to 85% of 1-RM

Muscle tone
60% to 80% of 1-RM

Muscle endurance
50% to 70% of 1-RM

Starting Weight

Beginners should start with a weight that is light so they can easily perform each exercise correctly. Resistance is increased gradually. Don't be in a big hurry to load up on resistance. If you give your body time to adapt, you will experience more progress, less muscle soreness, less frustration, and more enjoyment. You have plenty of time to add weight if you are *weight training for life*.

Repetitions

The resistance you choose will affect the repetitions you can perform:

Strength
1–6 repetitions

Muscle size
6–12 repetitions

Muscle endurance
12–20+ repetitions

Sets

The resistance and repetitions influence the number of sets you will be able to perform for each exercise:

Strength
4–8 sets

Muscle size
3–6 sets

Muscle endurance
2–4 sets

	Muscle Strength	Muscle Size	Muscle Endurance	Muscle Tone
Resistance	85% to 100% of 1-RM	70% to 85% of 1-RM	50% to 70% of 1-RM	60% to 80% of 1-RM
Repetitions	1 to 6 RM	6 to 12 RM	12 to 20+ RM	8 to 12 RM
Sets	4 to 8	3 to 6	2 to 4	1 to 3
Rest (between sets)	2 to 4 minutes	1 to 2 minutes	30 to 90 seconds	30 to 60 seconds

Table 16.1 Summary of Weight Training Guidelines

Rest

The amount of rest between sets is determined by what you are trying to develop:

Strength
2–4 minutes

Muscle size
1–2 minutes

Muscle endurance
30–90 seconds

Frequency

A muscle usually requires 2 or 3 days of rest to recover and adapt before it should be exercised again. Exercising a muscle 3 days per week with 48 to 72 hours of rest between training sessions works well for most weight trainers. Advanced weight trainers perform different exercises on different days, so they may exercise 4, 5, or 6 days a week; however, they do not exercise the same muscles two days in a row.

Fixed or Variable Exercise Load

A load is applied to each exercise in two basic ways—fixed or variable. With a *fixed load,* the resistance, repetitions, sets, and rest interval remain the same (fixed) during a training session for an exercise.

Example: Bench Press
150 pounds
10 repetitions
3 sets
1 minute rest between sets

With a *variable method* of loading, the resistance, repetitions, and rest interval change for each set of an exercise.

Example: Bench Press
150 lbs 10 reps 1 min. rest
170 lbs 8 reps 2 min. rest
190 lbs 6 reps 3 min. rest
210 lbs 4 reps 4 min. rest

Muscle Tone or Muscle Fitness

Beginners often say they just want to tone the muscles. They are not especially interested in developing strength, size, or endurance.

What is muscle tone? When the word "tone" is used in reference to muscle tissue, it refers to muscle tissue that is firm, sound, and resilient. This is in contrast to the loose, flabby, and weak muscle tone of the sedentary person. Although the former is desirable, measuring changes in muscle tone is rather difficult.

Whether a person chooses to train for strength, size, or endurance, it will result in an improvement in muscle tone. Also, if an individual chooses to train for muscle tone, it will lead to some improvement in strength, size, and muscle endurance. These improvements, however, will be more gradual and more difficult to measure.

Some guidelines for those who wish to train for muscle fitness or muscle tone are:

60% to 80% of 1-RM
8 to 12 repetitions
1 to 3 sets of each exercise
30 to 60 seconds rest between sets
3 days per week (every other day)

Although training for muscle tone is possible, the lack of measurable progress can result in a loss of motivation for beginners. Therefore, beginning weight trainers are advised to work toward changes in strength, size, or muscle endurance, which can be measured more easily. Measured progress is evidence that weight training is effective, and it serves as a motivating influence to continue.

Table 16.1 provides a summary of the weight training guidelines outlined above.

Suggested Lifetime Fitness Weight Training Programs

The following training programs are appropriate for adults as lifetime weight training programs:

1 × 15–20
1 × 8–12
2 × 10
3 × 10
3 × 8
3 × 10, 8, 6

3 × 20, 10, 5
DeLorme 3 × 10

The 1 × 15–20 workout is one in which you perform one set of each exercise and attempt to complete 20 repetitions. If you complete all 20 repetitions in good exercise form, you can increase the weight on that exercise for the next training session. You always should be able to complete at least 15 good repetitions. If you cannot complete at least 15 repetitions, the weight is too heavy. If you can complete more than 20 repetitions, the weight is too light.

The 1 × 8–12 workout is the same as the previous workout except that you should be able to get at least 8 repetitions, and you should increase the weight if you can get more than 12 good repetitions. This and the previous workout are two fast weight training programs for those who do not want to spend much time weight training.

The 2 × 10, 3 × 10, and 3 × 8 workouts can be performed using the same weight for two or three sets with a short 1- or 2-minute rest between sets. If you are able to complete all of the repetitions in every set, you can increase the weight for the next training session.

The 3 × 10, 8, and 6 workout consists of three sets. The first set calls for 10 repetitions, the second set, 8 repetitions. In the third set you perform 6 repetitions. Each set is done with a heavier weight.

The 3 × 20, 10, 5 workout includes three sets of each exercise. The first set calls for 20 repetitions. Twenty repetitions will provide a good warm-up, as well as a stimulus for developing muscle endurance. The second set calls for 10 repetitions. Ten repetitions will provide some stimulus for muscle endurance gain, some stimulus for muscle size gain, and some stimulus for strength gain. The third set calls for 5 repetitions. The first two sets should ensure that the muscles and joints are warmed up and ready for this heavier load. Five repetitions with a heavy resistance will provide a stimulus for strength gain.

The DeLorme 3 × 10 workout consists of three sets of 10 repetitions:

1st set: 10 reps with 50% of 10 RM

2nd set: 10 reps with 75% of 10 RM

3rd set: 10 reps with 100% of 10 RM

The first set of 10 repetitions should be performed with 50% of your 10-repetition maximum (10-RM). (Your 10-repetition maximum is the heaviest weight you can lift 10 times.) The second set of 10 repetitions should be performed with 75% of your 10-repetition maximum. The third set should be performed with 100% of your 10-repetition maximum. When you can complete 10 repetitions in the third set, the weight used in that set is raised for the next training session and the first two sets are adjusted according to this new 10-RM. You should be able to get about 8 repetitions in the last set with the new weight. Keep working with that weight until you can get 10 good repetitions. Then increase the weight again. You should never get fewer than 6 good repetitions in the last set. If you cannot get at least 6 good repetitions, you have increased the weight too much and should reduce the weight for the next training session.

The DeLorme method is fast and easy on weight-stack machines but involves quite a bit of weight-changing when using barbells, especially when alternating sets with a training partner. Based on the information presented in this chapter, complete "Planning Your Personal Weight Training Program" using the form provided at the end of this chapter.

A Simple Home Training Program for Busy People

This is a simple training program you can do at home. It takes very little time and very little money, but it can make a very big difference. The only equipment required is a set of two adjustable-weight dumbbells and a flat exercise bench. These items often appear inexpensively at garage sales. The eight exercises are as follows:

Chest Dumbbell Bench Press
Back One-Dumbbell Rowing

Shoulders Seated Dumbbell Lateral Raise

Arms (Biceps) Seated Dumbbell Arm Curls

Arms (Triceps) Seated One-Dumbbell Triceps Extension

Hips and Thighs Dumbbell Lunges

Lower Leg One-Dumbbell Calf Raise

Abdominals Crunches

Perform these exercises every other day. If it takes 1 minute to perform each exercise and 1 minute between exercises, to rest and change the weight for the next exercise, you would complete this workout in 16 minutes. Realistically, plan on 20 minutes, especially as the resistance increases. For better total fitness results, perform 20 minutes of continuous aerobic exercise on nonlifting days. Convenient, inexpensive aerobic exercises include walking, jogging, and stair-stepping at home.

If this is still too time-consuming, split the weight training program by performing the upper body exercises one day (the first five exercises) and the lower body exercises the next day (the last three exercises). The upper body workout would take approximately 10 minutes every other day, and the lower body workout would take about 6 minutes every other day.

During the first month, perform one set of 20 repetitions of each exercise. The second month, perform one set of 15 repetitions of each exercise. The third month, perform one set of 12 repetitions of each exercise. After 3 months, you might want to just maintain on this workout or you might want to try some of the other set and repetition combinations suggested in this chapter.

Dumbbell Bench Press
(see page 60)

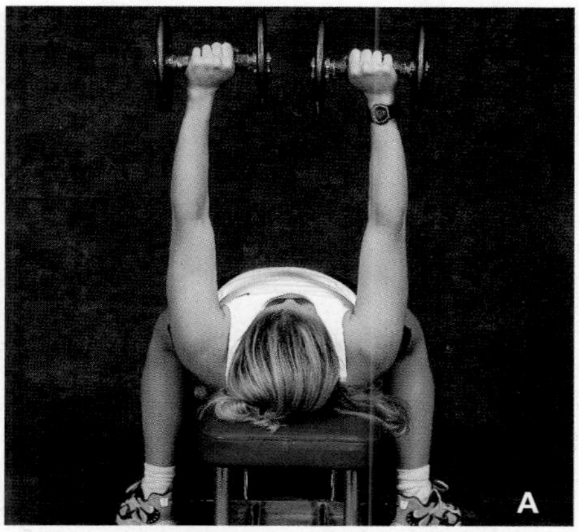

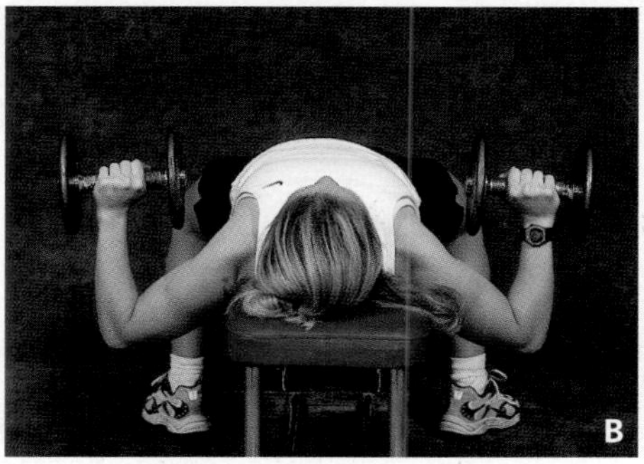

Photos Jon Kelley

One-Dumbbell Rowing
(see page 70)

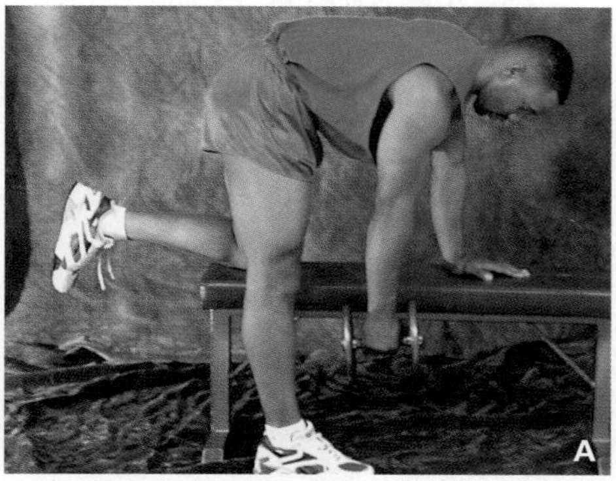

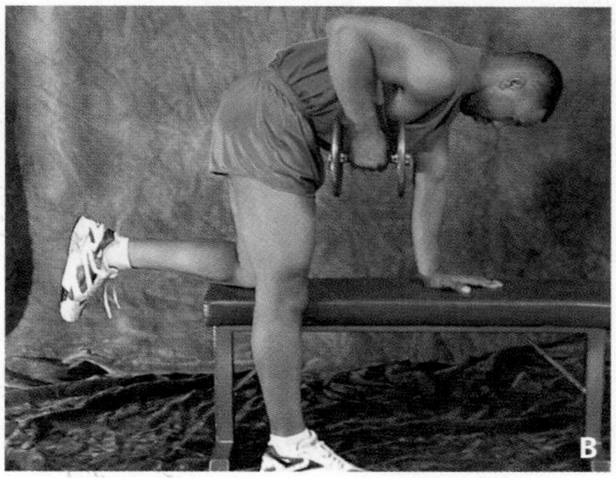

Photos Eric Risberg

Dumbbell Lateral Raise
(see page 82)

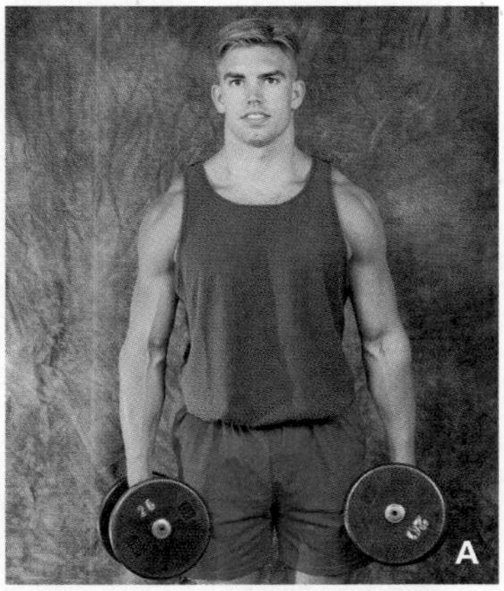

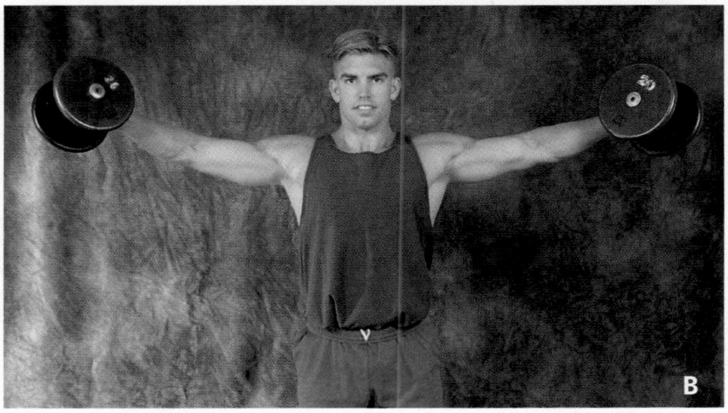

Photos Eric Risberg

Seated Dumbbell Arm Curl
(see page 88)

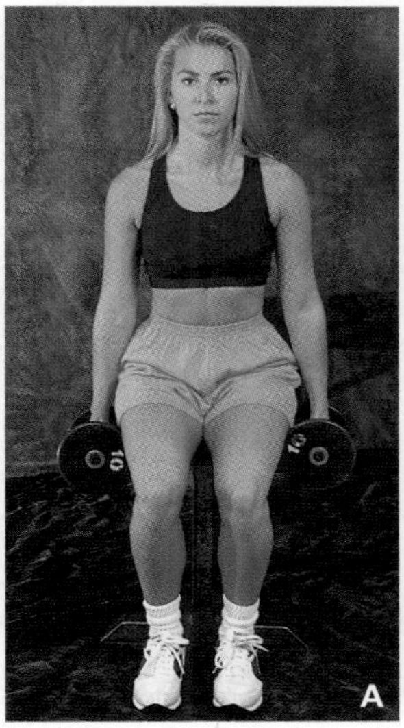

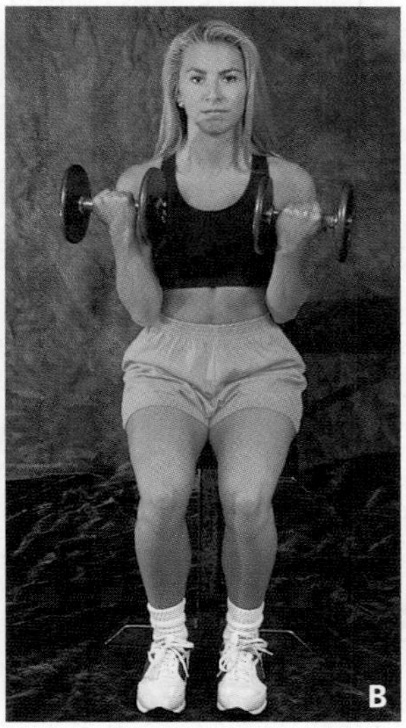

Photos Eric Risberg

Seated One-Dumbbell Triceps Extension
(see page 92)

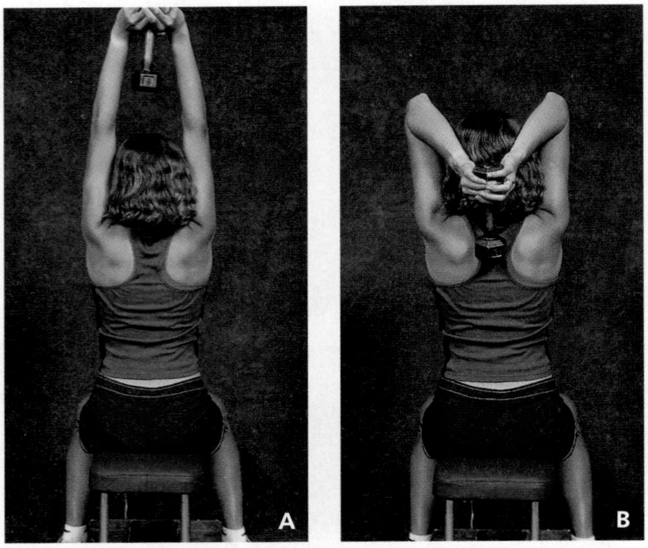

Photos Jon Kelley

Dumbbell Lunges
(see page 106)

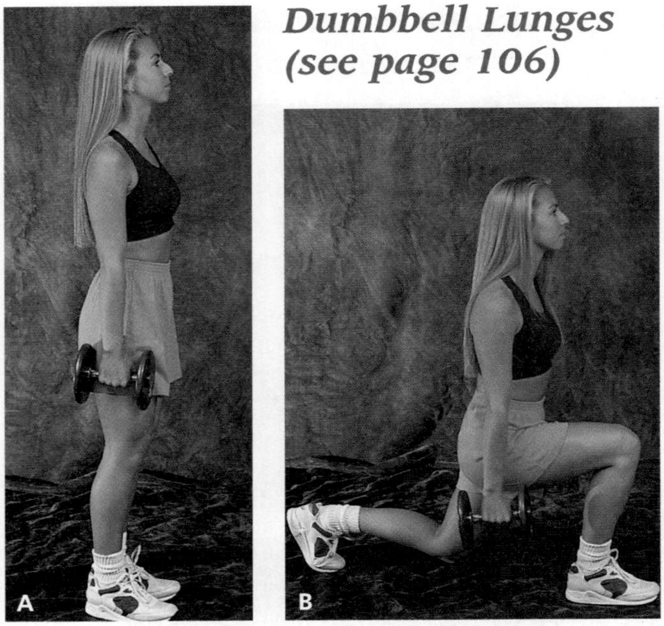

Photos Eric Risberg

One-Dumbbell Calf Raise
(see page 114)

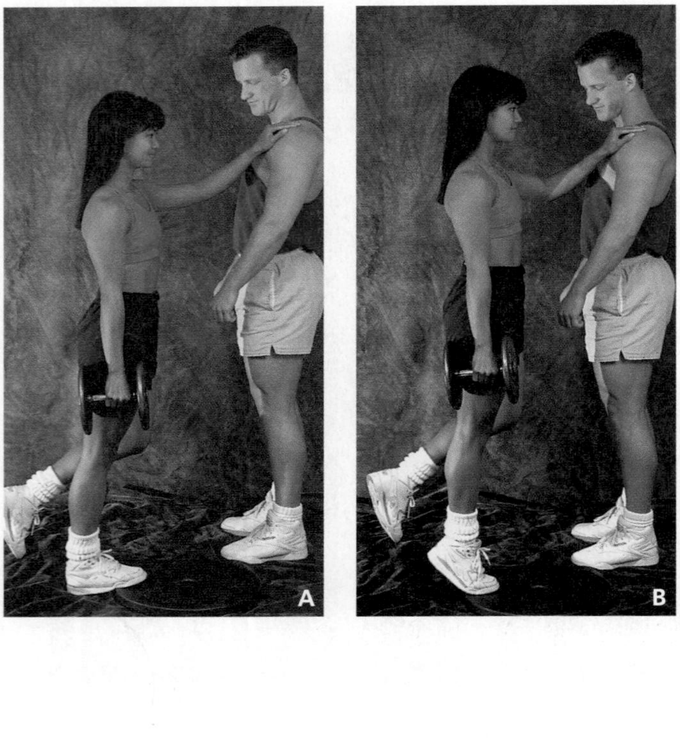

Photos Eric Risberg

Crunches
(see page 118)

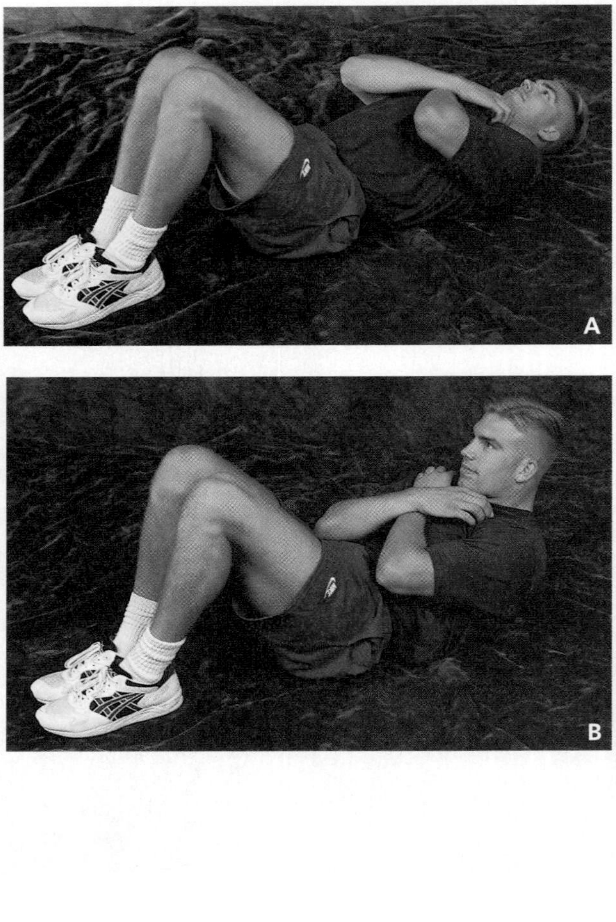

Photos Eric Risberg

Name ______________________________ Section ______________

Planning Your Personal Weight Training Program

Directions:

1. Read Chapter 16, Planning Your Personal Weight Training Program.
2. Plan a weight training program that is consistent with your goals from Chapter 15.
3. Refer to the exercise chapters for general body part and specific exercises.
4. Refer to Chapter 16 for resistance, repetitions, sets, rest, and frequency.

General Body Part	Specific Exercise	Resistance % of 1-RM	Repetitions	Sets	Rest Interval	Frequency Days/wk.

General Body Part	Specific Exercise	Resistance % of 1-RM	Repetitions	Sets	Rest Interval	Frequency Days/wk.

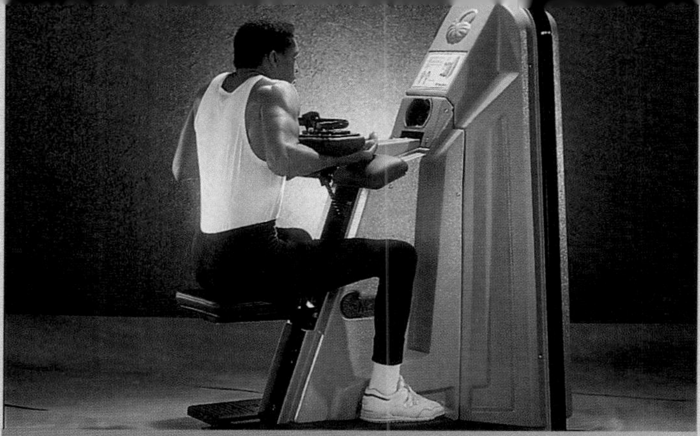

Photo © Nautilus Sports/Medical Industries, Inc.

17

Advanced Weight Training

The principle of progressive overload is worth repeating for advanced weight training. Also, some exercise routines have been developed specifically for advanced weight training. These include increased exercise intensity, total body and split routines, fixed systems, and variable systems. The chapter also explores some equipment options.

Progressive Overload

Progressive overload is the basis of all successful weight training programs. The muscles can be overloaded in many ways and depend upon all of the following variables:

- Which exercises are performed.
- How many total exercises are performed.
- How many exercises are performed for each body part.
- Order in which exercises are performed.
- Amount of resistance or weight used in each set.
- Number of repetitions per set.
- Number of sets per exercise.
- Amount of rest between sets.
- Frequency of training sessions.
- Method of progression.
- Whether the exercise load is fixed or variable.
- Whether the total body is exercised in each training session or is divided into a split routine.
- Exercise intensity.

These variables may be changed and combined in a seemingly unlimited number of ways. Some of the more common training programs are presented here to give you an idea of the variety available to you in weight training. All of these training programs represent different ways to arrive at the same thing: progressive overload.

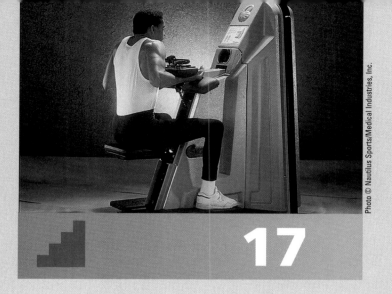

Beginning weight trainers gain on almost any weight training program. The greatest danger for beginners is overtraining. If you find yourself training very hard, not making any progress, and feeling tired all the time, you are probably overtraining. Try less exercise and more rest.

Humans cannot maintain absolute peak condition for very long—a few weeks at best. Therefore, highly trained advanced weight trainers, competitive lifters, and body builders use *periodization* or *cycling*. They divide the year into periods or cycles, then vary their training methods and intensity during the cycles so they reach their peak condition during their competitive season—and, it is hoped, for their most important contest of the year.

Increasing Exercise Intensity

As advanced weight trainers progress in their training, they increase the intensity of their exercise. The following are seven common methods of increasing exercise intensity. All these increase the risk of injury, so caution is advised.

Concentric Failure

Concentric failure requires weight trainers to perform repetitions until they cannot do another repetition while maintaining strict exercise form.

Forced Reps

Forced reps are repetitions performed after reaching concentric failure. When weight trainers cannot perform another repetition correctly by themselves, a spotter assists, as little as possible, to help them complete one or two more repetitions.

Negatives

Weight trainers can lower a heavier weight than they can lift. To perform *negatives*, spotters help them lift a weight and then allow the weight trainers to lower the weight by themselves. This advanced training method can result in extreme muscle soreness and is not recommended for beginning weight trainers.

Eccentric Failure

When weight trainers perform negatives (lower a weight) until they no longer can control the speed at which they lower the weight, they have reached *eccentric failure*. This is obviously dangerous and is not recommended.

Cheating

The use of body movement to get past the weakest point in the range of motion of an exercise is called *cheating*. Although most weight trainers cheat to make the exercise easier, it can be a useful means for advanced lifters to add to the overload.

Pre-Exhaustion

Performing an isolation exercise for a muscle and following this immediately with a compound exercise results in *pre-exhaustion*. The idea is to work the muscle to concentric failure with the isolation exercise, then force the muscle to continue working with the assistance of other muscles that are not exhausted.

Cycle or Periodization

Advanced lifters use training cycles or periods in which they vary the exercise intensity and volume to reach a peak during their competitive season.

Note: Beginning weight trainers do not need to use any of these methods of increasing exercise intensity as long as they are making progress.

Total Body and Split Routines

Beginners, fitness weight trainers, and more advanced weight trainers typically conduct their routines differently.

Total Body Training Routines

Beginners and fitness weight trainers often perform all of their weight training exercises at one time and repeat this procedure every other day. They exercise the total body in one training session.

Split Routines

As weight trainers advance and the total workload increases, many choose to split their exercises, performing part of them one day and the remainder on another day. One example is the 4-day split, in which half of the exercises are performed on Monday and Thursday and the other half on Tuesday and Friday. An example of a 4-day split is a push-pull routine in which the pushing exercises are performed on Monday and Thursday and the pulling exercises on Tuesday and Friday. Another example is to perform the upper-body exercises on Monday and Thursday and the lower-body exercises on Tuesday and Friday.

Some advanced body builders go to a 6-day split, in which they perform about a third of their exercises on Monday and Thursday, a third on Tuesday and Friday, and a third on Wednesday and Saturday. The ultimate split is the *blitz routine*, in which they exercise only one body part each day.

Fixed Systems

Fixed systems are those in which variables are not changed during a training session but a variable may be changed for the next training session. Fixed systems are of several types.

Simple Progressive System

A *simple progressive system* involves changing only one variable, such as the resistance. An example is performing one set of 10 repetitions of an exercise. If 10 repetitions are completed, the weight is increased for the next training session.

Double Progressive System

A *double progressive system* calls for changing two variables, such as resistance and repetitions. An example is performing one set of 12 repetitions. If 12 repetitions are completed, the weight is increased for the next training session and the repetitions are decreased to 8. The repetitions then are increased by one each training session until one set of 12 repetitions is completed with the new weight. Then the weight is increased and the repetitions are decreased again. This pattern—increasing the repetitions, then the weight—continues.

One Set to Failure

A variation of the double progressive system is *one set to failure*. In this system one set of each exercise is performed to the point at which the weight trainer cannot perform another repetition and still maintain correct exercise form. A weight is used that causes this failure to occur between 8 and 12 repetitions. After completing 12 repetitions, the weight is increased for the next training session.

Set System

The *set system* requires the lifter to perform more than one set of each exercise. In a fixed system the repetitions remain the same for each set. One example is three sets of 6 repetitions. When the weight trainer can perform 6 repetitions in all three sets, the weight is increased for the next training session. This is a good program when training with barbells because it reduces the amount of time spent changing weights.

Circuit System

In a *circuit system* a series of exercises is performed in a sequence or circuit, with one exercise at each station. The weight trainer moves from one exercise to the next, performing one set of each exercise until completing every exercise in the circuit once. The entire circuit then may be repeated. The circuit usually is completed one, two, or three times during a training session.

Circuit training often is used with a large group when time and equipment are limited. This is often the case with athletic teams. Circuit training allows a large number of people to get a good workout in a short time.

Aerobic Circuit System

In an *aerobic weight training circuit*, exercises are performed one immediately after the other with little rest between exercises. This is done to keep the heart rate elevated during the entire circuit and thereby produce a training effect for the cardiovascular system. An aerobic circuit training program may even add an aerobic exercise station between each weight training station.

Super Set System

A *super set* requires performing two exercises in a sequence, followed by a rest interval. Often, opposing muscle groups are exercised in this manner. For example, the first set might consist of barbell curls for the elbow flexors. The next set would be tricep extensions for the elbow extensors. Because these muscles work in opposition to one another, one is resting while the other is working. After one set of each exercise, there is usually a rest interval before repeating the sequence. This is a good way to reduce training time without reducing the amount of work completed during the training session. It is like a mini-circuit.

Giant Sets

Giant sets usually involve three to five exercises for the same muscle. One set of each exercise is performed with little or no rest between sets. After all of the exercises in the sequence have been performed, there is a rest interval before repeating the sequence. This is a highly advanced training system that some body builders use.

Rest-Pause System

The *rest-pause system* has many variations. Here is one: Perform an exercise to the point of temporary muscular failure, hold the weight while the muscle recovers slightly, perform another repetition, pause, do another repetition, pause, and continue until no more repetitions can be performed.

Variable Systems

In *variable systems* one or more variables are altered during the performance of one exercise.

Pyramid System

In a *pyramid system* the weight used for each set of an exercise is increased and the number of repetitions is decreased correspondingly. This allows the exerciser to proceed from a light weight to a heavy weight. This system is often used when training for strength. Some weight trainers choose to pyramid up only; others pyramid up to a heavy weight, then back down again.

Percentage System

The *percentage system* is a variation of the pyramid system. Multiple sets of an exercise are performed at various percentages of the 1-RM for that exercise. The percentages usually start low in the first set and increase in each of the subsequent sets.

DeLorme System

An additional system, most often used by beginners and those training for fitness, is the *DeLorme system*. This system consists of:

1st set:	10 reps	50% of 10-RM
2nd set:	10 reps	75% of 10-RM
3rd set:	10 reps	100% of 10-RM

Continuous Set System

In the *continuous set system*, weight trainers start with a weight they can use to complete a given number of repetitions—for example, 10 repetitions. After reaching the point at which they can do no more repetitions, the training partner quickly removes a small amount of weight while the weight trainer continues to hold the bar or stays in position on the machine. As soon as some weight has been removed, the exercise is continued until no more repetitions can be performed. Once again, the training partner removes a small amount of weight. This process continues until the weight trainer cannot do any more repetitions, even with the lightest weight.

Light to Heavy System

The *light to heavy system* is a variation of the pyramid and continuous set systems. The weight trainer starts with a light to moderate weight and performs 3 repetitions. The training partners quickly add a small amount of weight. After 3 more repetitions, they add weight again. This process continues until the weight trainer can perform only one repetition.

Tonnage System

The resistance and repetitions vary in the *tonnage system*, and the lifter keeps track of the total pounds lifted in a training session. Each weight lifted is multiplied by the number of repetitions completed with that weight. For example, 200 pounds times 10 repetitions equals 2,000 pounds, or 1 ton. The total number of pounds or tons lifted during a training session is added. The tonnage system is used most often by competitive weight lifters.

These are only a few of the methods that advanced weight trainers have used to overload their muscles. There are many more.

Training Equipment

Training equipment includes constant external resistance equipment, variable resistance equipment, and isokinetic equipment.

Constant External Resistance Equipment

Barbells, dumbbells, and some weight-stack equipment have a resistance that is constant—the weight remains the same throughout the exercise. Because of changes in leverage at the joints during movement through the full range of motion, this fixed weight is more difficult to lift at some joint angles and easier to lift at others.

With constant external resistance equipment, the weight trainer is limited to the heaviest weight that can be lifted through the weakest point in the range of motion. Two basic equipment design approaches have attempted to overcome this limitation: variable resistance equipment and isokinetic equipment.

Variable Resistance Equipment

Some weight-stack equipment has been designed so that as the leverage changes for the working muscles and joints, the exercise machine makes compensating leverage changes. When exercising with constant external resistance equipment, once the weight trainer can get past the weakest point in the range of motion, the rest of the exercise movement is fairly easy. With the compensating leverage change of *variable resistance equipment*, the muscle must continue to work hard throughout the full range of motion.

The weight in the stack lifted remains constant, but the leverage change in the machine makes the resistance greater at some joint angles and less at other joint angles. The intent of variable resistance equipment is to keep the muscles fully loaded throughout the full range of motion.

Isokinetic Equipment

Isokinetic equipment offers another solution to keeping the muscle fully loaded throughout the full range of motion. *Isokinetic* refers to constant motion or constant speed. True isokinetic exercise equipment limits the speed at which the exercise device will move. Therefore, a muscle can contract at its maximum force from full extension to full contraction without producing acceleration.

Which Type of Exercise Equipment is the Best?

So far, no one type of exercise equipment has been proven superior for the development of muscle tissue. Muscles don't know or care what type of exercise equipment is used to provide the resistance as long as they receive the same overload stimulus.

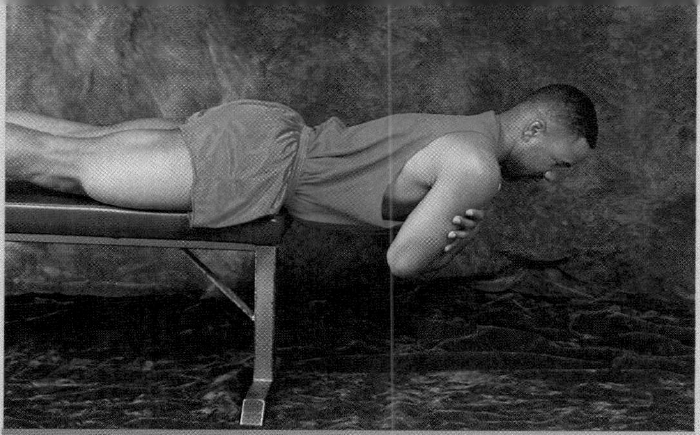

Eric Risberg

18

Weight Training for Life

Anyone can start a weight training program, and many do, but few stick with it. The following are some ideas, strategies, and tips for sticking with your weight training program and getting the results you want.

Transtheoretical Model of Behavior Change

Behavior change is usually a gradual process that involves several stages. Psychologists James Prochaska, John Norcross, and Carlo DiClemente have developed the Transtheoretical Model of Behavior Change, which describes six stages of change. Most people relapse from time to time.

1. *Precontemplation.* In this first stage you are not interested in changing. You may not know you need to change, or you may deny a need for change. If you are in this stage, you might say, "I **don't need or want** a weight training program."

2. *Contemplation.* In this second stage you have begun to recognize a need for change and you are beginning to consider a change. Perhaps you have noticed a loss of strength, vitality, or undesirable changes in your appearance and you have started thinking about an exercise program to build your strength, regain your vitality, or improve your appearance. If you are in this stage, you could say, "I **might** start a weight training program."

3. *Preparation.* In the third stage you are seriously planning to change a behavior within the next month. You might sign up for a weight training class, read a weight training book, join a fitness center, or start looking for a personal trainer. If you are in this stage, you might say, "I **will** start a weight training program."

4. *Action.* In this fourth stage you have made a commitment and have taken action. If you are in this stage, you might say, "I **do** have a planned weight training program and I lift weights at a regular time and place."

5. *Maintenance.* In the fifth stage you have maintained your behavior change for a long time. If you are in this stage, you might say, "I **have been** weight training on a regular basis for the last five years."

6. *Adoption.* In the sixth stage you have adopted a positive behavior and it has become part of your lifestyle. If you are in this stage, you might say, "I **am** a weight trainer." The behavior has become a regular part of your current lifestyle and your identity.

Relapse

Relapse is when the person returns to an old behavior. Relapse may set in at any level after precontemplation. Occasionally you will miss a workout or a week of weight training—everyone does. Life can be planned, but you need to be flexible enough to adapt to changes that occur. Sometimes in life you must bend with the wind, but you need to spring back as soon as the wind lets up a bit. Relapse is not failure. It is human. We can strive for perfection but must accept excellence. *Weight training for life* is a continuous process of starting over and adapting to change.

Changing your behavior is one of the most difficult challenges in life. It is stressful. If you change to healthier behaviors, however, you will become more resilient and better able to cope with change and stress. It is easier not to lift weights, but it is better to lift weights, to overcome resistance. It is easier not to learn, but it is better to continue learning. The path that is flat and level and easy does not lead to the top of the mountain. You cannot reach your full potential by taking the easy path. You cannot improve yourself or your life by staying on the easy path.

Tips for Sticking With It

The following are ideas that will help you adhere to your weight training program and get the results you want.

Motivation

Needs and wants motivate behavior. The depth of your desire to meet a need or want determines the strength of your motivation. Once you reach your goal, it loses its power to motivate. After all, now you have what you want. To be motivated to continue weight training, you need to set new goals. The new goal could be further improvement, or it could be to maintain what you have achieved.

Enjoyment

Enjoyment is extremely important in sticking with your weight training program. Most people seek pleasure and avoid pain. We find time for the activities we enjoy and find excuses to avoid the activities that are difficult and painful for us. If you enjoy weight training, you will find a way to do it on a regular basis. If you design a personal weight training program for yourself that is a long, boring, terrible, painful experience, you will find excuses to avoid it. Different people find enjoyment or satisfaction in exercise in different ways. Some of the things that bring enjoyment to weight training are improvement, challenge, excitement, relaxation, competition, and social interaction.

Importance

Regular lifelong weight trainers have a common belief that weight training is good for them. A lot of evidence supports that belief. If you haven't read the evidence yet, maybe you should start now. To continue regular weight training, you must believe that the benefits you receive from your program are worth the time, effort, energy, and money you put into it.

Priority

To stick with your program, you must place a high priority on it. Build it into your schedule and stick with the time you have set for training. You will always be able to find other things you could do during that time, but don't allow those other things to replace your training time.

Time

We all have the same amount of time each year, each month, each week, and each day. Some people make time for exercise, and some claim they don't have time to exercise. Surveys have indicated that the average American watches three to four hours of television each day, and yet these same people claim they don't have time to exercise. Clearly, for most people exercise is not a question of time but, instead, one of priorities. Schedule your weight training time and stick with it.

Record

Improvement is a powerful motivator for most people. Write down the relevant information from each weight training session. These records will provide visible evidence of your improvement and of your ability to stick with a weight training program.

Reward

Regular weight trainers get a sense of satisfaction, an intrinsic reward, from regular exercise sessions. As a beginner, however, you may benefit from extrinsic rewards. You might want to promise yourself something for reaching a goal you have set for yourself. Of course, it should be a healthy reward, and you should get it only when you reach your goal.

Knowledge

The more you learn about weight training, the more you understand the benefits, the more you know about correct technique, the more you know about designing programs, the more likely you are to continue. Most people want to be good at something. If you are willing to learn, and to stick with your training, you can become good at weight training.

Social Interaction

Some people enjoy the social benefits of weight training. They like to exercise with a friend or a small group. They enjoy the new friends they meet when they are weight training. If you meet people while you are weight training, you instantly have something in common, and a topic of conversation, with them.

Support

Share your new weight training goals and your new weight training program with people you know who will be supportive. Get support from as many people as you can. Once you tell a large number of people you are going to do something it becomes harder to quit and easier to continue.

Identity

When you become a regular weight trainer, it becomes a part of your identity. Once it is a part of who you are and what you do, it is easier to stick with it and harder to quit. Friends and family no longer ask if you are going to work out, they know when you are going to work out.

Place

If you like the place where you exercise, you will want to go there. If you don't like the place where you do your weight training, you will not want to go there. Therefore, you should find or create a pleasant place to do your weight training.

Convenience

If weight training is too inconvenient, you are more likely to quit, so you should seek ways to make weight training as convenient as possible. Identify the obstacles to regular weight training, and begin to eliminate them one by one.

Instruction

Most people get satisfaction from doing something well. Getting good instruction whenever you start a new activity is usually an excellent investment of your time and money. Excellent instruction gets you past the awkward beginner stage more quickly. Getting good weight training instruction when you are beginning will get you past the beginner stage more quickly and will help you avoid mistakes.

Variety

Weight training programs offer a wide variety of options. Some people prefer a highly structured routine that almost never changes. They like to do the same exercises in the same order at the same time on the same days for years. Others like to do something different during every training session. Most people are somewhere in between. They like to follow an exercise plan for 6 weeks or 8 weeks or 12 weeks or some other block of time, then change their program for the next block of time. You need to determine what works best for you—what keeps the training fun and interesting for you.

Fitness

If you can stick with a weight training program long enough to reach a fitness level you are proud of, you are more likely to continue to train for the rest of your life. It is much easier to maintain a higher level of fitness than it is to get there in the first place.

Success

You can learn to set reasonable goals. You can learn to plan weight training programs to reach your goals. You can learn to stick with your weight training program. You can improve your fitness level. You can achieve success through weight training.

Appearance

In our society, appearance is important. We are bombarded by daily messages—from movies, television, and advertising—that looking good is important. Although it is okay to want to improve your appearance and look good, self-worship is not attractive. One of the most effective and efficient ways to improve your appearance is weight training.

Image

Your body image is how you see yourself. Most people have a subconscious drive to maintain a body that is consistent with their body image. This does not mean a perfect body. Even if we could come to some general agreement of what the perfect body would look like, training for perfection is unrealistic and unattainable. Instead, we should train for a healthy body image. Although you cannot change your genetic body type, you can make the most of what you have.

Regularity

The greatest benefits of weight training come from making regular training a lifelong habit. Losers weight train too hard for a short time, then quit and do nothing for a long time. They may start again, but they generally train too hard again for a short time, then quit again. Winners persevere and are consistent in their training. They generally train at a more moderate pace and design programs that are realistic, lifetime weight training programs. Will you choose to be a winner or a loser?

Habit

Your body adapts gradually to weight training. Healthy weight training is a healthy lifestyle habit much like brushing your teeth. It is most effective if it is done regularly and continuously as a part of the routine of living. Good habits bring good results.

Weight Training for Life

If you don't take care of your body where will you live? Do you know people who take better care of their house or car than their body? You may live in many houses and drive many cars in your lifetime, but you only get one body to live in for your entire life. Take good care of it by *weight training for life*.

Place a checkmark by the tips for sticking with it that you believe will help you the most with weight training for life.

___ Motivation
___ Enjoyment
___ Importance
___ Priority
___ Time
___ Record
___ Reward
___ Knowledge
___ Social Interaction
___ Support
___ Identity
___ Place
___ Convenience
___ Instruction
___ Variety
___ Fitness
___ Success
___ Appearance
___ Image
___ Regularity
___ Habit

Internet Sites

Internet sites and addresses tend to appear and disappear rather quickly. Although these were active sites when the manuscript was submitted, they may have changed or disappeared by the time this book is published or by the time you read it.

Aerobic and Fitness Association of America
http://www.afaa.com

American Alliance for Health, Physical Education, Recreation and Dance (AAHPERD)
http://www.aahperd.org

American College of Sports Medicine (ACSM)
http://www.acsm.org

American Dietetics Association
http://www.eatright.org

American Heart Association
http://www.americanheart.org

American Medical Association
http://www.ama-assn.org

American Running and Fitness Association
http://www.arfa.org

Ask the Dietitian
http://www.hoptechno.com/rdindex.htm

Bodybuilding
http://www.bodyforlife.com/

Bodybuilding
http://www.muscle-fitness.com

Center for Science in the Public Interest
http://www.cspinet.org

Centers for Disease Control and Prevention
http://www.cdc.gov

CNN's Health Report
http://www.cnn.com/Health

Diet Analysis Web Page
http://dawp.futuresouth.com/

Dietary Guidelines
http://www.nal.usda.gov/fnic/dga/index.html

Dr. Koop's Community
http://www.drkoop.com

Duke University Diet
and Fitness Center Home Page
http://dmi-
www.mc.duke.edu/dfc/home.html

Exercise Library
http://fitnesslink.com/mind/all-mind.shtml

Fast Food Finder
http://www.olen.com/food/

FDA Center for Food Safety
and Applied Nutrition
http://vm.cfsan.fda.gov/list.html

FitnessLinks to the Internet
http://www.fitnesslink.com/links.htm

Fitness World
http://www.fitnessworld.com

Food and Nutrition Center,
U.S. Department of Agriculture
http://www.nal.usda.gov/fnic

General Nutrition Site
http://www.healthy.net/index.html

Health A to Z
http://www.HealthAtoZ.com

Healthfinder
http://www.healthfinder.gov

Healthy People 2001
http://odphp.osophs.dhhs.gov/pubs/hp2001/

Interactive Food Guide Pyramid
http://www.nal.usda.gov:8001/py/pmap.htm

Internet Fitness Resource
http://sickbay.com/netsweat

Mayo Clinic Health Information
http://www.mayo.ivi.com

Meals Online
http://www/meals.com

Medscape
http://www.medscape.com

National Bodybuilding
and Fitness Magazine
http://nbaf.com/nbaf/hom.html

National Health Information Center (NHIC)
http://nhic-nt.health.org/

National Institutes of Health
http://www.nih.gov/health/

Nutrition Sites on the Internet
http://wce.uwyo.edu/
wctl/high/nutr/default.html

Olympic Lifting
http://www.lifttilyadie.co

Olympic Lifting
http://www.goheavy.com/olympic

Physical Activity
and Health Network (PAHNet)
http://www.pitt.edu/~pahnet/

Pointer to Frequently Asked
Questions about Weight Lifting
http://www.imp.mtu.edu/~babucher/
weights/pointer.html#FAQs

Power Lifting
http://www.powerlifting.com

Power Lifting
http://www.drsquat.com/

Powerlifting Competition—
Frequently Asked Questions
http://www.cs.unc.edu/~wilsonk/power.
faq.html

President's Council on
Physical Fitness and Sports
http://www.hoptechno.com/book11.htm

Shape Up America!
http://www.shapeup.org

Stanford Health Link
http://healthlink.stanford.edu/

Strength Training Muscle Map
and Explanation
www.global-
fitness.com/strength/s_map.html

Stretching Information
http://www.enteract.com/~bradapp/docs/
rec/stretching_1.html

Ten Tips to Maximize Your Weight Training
www..vitality.com/vfm/weight_train.html

USA Weightlifting
http://www.usaw.org-usa

USDA Food and
Nutrition Information Center
http://www.nalusda.gov/fnic/

United States Olympic Committee
Sports from A to Z
http://www.olympic-usa.org/sports/

Virtual Vegetarian
http://www.vegetariantimes.com/

Weight Lifting: Olympic Style
http://www.waf.com/weights/index.htm

Weight Management
http://www.wellweb.com/nutri/weight_
management.htm

Welcome to the National Strength and
Conditioning Association
http://www.colosoft.com/nsca/

Worldguide Forum on Health and Fitness
http://www.worldguide.com/Fitness/hf.html

Yahoo Health Directory
http://www.yahoo.com/health

References and Suggested Readings

Aaberg, E. *Resistance Training Instruction*. Champaign, IL: Human Kinetics, 1999.

Allsen, P. E. *Strength Training: Beginners, Bodybuilders, and Athletes* (2d edition). Dubuque, IA: Kendall/Hunt Publishing, 1996.

Alter, M. J. *Sport Stretch* (2d edition). Champaign, IL: Human Kinetics, 1998.

American College of Sports Medicine. *ACSM's Resource Manual for Guidelines for Exercise Testing and Prescription* (3d edition). Philadelphia: Lippincott/Williams & Wilkins, 1998.

American College of Sports Medicine. *ACSM's Guidelines for Exercise Testing and Prescription* (6th edition). Philadelphia: Lippincott/Williams & Wilkins, 2000.

American College of Sports Medicine. "Exercise and Physical Activity for Older Adults." *Medicine and Science in Sports & Exercise,* Vol. 30. No. 6., pp. 992–1008. 1998.

American College of Sports Medicine. "The Recommended Quantity and Quality of Exercise for Developing and Maintaining Cardiovascular and Muscular Fitness, and Flexibility in Healthy Adults." *Medicine and Science in Sports & Exercise,* Vol. 30. No. 6., pp. 975–991, 1998.

Anderson, B., Burke, E., and Pearl, B. *Getting in Shape*. Bolinas, CA: Shelter Publications, 1994.

Baechle, T. R., and Earle, R.W. *Essentials of Strength Training and Conditioning* (2d edition). Champaign, IL: Human Kinetics, 2000.

Baechle, T. R., and Earle, R. W. *Fitness Weight Training*. Champaign, IL: Human Kinetics, 1995.

Baechle, T. R., and Groves, B. R. *Weight Training: Steps to Success* (2d edition). Champaign, IL: Human Kinetics, 1998.

Bennett, J. *The Basics of Weight Training Workbook*. Boston: Allyn & Bacon, 1995.

Boyle, M.A. *Personal Nutrition*. Belmont, CA: Wadsworth/Thomson Learning, 2001.

Brzycki, M. *A Practical Approach to Strength Training* (3d edition). Indianapolis: Masters Press, 1995.

Cissik, J. M. The Basics of Strength Training. New York: McGraw-Hill Higher Education, 1998.

Fahey, T. *Basic Weight Training for Men and Women* (4th edition). Mountain View, CA: Mayfield Publishing, 2000.

Fahey, T., and Hutchinson, G. *Weight Training for Women*. Mountain View, CA: Mayfield Publishing, 1992.

Faigenbaum, A., and Westcott, W. *Strength and Power for Young Athletes*. Champaign, IL: Human Kinetics, 2000.

Field, R. W., and Roberts, S. O. *Weight Training*. Boston: WCB/McGraw-Hill, 1999.

Fleck, S. J., and Kraemer, W. J. *Designing Resistance Training Programs* (2d edition). Champaign, IL: Human Kinetics, 1997.

Hales, D. *An Invitation to Fitness and Wellness*. Belmont, CA: Wadsworth/Thomson Learning, 2001.

Hoeger, W. W. K. *Lifetime Physical Fitness and Wellness* (6th edition). Belmont, CA: Wadsworth/Thompson Learning, 2000.

Hoeger, W. W. K., and Hoeger, S. A. *Principles and Labs for Fitness and Wellness* (6th edition). Belmont, CA: Wadsworth/Thompson Learning, 2002.

Hoeger, W. W. K., Turner, L. W., and Hafen, B. Q. *Guidelines for a Healthy Lifestyle* (3d edition). Belmont, CA: Wadsworth/Thomson Learning, 2002.

Howley, E. T., and Franks, B. D. *Health Fitness Instructor's Handbook* (3d edition). Champaign, IL: Human Kinetics, 1997.

Kraemer, W. J., and Fleck, S. J. *Strength Training for Young Athletes*. Champaign, IL: Human Kinetics, 1993.

Kubik, B. D. *Dinosaur Training: Lost Secrets of Strength and Development*. Louisville, KY, 1996.

Moran, G. T., and McGlynn, G. *Dynamics of Strength Training and Conditioning* (3d edition). New York: McGraw-Hill Higher Education, 2000.

NSCA Certification Commission. *Exercise Technique-Checklist Manual*. Lincoln, NE: NSCA Certification Commission, 1997.

O'Connor, B., Simmons, J., and O'Shea, P. *Strength Training Today* (2d edition). Belmont, CA: Wadsworth/Thompson Learning, 2000.

Peterson, J. A., Bryant, C. X., and Peterson, S. L. *Strength Training for Women*. Champaign, IL: Human Kinetics, 1995.

Roberts, S. O., and Pillarella, D. *Developing Strength in Children: A Comprehensive Guide*. Reston, VA: American Alliance for Health, Physical Education, Recreation and Dance, 1996.

Trestrail, R. T. *Weight Training: A Practical Approach to Total Fitness*. Dubuque, IA: Kendall/Hunt Publishing, 1999.

Westcott, W. L., and Baechle, T. R. *Strength Training Past 50*. Champaign, IL: Human Kinetics, 1998.

Index

Abdominal muscles, 126
Actin, 13
Action stage of transtheoretical model, 158
Adoption stage of transtheoretical model, 158
Advanced weight trainers/training, 147, 153
Aerobic exercise, 148
  and the "ab solution," 126
  calories expended through, 2, 8
  circuit system of, 155
  and weight loss, 47
Aging, and exercise, 4, 9
Alcohol consumption, 50, 131
American Dietetic Association, 47
American Heart Association, 41
Amino acids, 43, 47
Anabolic steroids, 49–50
Anemia, iron-deficiency, 40
Appearance, 3, 5, 9, 21, 131, 159
Arm exercises, 87
Athletes, 2, 8, 17
  strength, 131, 146
Atrophy, muscle, 7, 15
Attitude, 1, 34, 140
Autosuggestion, 140

Back, 146
  exercises for, 69, 124, 146
  injury, 31, 70
Barbell(s), 13, 14, 28, 29, 31, 148, 156
Barbell Bent-Arm Pullover exercise, 66
Barbell Curl exercise, 88
Barbell Reverse Curl exercise, 90
Barbell Squat in Power Rack exercise, 103
Beginning weight training, 32, 33–34, 128, 130, 146, 154
Behavior change, 157
  transtheoretical model of, 167
Belief, 140
Bench Dips exercise, 94
Bench press, 2, 60, 146, 147
Bent-Arm Flyes, 64
Blitz routine, 154
Body
  composition, 9
  image, 159
  movement, 11, 12, 13, 22
  weight, measuring, 131
Body builders, 2, 9, 17, 50, 131, 146, 154
Boss Dip Machine exercise, 95
Body fat, 2, 5, 7, 8, 126, 130
Body Master Leg Curl Machine exercise, 111
Body Master Leg Extension Machine exercise, 110
Body Master Machine Flyes exercise, 64
Body Master Triceps Extension exercise, 97
Body position
  on arm curl machines, 25
  in clean lift, 31
  on weight machines, 25
Body weight, measuring, 131
Boss Dip Machine exercise, 95
Boss Incline Bench Press Machine exercise, 63
Boss Overhead Press Machine exercise, 79
Boys, weight lifting for, 3
Breathing, 9, 21, 24, 28, 33, 126
  deep, 126

Calcium, 40
Calf Press on Body Master Leg Press Machine, 114
Calf Press on Cybex Leg Press Machine, 115
Calories, 39, 126
  and caloric values of food, 40 (Figure 7.1) 40, 41
  expended through exercise, 2, 7, 8
Carbohydrates, 41, 45
Cardiovascular
  development, 8, 155
  endurance, 9
Centers for Disease Control and Prevention (CDC), 4
Cheating, 154
Chest exercises, 59
Chin-ups, 72
Cholesterol, blood, 41
Circuit training, 9, 146, 155
Circumference measurements, 130
Clean lift, 31, 32
Clean-and-jerk lift, 2
Close-Grip Bench Press exercise, 96
Clothing during exercise, 21, 22 (Figure 5.1)
Compound exercises, 146
Concentration, 24
Concentric
  contraction, 14
  failure, 154
  phase of exercise, 22, 57
Constant external resistance equipment, 156
Contemplation stage of transtheoretical model, 157
Continuous set system, 156
Contractility, 11
Coordination, 9
Crunches, 118, 150
Curl-ups, 118
Cybex Abdominal Machine exercise, 119
Cybex Back Extension machine exercise, 125
Cybex Hip Extension Machine exercise, 108
Cybex Incline Bench Press Machine exercise, 63
Cybex Leg Extension Machine exercise, 110
Cybex Leg Press (Plate-Loaded Machine) exercise, 105
Cybex Leg Press (Weight Stack Machine) exercise, 104
Cybex Seated Back Extension Machine exercise, 125
Cybex Seated Chest Press Machine exercise, 61
Cybex Seated Lateral raise Machine, 83
Cybex Seated Rowing Machine exercise, 71
Cybex Standing Calf Raise Machine exercise, 113
Cybex Triceps Extension Machine exercise, 97
Cybex Weight-Assisted Parallel Bar Dips exercise, 95
Cybex Weight-Assisted Pull-up Machine exercise, 73
Cycling, 154

DCER, 14
Dead Lift exercise, 103
Dead lift, 2, 31, 103
Death, premature, 4
Deep-breathing, 126
DeLorme, Thomas, 2
  system, 156
  workout, 148
DiClemente, Carlo, 157
Diet, balanced, 40, 43 (Figure 7.3), 45, 48
Dietary Guidelines for Americans, 45, 46 (Table 7.2)
Disabilities, people with, 2, 4
Double progressive system, 155
Drugs, 49–50, 131
Dumbbell(s), 18, 19, 29, 31, 148, 156
Dumbbell Bench Press, 54, 149
Dumbbell Bent-Over Lateral Raise exercise, 85
Dumbbell Front Raise exercise, 84
Dumbbell Lateral Raise exercise, 82, 149
Dumbbell Lateral Raise, 76
Dumbbell Lunges, 150
Dumbbell Straight-Arm Pullover exercise, 66
Duration of exercise, 3
  in stretching, 19

Eccentric
  contraction, 14
  failure, 154
  phase of exercise, 22, 57
Elasticity, 11
Electrolytes, 47
Emotional development, 5
Endomysium, 12
Endurance
  cardiovascular, 9
  muscular, 2, 16, 130, 137 (log), 146
  and resistance, 146
Energy, 2, 39, 40, 41, 43, 47. *See also* Calories
Enjoyment of exercise, 158
Epimysium, 12
Equipment
  constant external resistance, 156
  isokinetic, 156
  variable resistance, 156
  weight-stack, 156
Evaluating progress, 131
Excitability, 11
Exercise(s)
  aerobic, 8, 47, 148
  aging and, 4
  for back, 69, 124,146
  for beginners, 33 (Table 6.1)
  cardiovascular, 4
  for children, 3
  clothing for, 21
  compound, 146
  concentric phase of, 22
  eccentric phase of, 22
  duration of, 3, 19
  during pregnancy, 3
  flexibility, 4
  form, 22, 23 (Figure 5.1), 28, 33, 128, 130, 154
  high-impact, 3
  high-intensity, 3, 41
  intensity of, 18–19, 154
  machine, 24–28
  during pregnancy, 3
  stretching, 18–20
  technique, 3, 33, 34
  vigorous, 19
Extensibility, 11
Extension, 12, 18

Fat, body, 2, 5, 7, 8, 130
  estimating, 131
Fat, dietary, 41, 45
  content of selected foods (Figure 7.2), 42
Fat-loss programs, 2, 8
Fat-soluble vitamins, 40, 41
Fiber
  dietary, 41
  muscle, 12, 13
Fine motor coordination, 9
Fitness, physical, 2, 5, 31, 159
  in children, 3
  muscle, 147
Fixed load, 147
Fixed systems, 155
Flexibility, 4, 8, 9, 18, 22, 25, 47
Flexion, 12, 18
Food guide pyramid, 43-44 (Figure 7.4), 45
Forced reps, 154
Free weights, 29, 31
Frequency, 131, 147
  for beginning weight trainers, 32
  of stretching, 19

Genetic potential, 131
Giant sets, 155
Goals
  setting, 139–140
  weight training, 5, 9, 34, 48, 145–147
  worksheet, 143
  written, 141
Grip(s)
  with back exercises, 146
  with barbells/dumbbells, 31
  mixed, 30
  pronated, 30
  supinated, 30
Gulick tape measure, 130
Gymnasts, 8

Hack Squat Machine, 107
Hammer Strength Arm Curl Machine exercise, 89
Hammer Strength Bent-arm Pullover Machine exercise, 67
Hammer Strength Overhead Press Machine, 79
Hand-spacing, 30–31
Hanging Knee Raises exercise, 123
Hanging Reverse Crunches exercise, 123
Happiness, 140
Health 9, 34
  benefits of physical activity, 4
Health-related physical fitness, 9, 10
Healthy eating, 1, 8, 34, 47, 126
Heart disease, 41
Hernia, 9
Hip Extension Machine exercise, 109
Hip extension(s), 8
Hormones, 3, 8
Hypertrophy, 15

Incline Bench Press exercise, 62
Incline Dumbbell Curl exercise, 90
Injuries, 9, 34
  back, 31
  risk for, 2, 5, 17, 18, 19, 22, 24, 25, 26, 28, 128
  soft-tissue, 18
  youth, 3
Intensity
  of exercise, 3, 18–19, 131, 154
  isolated, 24
Iron, 40

Isokinetic
- contraction, 14
- equipment, 156

Isometric contraction, 13
Isotonic contraction, 13–14

Joints, 8, 12
- range of motion, 8, 11, 18
- strength, 2

Junk food, 43

Lat Pulldown Machine exercise, 73
Lean body mass, 47–48
Leg exercises, 101
Leg Press Machine, 107
Lifestyle, 1, 139
- healthy, 34, 160
- sedentary, 4, 147

Lift
- clean, 31
- clean-and-jerk, 2, 3
- dead, 2, 31
- 1-RM, 128
- overhead, 3

Lifting technique, 9, 33
- and spotting, 27–28, 32

Ligaments, 18
Light to heavy system, 156
Lipids, 41
Low Pulley Curl exercise, 91
Low Pulley Shoulder Shrug exercise, 75
Low Pulley Upright Rowing (Curved Bar) exercise, 81
Low Pulley Upright Rowing (Straight Bar) exercise, 81
Lunge exercise, 106
Lying Barbell Triceps Extension exercise, 96

Machines
- advantages of, 29
- cleaning, 26
- exercises using, 24–28
- safety when using, 27–28

Maintenance stage of transtheoretical model, 158
Measurements
- body weight, 131
- circumference, 130
- muscle endurance, 130
- muscle size, 130, 133 (log), 133
- skinfold, 131
- strength, 128, 135 (log)

Medical clearance, 21
Men, weight training for, 3, 8
Mental development, 5
Metabolic rate, 2, 7
- basal, 48
- resting, 8

Metabolism, 39, 48
Military Press exercise, 78
Minerals, 40, 45
Mobility, 11
- and aging, 4

Motivation, 127, 131, 147, 158
Motor
- nerves, 14, 15
- unit, 14–15

Movement, body, 11, 12, 13, 22
- speed of, 25

Muscle(s)/muscular, 7, 15
- abdominal, 126
- cardiac, 12
- contraction (Figures 3.2 and 3.3), 13
- endurance, 3, 16, 146
- fibers, 12, 13, 14–15
- involuntary, 11, 12
- major, 4, 58
- mass, 4, 9
- opposing, 2, 8, 18, 146
- size, 2, 3, 7, 16, 130, 146
- skeletal, 3, 11, 12 (Figure 3.1)
- smooth, 12
- tissue, 11
- tone, 146, 147

Muscle-bound, 8
Muscular endurance, 9
- measuring,130, 137 (worksheet)

Muscular strength, 9
Musculoskeletal system, 12
Myofibril, 13
Myofilaments, 13
Myosin, 13

National Academy of Sciences, 40
National Center for Health Statistics, 47
National Strength and Conditioning Association, 3, 57
Nautilus Abdominal Crunch Machine, 119
Nautilus Arm Curl Machine exercise, 89
Nautilus Leg Press Machine exercise, 105
Nautilus Pullover Machine exercise, 67
Nautilus Seated Leg Curl Machine exercise, 111
Nautilus Seated Rowing Machine exercise, 71
Nautilus 10-Degree Chest Machine exercise, 65
Nautilus Triceps Extension Machine exercise, 93
Negatives, 154
Norcross, John, 157
Nutrients, 8, 39, 43
- essential (Table 7.1), 45
- supplementation, 45, 47

Nutrition, 8, 34, 39, 131

Obesity, 47, 48
Olympic lifters, 2, 9, 17
One-Dumbbell Calf Raise exercise, 114, 150
One-Dumbbell Rowing, 149
One-repetition maximum (1-RM), 3, 128, 130
One set to failure, 155
Osteoporosis, 40
Overhead Press exercise, 78
Overhead
- lifts, 3
- press, 24, 31

Overload, principle of, 16, 145–146, 153
Overtraining, 32–33, 154

Parallel Bar Dips exercise, 94
Patients, 2
Pec Deck Machine exercise, 65
Percentage system, 156
Percent body fat, 131
Perimysium, 12
Periodization, 154
Persistence, 141
Personal Weight Training Program (worksheets), 151
Physical activity
- for older adults, 4
- vigorous, 4, 17
- for weight loss, 48

Physical Activity and Health (Surgeon General's Report), 4
Physical development, 3, 5
Physical fitness, 2, 31
- in children, 3
- health-related, 9, 10 (Table 2.1)

Plan, written, 140
Positive thinking, 140, 141
Posture(s), 21
- exercises for, 126

Power lifters, 2, 9, 17
Preacher Curl exercise, 91
Precontemplation stage of transtheoretical model, 157
Pre-exhaustion, 154
Pregnancy, exercise during, 3
Preparation stage of transtheoretical model, 157
Prochaska, James, 157
Procrastination, 141
Progress, evaluating, 131
Progression, principle of, 16, 145
Progressive overload, 146, 153
Progressive resistance, 1, 126
Prone Bench Press Machine exercise, 61
Proteins, 43, 45
- supplementation, 47

Pull-ups, 72
Pyramid system, 155

Range of motion, 8, 11, 18, 22
- on machines (Figure 5.7), 25

Recommended body weight, 48
Record keeping, 128 (Figure 14.1), 129 (Figure 14.2), 158
Rehabilitation, 2
Relapse, 158
Repetition maximum, 128
Repetitions, 130, 146, 147, 154
Resistance, 4, 32, 34, 131, 146, 147
- equipment, 156

Rest, 8, 34, 39, 48, 131
- between sets, 147

Rest-pause system, 155
Reverse Wrist Curl exercise, 99
Rowing, 70, 126

Sacromeres, 13
Safety, 3, 9, 21, 24
- for beginners, 33
- grip, 30
- in machine weight training, 27–28, 29

Salt, 45
Saturated fats, 41, 45
Seat belts, 25
Seated Calf Raise exercise, 115
Seated Dumbbell Arm Curl, 149
Seated Dumbbell Curl exercise, 88
Seated One-Dumbbell Triceps Extension, 150
Seated Reverse Crunches exercise, 122
Secondary gender characteristics, 3
Self-esteem, 3
Sets, 131, 147
Set system, 155
Shoes, 22
Shoulder exercises, 77
Shoulder Shrug exercise, 74
Simple progressive system, 155
Sit-ups, 8, 120
Size, measuring muscle, 130, 133 (worksheet)
Skeletal muscles, 3, 11, 12 (Figure 3.1)
Skinfold measurements, 131
Sleep, 48
Smoking, 50
Snatch lift, 2
Social
- benefits of weight training, 159
- development, 5

Specificity, principle of, 16, 145
Speed of movement, 25
Spiritual development, 5
Split routines, 154
Sports, 9
- drinks, 47
- performance, 3, 8

Spot reducing, 8, 47
Spotting/spotter, 3, 21, 26–28 (Figures 5.9, 5.10, 5.11), 128, 154
- guidelines for, 27

Squat 2, 102, 146
Squat Machine exercise, 104
Standing Calf Raise exercise, 112
Static stretch, 18
Step Up exercise, 106
Steroids, anabolic, 49–50
Strength, 2, 3, 8, 9, 16
- abdominal muscle, 126
- and aging, 4, 9
- grip, 146
- measuring, 128, 135 (log)
- and resistance, 146
- training, 47

Stress, 5
Stretch(ing), 12, 17, 18–20
- duration of, 19
- guidelines, 18
- static, 18

Subconscious mind, 140
Success
- achieving, 139–140, 159
- steps to, 141

Sugars, 41, 45
Super set, 155
Supplementation, nutrient, 45, 47
Surgeon General's Report on physical activity and health, 4

Tape measure, 130
Technique, correct, 3, 9, 33, 34
Tendons, 12, 18
Tension, muscle, 13, 18–19. *See also* Stress
Testosterone, 3, 8, 15
Tobacco, 50, 131
Tone, muscle, 146, 147
Tonnage system, 156
Total body training routines, 154
Trace minerals, 40
Training
- equipment, 156
- partner, 26

Transtheoretical model of behavior change, 157
Triceps Extension exercise, 92
Triceps Pushdown exercise, 93
Trunk exercises, 117
Tuck-Ups exercise, 121

U.S. Department of Agriculture, 40, 43, 45
U.S. Department of Health and Human Services, 40, 45
Universal Heel Raise Machine, 113
Upright Rowing exercise, 80

Variable
- loading, 147
- resistance equipment, 156
- systems, 155

Vigorous exercise, 4, 17
Vitamins, 40, 45

Warm-up, 17–18, 19, 28, 128
Water, as nutrient, 39–40, 45, 47
Water-soluble vitamins, 40
Weight gain, 47
Weight management/control/loss, 4, 47–48
Weight trainers, 2, 8
- advanced, 147, 153
- beginning, 33–34, 128, 130, 146, 154

Weight training, 4, 18, 127, 147, 153
- for athletes, 8
- definition of, 1
- goals, 141
- guidelines for, 147 (Table 16.1)
- for men and women, 3
- in older adults, 4
- programs, 147–148, 151
- time required for, 9

Weight, measuring, 131
Weight-stack equipment, 156
Women, weight training for, 3, 8
Work-rest principle, 146
Wrist Curl exercise, 98

Photo Credits

Eric Risberg, v, vi, 1, 11, 17, 18, 19, 21, 22, 23, 24, 25, 26, 27, 29, 30, 31, 32, 59, 60, 62, 63, 64, 66, 69, 70, 71, 72, 73, 74, 75, 77, 78, 80, 82, 83, 84, 85, 87, 88, 90, 91, 92, 94, 95, 96, 98, 99, 102, 104, 106, 108, 112, 113, 114, 115, 117, 119, 120, 121, 122, 123, 124, 125, 127, 145, 149, 150, 157

©Fitness & Wellness, Inc., vii, 39, 41, 47

Jon Kelly, vii, 7, 57, 63, 64, 73, 79, 80, 81, 89, 94, 95, 97, 98, 99, 103, 106, 107, 110, 111, 112, 114, 139, 149, 150

Kristin Dilworth, 17, 20, 22, 25, 28, 49, 61, 67, 79, 81, 91, 93, 97, 104, 105, 109, 110, 118, 125

©Nautilus Sports/Medical Industries, Inc., vi, 61, 65, 67, 71, 75, 89, 93, 101, 105, 111, 119, 153

©Universal Gym Equipment, Inc., 65, 113